COLON & RECTAL CANCER

A Comprehensive Guide for Patients & Families

COLON & RECTAL CANCER

A Comprehensive Guide for Patients & Families

Lorraine Johnston

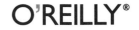

Beijing • Cambridge • Farnham • Köln • Paris • Sebastopol • Taipei • Tokyo

Colon and Rectal Cancer: A Comprehensive Guide for Patients and Families
by Lorraine Johnston

Copyright © 2000 O'Reilly & Associates, Inc. All rights reserved.
Printed in the United States of America.

Published by O'Reilly & Associates, Inc., 101 Morris Street, Sebastopol, CA 95472.

Editor: Linda Lamb

Production Editor: Claire Cloutier LeBlanc

Printing History:

> January 2000: First Edition

The O'Reilly logo is a registered trademark of O'Reilly & Associates, Inc. Many of the designations used by manufacturers and sellers to distinguish their products are claimed as trademarks. Where those designations appear in this book, and O'Reilly & Associates, Inc. was aware of a trademark claim, the designations have been printed in caps or initial caps.

This book is meant to educate and should not be used as an alternative for professional medical care. Although we have exerted every effort to ensure that the information presented is accurate at the time of publication, there is no guarantee that this information will remain current over time. Appropriate medical professionals should be consulted before adopting any procedures or treatments discussed in this book.

Library of Congress Cataloging-in-Publication Data:

Johnston, Lorraine.
    Colon & rectal cancer: a comprehensive guide for patients and families / Lorraine
        Johnston,—1st ed.
      p. cm.—(Patient-centered guides)
    Includes bibliographical references and index.
    ISBN 1-56592-633-1 (pbk.: acid-free paper)
1. Colon (Anatomy)—Cancer—Popular works. 2. Rectum—Cancer—Popular works.
I. Title: Colon and rectal cancer. II. Title. III. Series.
RC280.C6 J64 2000
616.99'4347—dc21

                                                   99-053773

This book is printed on acid-free paper with 85% recycled content, 15% post-consumer waste. O'Reilly & Associates is committed to using paper with the highest recycled content available consistent with high quality.

To my wonderful husband, Larry

Table of Contents

Preface

He who has begun has half done.

—Quintus Horatius Flaccus

IN THE FACE OF FEAR, YOU'VE CHOSEN TO EDUCATE YOURSELF about colorectal cancer and its treatments—a courageous and positive approach to moving past a dreadful event. This book will help you do so.

By enabling you to build a frame of reference from sound, current medical information, we'll help you understand the decision-making process needed to make appropriate choices about your medical care.

There's a great deal of promising information we can share with you about colorectal cancer, ranging through information about evaluating and choosing treatments; ways to locate and track new treatments being developed; preparatory information about tests and procedures; survivor experiences with keeping or losing friends; perspectives on handling employers, insurance companies, and the Social Security Administration; and so on. Did you know, for example, that you can find information about the dosage, mode of action, and side effects of medications being recommended for your treatment? That charitable groups exist expressly to fly you and your family, free of charge, to a distant cancer center where you might plan to be treated? And that if you're being treated away from home, the American Cancer Society's Hope Lodge network can provide you and your loved ones with rooms free of charge?

Sources of information

The chief resources used in developing this book were the journals and texts of Western medicine, which are summarized and presented to you in language understandable by those without a medical background. Appendix A, *Resources,* discusses references that can be accessed using a computer and the Internet, such as the National Cancer Institute's grand-daddy of all cancer information databases, and Medline, the National Library of Medicine's database of more than 9 million published medical research papers.

This book cannot substitute for up-to-date oncology training and good medical care. You should always consult with specialists in colorectal cancer before making decisions about your care.

Several chapters that are of interest to all cancer survivors, such as the chapters on stress, traveling for care, and clinical trials, were reused from my first book about lymphoma with appropriate changes made for colorectal cancer survivors.

Many colorectal cancer survivors generously volunteered to tell of their experiences with diagnosis, surgery, chemotherapy, radiotherapy, employment, and financial issues, and the emotional flotsam that might accompany any of these. Their words are included throughout the text, and serve as an anchor to reality and an inspiration for the rest of us.

Who should read this book?

If you were diagnosed recently, this book can help you understand what tests and treatments you'll encounter in the following months. We also discuss the emotional aspects of each experience: the shock and isolation of diagnosis and the reactions that follow, the fear of upcoming treatments, and the anxiety associated with waiting to see if treatment is successful.

If you are a long-term survivor of colorectal cancer, we provide the information you need to make sense of the possible long-term physical and emotional consequences of disease and treatment that you may be experiencing, such as dealing with an ostomy or with continued fatigue, as well as the information that some of you may need concerning recurrence of disease and its treatment.

If you're a caretaker of someone with colorectal cancer, the collective and pragmatic wisdom in this guide will enable you to make the most of your caretaking and advocacy efforts. It will assist you in relaxing and staying healthy so that you can best care for your loved one, both emotionally and instrumentally. We can help you understand and respond appropriately to the reactions of your loved one and yourself to the unique stressors that a cancer diagnosis entails.

Who should not read this book?

If you have not yet obtained a firm diagnosis of colorectal cancer, please do not read this guide until your doctors have clarified your circumstances. Symptoms that mimic colorectal cancer such as rectal bleeding are attributable to several other disorders. You should seek appropriate treatment for these conditions from a qualified physician.

If you have other cancers such as intestinal lymphoma, carcinoid tumors, sarcoma, anal cancers such as basal, squamous, or epidermoid carcinoma, anorectal melanoma, or malignancies of the gastrointestinal tract other than colorectal cancer, this book contains information that is not correct for your circumstances.

If you need detailed information about screening for colorectal cancer, see the American Cancer Society's 1999 book *Colorectal Cancer: A Thorough and Compassionate Resource for Patients and Their Families.* We have included a page in the back of this book that summarizes screening information. You might wish to photocopy and share this page with family and friends.

How to read this book

We've organized this book carefully to make the best use of what might be the prioritized time and energy of colorectal cancer survivors and those who look after them. The format of this book follows the path of your experience with colorectal cancer: symptoms, testing and diagnosis, surgery and hospitalization, treatment, long-term effects, and so on. We try to provide you with digestible amounts of information that you'll need at each stage of awareness and treatment. In fact, you might do well to consider reading only the chapters that are meaningful to you at a given point in order to avoid information overload. We believe that this method of organization will enable you to locate the information you need most in a timely manner.

A chapter is devoted to stress and its sometimes surprising effects on the immune system. We offer a variety of ways to cope with stress, and insights into making challenging experiences work in your favor. Moreover, in appropriate chapters, we discuss the impact of stress at that stage, and its possible effect on your well-being.

A glossary of medical terms related to colorectal cancer is included. Many general resources are provided in the appendixes.

Particular care has been taken to create a truly useful index. We suggest checking the index in order to locate a topic of your interest that appears not to be addressed by chapter subheadings.

You might find it upsetting to read about treatment options that don't apply to your situation, or to read ahead about the possibility of recurrence or disease progression. Don't feel that you have to read about everything all at once. Not all parts of this book will apply to you. Read only what will be helpful to you at a given stage.

Finally, we encourage you to mix humorous readings and other lighthearted distractions with your serious readings and considerations.

The author and contributors

My family has had several annealing experiences with cancer, including lymphoma, gastric cancers, and colorectal cancers. I have a degree in life sciences, but none of my scientific training prepared me to cope with cancer in my family. I hope I can help you feel better by sharing information about colorectal cancer, and, most significantly, by empowering you to find even more information.

The compelling voices in this resource guide are the many survivors of colorectal cancer, from those treated for local disease with colonoscopic surgery, to those who are long-term survivors of multiple surgeries, chemotherapy, and radiotherapy. The distillation of their experiences is intended to help you know what to expect in advance, to know where to find the best information for your circumstances, and to know that you are not alone.

Some of our contributors have used their real names, but some, in order to preserve their privacy, have chosen aliases or have used first names only. The italicized portions of the text are their thoughts, their feelings, their wisdom, their own words.

Acknowledgments

My first and greatest thanks go to my husband Larry, who is my role model for cancer survivors. His fortitude, determination, rollicking sense of humor, uncompromising sense of integrity, selflessness, and intelligence are an unending inspiration to me. In the year it took to write this book, he over-looked dust bunnies as large as our cats and ate many carry-out meals.

Special thanks are offered to Betty C., Chris Davies, Denise Suhrie, Max Holstein, Jeanne O'Neill, JouAnn, Kathy W., Lorraine, Linda Smith, Marsha S. Center, RDH, Myra, Nan Suhadolc, MSW, LCSW, Paul "Still Breathing" Lusczynski, Pat Behymer, Pete Potter, Peter, Pati, Randall White, Richard S., Susan E., Sue L. Browne (author of a book of cancer success stories), Dixie T., and to my other contributors who wish to remain anonymous. These brave people trusted me with their deep feelings and confidential experiences so that others will have an easier time facing the unknown. I've carefully preserved their words as offered. The genuineness and spontaneity of their thoughts and feelings communicate to the reader in ways I cannot. Several of them also agreed to review this text in advance, offering a fresh eye and valuable first-person insights that I'd have missed.

My heart aches as I thank the family of Shelly Weiler, who passed away in February 1999 when this book was being written. Shelly's family generously consented to my using his words at a time when many other families would have considered my asking an intrusion. He taught the rest of us how to live with cancer: with humor, intelligence, spirit, and with great honesty and integrity. Shelly's story is interwoven throughout this book, and he is greatly missed.

To Susan E. and to a certain family who wishes to remain anonymous, both of whom lost loved ones to colorectal cancer, I extend my most humble thanks and sorrow. You allowed me to probe painful memories much too soon after devastating losses. Please take some measure of comfort in knowing that we won't forget your loved ones, and that others will learn from your experiences.

To Bill Glenning, who runs the ACOR colon cancer discussion group on the Internet, I offer thanks and congratulations for being a tough long-term colorectal cancer survivor, and for keeping a firm but very loving hand on the tiller of our group. I thank Gilles Frydman for sponsoring all of the ACOR discussion groups.

My editor, Linda Lamb, continues to offer unerring guidance regarding the material cancer survivors will need to sustain them on their life journey. Her patience and tact, her flawless perspective, her willingness to log countless hours reviewing my work to ensure that answers are provided for cancer survivors are truly priceless. Working with her is a joy.

Carol Wenmoth, editorial assistant, is a beacon on the writer's horizon. Her experience in publishing benefits writer and reader alike. Carol oversees the complexity of a book's creation with ease; she shares her expertise kindly and willingly; her memory for detail is phenomenal. She made writing this book easy for me, and I thank her.

Medical reviewers

Several specialists reviewed the chapters of this book that are medically intense. If this book is a useful guide, it is so because of their efforts.

In daily life and in the medical literature, medical experts do not always agree. Not surprisingly, some of our medical reviewers disagreed on certain parts of this book. When a consensus of opinion was clear, I included the agreed-upon facts; when not, I stated that differences of opinion exist on a given topic. Every effort was made to clarify obscure topics and provide correct and current information. Any errors that remain in this book are mine.

I thank Costas Giannakenas, MD, PhD, Nuclear Physician, of the University of Patras Medical School, Greece, for his very thorough medical review of the chapters on modes of treatment, side effects, and late effects, and for fielding my many questions. In the years since my husband's diagnosis and treatment, Dr. Giannakenas has been kindly, tactfully, and consistently ready to help me understand medical issues surrounding cancer. I could not ask for a better mentor.

Charles A. Padgett, MD, a medical oncologist at Good Samaritan Hospital in Baltimore, Maryland, reviewed the chapter on modes of treatment, answered my many questions on this and numerous other medical topics, and has in general been our lifeline since my husband's illness in 1990. He typifies the doctor that all of us hope to have at our worst moments: a person of high medical and personal standards, of goodwill and gentleness, possessed of a sturdy sense of humor.

Paul Ian Tartter, MD, FACS, associate professor of surgery and chief of breast surgery at Mount Sinai School of Medicine, New York, kindly reviewed the chapter on prognosis, offering his corrections and suggestions.

I thank Jill D. Brensinger, MS, genetics counselor at the Johns Hopkins Hereditary Colorectal Cancer Registry, who reviewed Chapter 3, in which risk factors for colorectal cancer and the familial colorectal cancer syndromes are discussed. Ms. Brensinger's good eye and sound background in cancer genetics serve the reader in good stead.

Asnat Groutz, MD, of the Department of Obstetrics and Gynecology, Lis Maternity Hospital, Sackler Faculty of Medicine, Tel Aviv University, Israel reviewed Chapter 18, *Sexuality, Fertility, and Pregnancy*. Dr. Groutz, who is doing a fellowship with Jerry Blaivas, MD, FACS, Clinical Professor of Surgery at Cornell University Medical College, offered corrections, insights, and suggestions that are very much appreciated.

Several delightful, tactful, and extraordinarily generous medical doctors reviewed the chapter on modes of treatment and, in some cases, discussed issues with me by phone. Their insights, corrections, and suggestions are beyond measure. They are:

Kirby Bland, MD
J. Murray Beardsley Professor and Chairman
Department of Surgery
Brown University School of Medicine
Providence, Rhode Island

Dennis Devereux, MD
Mid-Hudson Valley Center
Poughkeepsie, New York

Garner P. Johnson, MD, FACS
Assistant Professor of Surgery
Albany Medical College
Albany, New York

Mohammed Mohiuddin, MD
Professor and Chairman
Department of Radiation Medicine
University of Kentucky
Lexington, Kentucky

James Muchmore, MD
Associate Professor, Surgery
Tulane University Medical Center Hospital
New Orleans, Louisiana

Stephen S. Schild, MD
Assistant Professor of Oncology
Mayo Medical School
Rochester, Minnesota

Karen Seiter, MD
Associate Professor of Medicine
New York Medical College
Valhalla, New York

Raymond Staniunas, MD, FACS
Assistant Professor of Surgery
Case Western Reserve
Cleveland, Ohio

Timothy Yeatman, MD
Assistant Professor of Surgery
H. Lee Moffitt Cancer Center and Research Institute
University of Southern Florida
Tampa, Florida

I am especially grateful to those individuals who diligently reviewed the entire manuscript, offering many insights, suggestions, corrections, and copious explanations throughout. Their efforts were not only a great service to me, but a crucial service to readers.

In this second book, I again thank cancer researchers in the United States and elsewhere who, though often underpaid and unrecognized, have devoted their lives to caring about our well-being and our outcomes. Thanks to the effort and altruistic collaboration of cancer researchers all over the world, we are witnessing and benefiting from robust progress in the understanding and treatment of cancer.

CHAPTER 1

Symptoms, Diagnosis, and Staging

*To learn how to treat a disease, one must
learn how to diagnose it. The diagnosis is the
best trump in the scheme of treatment.*

—Jean Martin Charcot

EACH OF US HAS HAD A UNIQUE EXPERIENCE WITH SYMPTOMS—or the absence of them—and with diagnosis. We might have had a lengthy, emotionally depleting diagnostic experience, perhaps just a few symptoms, or a diagnosis out of the blue when a fecal occult blood test or colonoscopy found a problem.

Before we discuss symptoms, diagnosis, and staging in greater depth, it's important to note that the process of discovery of a cancer is, by most people's accounts, associated with great emotional upheaval. There may be a few of us who are so highly evolved spiritually, or who have lived so full a life, that we accept a cancer diagnosis with equanimity, but this is not the case for most of us. At the end of this chapter we discuss the emotional tumult associated with diagnosis and the range of responses that people may have.

Please note that it may not be useful to read this material if you have not yet received a confirmed diagnosis of colorectal cancer, as the symptoms associated with colorectal cancer also are associated with various noncancerous diseases.

Symptoms

Because the experience of colorectal cancer might begin with symptoms that you or your doctor may notice, we too begin by describing symptoms, although many people are diagnosed with colorectal cancer as part of a routine examination, without any symptoms being present.

Symptoms of colorectal cancer may appear suddenly, or may develop gradually over a period of time:

- Changes in bowel movements:
    - Narrowing of stools
    - Red, bloody bowel movements, perhaps with blood clots
    - Black, tarry bowel movements
    - Bowel movements containing mucus as well as blood
    - Persistent diarrhea
    - Constipation
    - Total bowel obstruction, characterized by extreme pain
- Bowel perforation, accompanied by fever and pain
- Rectal bleeding between bowel movements
- Abdominal pain and cramping, either chronic or acute
- Distention of the abdomen
- Nausea
- Vomiting
- Weight loss
- Fatigue
- Anemia (low red blood cell counts)
- A sense that the bowel hasn't completely emptied
- An ongoing urgent feeling to empty the bowels
- Vaginal fistulas, that is, tubes that form between the vagina and colon or vagina and bladder as the result of a disease process
- Pain in the tissue between the anus and vagina, or between the anus and scrotal sac
- Urinary tract symptoms such as pain, blockage, or urge to urinate

When colorectal cancer is advanced, jaundice, back pain, and cough also may be present.

A survivor of stage I colon cancer describes his journey through symptoms and diagnosis:

> As a child, I tended to always have a nervous stomach that would turn into diarrhea. I remember this as early as fifth grade. When I was a sophomore in college, I began to have bloody diarrhea. After a month of this I came home one evening and slept for two days, only getting up to go to the bathroom. I was hospitalized and diagnosed with ulcerative colitis. I was hospitalized three times over the next year and a half. I lost a lot of blood and was anemic and received a total of eleven units of blood during that time frame, some while I was in the hospital and some on an outpatient basis.

> The doctor asked if I had been traveling outside the country and picked up something that way. My original doctor, when admitted to the hospital, was a surgeon. I felt like hell. They discussed the "cure" with the doctor and decided to wait and get some other opinions. The other doctors felt that of course a surgeon wants to remove the problem. I found out that 20+ years later, that is the only cure.

> As time passed, I learned to live with constant diarrhea. I learned to plan my life around urgent needs to use the bathroom. I always knew where a bathroom was, and if there wouldn't be one, I wouldn't go. My job requires a lot of travel, so checking out my new surroundings for the nearest bathroom became part of my travel plans. There was always a certain amount of stress while flying: Will I have to go the restroom? Will the seatbelt light be off? If I wait until I get to the terminal, will I make it?

> Early on I tried all the medications for ulcerative colitis. On one trip to the hospital they tried a sulfa drug (asulfidine) and I was allergic to it. I was to take it before I ate and it would kill my appetite. I wasn't overly heavy at the time and I lost a lot of weight. The nurses stopped weighing me at around 118 pounds. I am 5'10". My weight started returning as soon as I stopped the medication. I gained two pounds per day until I reached 145 by eating a full meal every two hours.

> I tried prednisone and, as for many people, it helped for a while. I have scars on my back from the acne that was stimulated at certain levels of the drug.

It took about two or three years before I sort of got it under control. I didn't like doctors telling me I needed to have my colon removed, so I stopped going to see them. I went to a few different gastroenterologists over the years, and seven to ten years ago I started seeing the same one on a less-than-more regular basis. Why go when all he would do was tell me how bad things were?

I don't remember how long the doctors were using the term "dysplasia." I know my current doctor discussed my situation with some of his medical colleagues. Their immediate response was to recommend removing my colon because of the damage to it.

When I was in my late thirties, after years of good spells, bad spells, and trying to make things better by choosing foods that seemed to help and using allergy medicines (my nose and my intestines seemed to work together), I decided to have a colonoscopy. The doctor who analyzed the findings said that my colon couldn't possibly be in worse shape, and that I should consider having a total colectomy immediately. He biopsied some tissue from random locations and found low- to high-grade dysplasia. I was reminded/told that these were precancerous cells. I was also told that I had a 100 percent chance of having colon cancer with the activity of the disease and the damage that had been done. With the damage to the tissue, the expected time frame for cancer was after 20 to 25 years of active ulcerative colitis. He gave me a medication without first telling me how sick it would make me feel: 6MP—a form of chemotherapy, if I remember correctly. I had terrible side effects. I later reviewed the information paper for the drug and I had had just about all of the side effects.

My wife and I talked it over, and decided that alternative medicine might have something less harsh, less drastic, to offer, but after trying a few remedies without much change for the better, I realized surgery probably was the best choice.

My wife and I continued to talk over what was best, and we felt sure I was doing the right thing. She would have pushed me sooner had she known the odds of cancer.

Diagnosis

The most accurate way to diagnose a colorectal cancer is by biopsy, either with a colonoscope or during surgery, but a number of tests might be suggested before colorectal cancer is suspected and definitively diagnosed:

- Blood tests to count the number of red blood cells, white cells, and platelets.
- Blood tests for liver and kidney function.
- Digital rectal examination for rectal and low colonic tumors.
- Radiographic studies (x-rays) of the bowel using barium (single contrast), or barium and air (double contrast).
- Colonoscopy, a procedure using a miniature camera and a light source fastened to a very long flexible tube to visualize the inside of the colon. Surgical instruments can be passed through the tube.
- Sigmoidoscopy, a procedure using a miniature camera and a light source fastened to a flexible tube to visualize the inside of the rectum and the last portion of the colon beyond the rectum. Surgical instruments can be passed through the tube.
- Hydrocolonic ultrasonography (sonogram, ultrasound) of the colon.
- Ultrasonography of the liver.
- Needle aspiration of fluid in the abdomen or chest to search for cancer cells.
- Computed tomography (CT), numerous thin x-ray images assembled into a detailed image by computer.
- Magnetic resonance imaging (MRI), a mapping of tissues that respond differently to magnetic waves.
- Positron emission tomography (PET), an assessment of the uptake of radioactive glucose by tissue suspected to be cancerous (often, cancerous tissue metabolizes glucose more rapidly than healthy tissues).

The practical details associated with experiencing these tests are described at length in Chapter 5, *Tests and Procedures*.

If various tests and imaging studies reveal no suspected area of disease that appears to involve the full thickness of the colon wall, or that has spread outside the colon, tissue may be simply collected with a colonoscope and biopsied.

If blood tests, imaging studies, or colonoscopy reveal the possibility of disease beyond that accessible and removable with a colonoscope, a more extensive surgery might be planned.

> *My story begins with denial and fear. I had rectal bleeding for a few months, but just kept delaying going to the doctor. Surely it's hemorrhoids. But then I gradually began having frequent bowel movements and finally made an appointment. Well, it was fast and furious from that moment on. Blood work found anemia, a colonoscopy found a tumor in the rectosigmoid junction. My team of doctors who worked together to form a plan included my GI doctor, radiology oncologist, oncologist, and surgeon. Then CAT scan, chest x-rays. I quickly began chemotherapy-enhanced radiation, 27 sessions with a 6-week break, before the resection surgery.*

CEA blood testing

Blood tests for nonspecific cancer markers such as carcinoembryonic antigen (CEA) or experimental cancer antigens such as CA19-9 might be done as part of a diagnostic workup. At this time, however, blood tests alone cannot confirm the presence of disease, as other non-cancerous conditions also cause these blood markers to emerge or rise. Instead, these blood tests are done to establish levels of antigen markers that can be used as a baseline for subsequent testing. In some patients, for instance, CEA levels drop to normal levels after surgical removal of all visible disease; thus, a persistent rise in CEA after surgery might, in some patients, indicate a return of disease.

Colonoscopy

Among all of the above tests, colonoscopy is, at this time, considered the best test for assessing the entire colon, because it provides the best visibility of internal surfaces of the colon and can collect tissue samples for analysis:

- These tissue samples may be assessed as fully encapsulating the cancer, with boundaries of healthy tissue called clear margins. This is a typical finding when precancerous colon polyps, called adenomatous polyps, are removed in the early stages before they have fully converted to cancers.

- If biopsy of tissue collected by colonoscopy reveals a more advanced evolution to cancer, however, or reveals surgical margins that were not composed entirely of healthy tissue, a more extensive surgery may be planned.

It's important to keep in mind that colorectal cancers that lie flat or are covered by healthy tissue might be missed during colonoscopy.

Surgical diagnosis

If tests aimed at identifying a suspicious mass reveal disease beyond that treatable with colonoscopy, the next step, both for diagnosis and for cure, is removal of the diseased area by surgery.

At this point your doctor will discuss choosing a surgeon. Initially, you may feel comfortable with whomever he or she recommends, but it is in your best interest to research independently the choice of a surgeon—see Chapter 2, *Finding the Right Treatment Team.*

Surgery may be traditional open surgery, or it may be laparoscopic surgery involving a few very small surgical openings through which surgical instruments are passed via an endoscope, a long tube that also contains a camera and light source. At the time of this writing, most surgeries for colorectal cancer are open surgeries, as the rate of cure with laparoscopic surgery remains unclear.

During an open surgery, the surgeon will examine the areas of colon, rectum, and surrounding tissue that were highlighted during imaging studies, as well as more distant organs such as the liver, stomach, spleen, and pancreas. Examination will be visual but may be supplemented by ultrasound, by colonoscope, or by radioimmunoguided (RIG) technique. RIG surgery involves injection prior to surgery of a safe radioactive substance that collects more readily in cancerous tissue, and is subsequently detected during surgery using a hand-held gamma counter. A detailed discussion of surgical theory and technique is provided in Chapter 6, *Modes of Treatment.*

All suspicious tissue will be removed by the surgeon and sent to the pathology laboratory for analysis.

Cure or palliation?

Surgery for colorectal cancer is not done simply to collect samples for biopsy. Once surgery is deemed necessary for suspected colorectal cancer, the intent is to remove as much diseased tissue as possible, striving for cure. This means that, in some cases, heavily diseased organs, or organs entwined with cancerous tissue, may be removed entirely, not just sampled for biopsy. Nearby organs such as the bladder, ovary, lymph nodes, and blood vessels, as well as portions of the liver, are most likely to be affected in this way.

In some cases, diagnostic tests reveal so much disease that surgery could never remove all disease. In other cases, the patient may be too frail to survive an extensive surgical procedure and its long-term recovery and side effects. In these instances, limited surgery, or chemotherapy or radiotherapy without surgery, may be used to relieve symptoms or to halt the spread of disease. Treatment aimed at reducing the patient's discomfort instead of providing a cure is called palliative treatment.

Misdiagnosis, delayed diagnosis

Unfortunately, certain groups of people are more frequently misdiagnosed, and certain tests can be erroneous or inconclusive:

- Very young people with colon cancer—children and teens—frequently are not diagnosed until disease is far advanced because the medical community sometimes attributes their symptoms to other causes more typically found in their age group.

- Colon cancer arising during pregnancy frequently produces symptoms such as nausea that are mistaken for the normal physical consequences of pregnancy. This can result in delayed diagnosis.

- Those with disease that does not begin with copious and distinct, visible polyps might be assessed as cancer-free when colonoscopy reveals no polyps, unless they are aware of and inform their physicians of any family history of disease.

- Incomplete imaging of the colon by barium enema or by colonoscopy is possible. During colonoscopy, the full length of the colon—that is, beyond the colon into the final portion of the small intestine—must be accessed and visualized.

- Reliance only upon blood markers such as CEA to detect or track disease is not recommended, as these markers can remain low or normal in the presence of certain types of colorectal cancers.

- Colon cancer that arises in the appendix may be incorrectly diagnosed as appendicitis until disease has spread to other organs.

- Bleeding hemorrhoids may mask symptoms of rectal cancer.

- Polyps that lie flat—sessile polyps—may be missed entirely during colonoscopy, or may be incompletely biopsied.

I'm a 44-year-old female who, in March of 1998, went in for a yearly checkup. I thought I had hemorrhoids. Well, guess what? I had a 7-centimeter tumor very low in my rectum. The women's health specialist brought in a doctor to confirm that she was feeling polyps, not stool! He concurred with her and they decided I needed to see a GI doctor as soon as possible. Both left the room, and one made a call to my primary doctor and the other to a GI doctor.

I was seen for a consultation two days later, on a Friday, by the GI doctor. He did a quick exam and told me I needed a colonoscopy, but he knew he would not be able to remove the polyp as it was too large. I had the colonoscopy the next Tuesday where he confirmed even without the biopsy back that I had colorectal cancer and needed surgery as soon as possible.

I was then scheduled for a CT scan that very next Friday! I was also able to see the surgeon that same day. He looked at the CT scan and, after examining me, decided he needed to do a sigmoidoscopy to look for himself. He determined that he couldn't do surgery safely without trying to shrink this large tumor first. So he made calls to both a radiation and medical oncologist to set up appointments for me.

The radiation doctor first told me she'd like to do five weeks of radiation to try and shrink the tumor. I told her maybe it would just disappear with radiation and she said, "No, honey, we are only going for shrinkage."

I then saw the medical oncologist who did not receive all the information from the other doctors, as I was seeing everyone so close together everything didn't get transferred fast enough. He was concerned about my liver. Turns out there were what looked like spots of cancer there also.

I was either going to be admitted in the morning to get a central line inserted in my chest to receive continuous chemotherapy or needed to have a liver biopsy first. He couldn't reach the other doctors to consult while I was there so he said he'd call me later in the day to let me know what to do.

When he called, they had decided the spots were probably just shadows, not cancer. I went in on Thursday morning and got my central line. All went smoothly, not any real pain, just a little discomfort for a few days. Friday I got marked for radiation; now I have permanent tattoos. I told the tattoo artist he needed to learn a better design than just a dot here and there! Monday came, and I received my first radiation treatment that took all of about four minutes. It took longer to get there and change than the treatment took. I was radiated in four spots.

I also went up to short stay where they administer chemotherapy at my HMO and was hooked up to my continuous 5-FU pump, which I just carried around in a fanny pack. I went for radiation 5 days a week and had the chemo 24 hours a day, 7 days a week for the 5 weeks. I went in once a week to have the 5-FU refilled.

I had very few side effects doing this. Fatigue was the biggest for me. Some diarrhea and nausea were controlled with medications. I did not get the mouth sores they predicted, but did use Biotene toothpaste and mouthwash as recommended. I also took two vitamin B6 tablets a day to prevent me from getting what I think is referred to as hand and foot syndrome. This pretty much prevented that from happening. During the last week I did get quite ill with GI tract pain, and was not able to eat at all. I went on pain pills for a week and recovered nicely.

About five weeks after ending this chemotherapy, I had surgery from which I was expecting to come out with a permanent colostomy due to the location of my tumor. In order to put me back together, the doctor needed to have a 2-cm margin of good tissue that he knew he didn't have. However, during surgery they did a quick freeze of the remaining tissue and it was clean, so he decided to put me back together with staples. This procedure has only been used in the US for about six years, so I'm fortunate to be able to have this done and not have a colostomy at all.

Shelly's story

Shelly Weiler was diagnosed with stage IV colon cancer in 1998. Sadly, he passed away in February 1999, but his life and his experience were nonetheless meaningful because he showed us how to confront cancer with honor and integrity. Shelly's story and the stories of others who have survived are interwoven throughout this book.

In this passage, Shelly tells of his first experiences with diagnosis:

> I had two successive years where I was told my blood work from my annual physical was normal. When we got a copy of the blood work before my diagnosis, my urologist, the doctor who diagnosed the disease, said to me "Shelly, you know you have an iron deficiency?" Why didn't my ex-primary pick up on it? Did he read the blood results at all, or was he too busy taking care of his personal business while my blood test rested on his desk? Not only was he not sensitive about colon cancer, he was not sensitive about patient needs. To be frank and honest with everyone, if I had him in front of me now, I'd rip his eyes out.
>
> What we need to do is make these idiots that call themselves doctors accountable. Short of suing the bastards we could report them to the medical boards of their states and also let the AMA know how they malpractice.
>
> I am very bitter about this because my ex-primary pooh-poohed my symptoms for over a year. Even when I finally complained of constipation he said that it was because of the Prevacid I was taking for acid reflux disease, something he diagnosed without doing an upper GI or any other testing. The man should be barred from practicing medicine.
>
> I have a friend who was also diagnosed with colon cancer at the age of 29. Thank God, after a year of intensive chemotherapy, she has been clear for five years. She was lucky. Her father is an internal medicine specialist and she told him of her symptoms. It was caught early before infiltrating other organs. Not all of us are that lucky. Not all of us have fathers who are doctors. Not all of us have doctors who know their ass from their elbow.

Staging and grading colorectal cancer

Even after surgery is performed and a colorectal cancer is confirmed, there may be some question about which type of colorectal cancer exists, its degree of aggressiveness, called grade, and the stage of its progression.

It is most important that your disease be correctly identified, graded, and staged so that the best treatment can be planned. All biopsies of tumor tissue should be reviewed by an experienced pathologist to be certain that type and grade are correctly identified.

> *I was in the hospital for eight days after surgery only to find out during this time I did have stage III cancer due to the fact that eight of the ten lymph nodes they tested were positive for cancer. I went home to recover and was scheduled to begin 5-FU and leucovorin in about four weeks. About two weeks after surgery I had terrible GI pain and was admitted with a kink in my bowel that worked its way out without surgery or even a nasogastric tube! I did begin treatments the beginning of July. This was five days in a row every four weeks for four courses ending in late September.*

Brief definitions of stage and grade are:

*   Staging describes how far disease has spread from its original site. Staging for many, but not all, cancers consists of stages I through IV. Colorectal cancer also includes a staging level of 0 to indicate a very early tumor that has virtually no effect on any other nearby tissue.

*   Grading describes how aggressive the tumor is, and often is related to type.

Staging your disease

Staging is a way of describing how far disease has spread from the original tumor, and how much of the body is affected by colorectal cancer.

Knowing your staging information gives you a way to compare your diagnosis and recommended treatment to reports in the literature or descriptions of clinical trials. It also gives you the vocabulary you need to speak with medical professionals who might not already be familiar with your case.

Several attempts have been made to stage the colorectal cancers in a way that is meaningful to the treatment chosen and the best outcome. Currently, the TNM system is favored by most cancer treatment centers. Ask your oncologist what standard was used to assess the spread and effects of your disease—Dukes, MAC, or TNM.

Moreover, many oncologists and institutions incorporate other clinical measures—age, ability to do normal everyday things, tumor size—to discuss more accurately the effect of disease.

TNM staging definitions

The definitions of staging that follow are organized by the TNM staging system within the two broad categories of colon and rectal cancer. The following definitions have been adapted from the National Cancer Institute's physicians' treatment statements for colon and rectal cancer. Because staging is based on penetration of the tumor through the bowel wall, these definitions will be easier to understand if you refer to Figure 1-1.

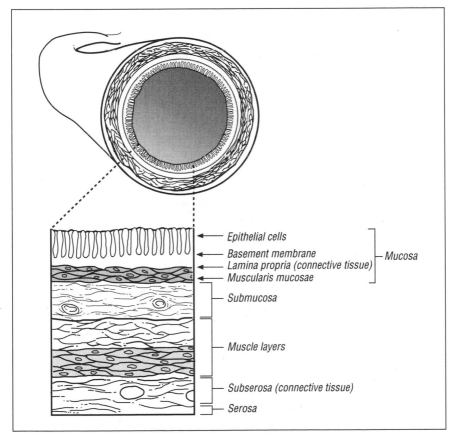

Figure 1-1. Cross-section of the colon

Going outward, the layers of the bowel are:

- Mucosa, comprised of:
  - Epithelium
  - Basement membrane
  - Lamina propria
  - Muscularis mucosae
- Submucosa
- Muscularis propria
- Subserosa
- Serosa, an additional outer layer in areas of the peritoneal cavity where the bowel is freely moving

T indicates the status of the primary tumor:

- TX: The primary tumor cannot be assessed.
- T0: No evidence of a primary tumor can be found.
- Tis: Carcinoma in situ (tumor in place): an intraepithelial tumor or an invasion of the lamina propria. Tis includes cancer cells entirely contained within the glandular basement membrane (intraepithelial) or lamina propria (intramucosal) with no breach through the muscularis mucosae into the submucosa.
- T1: Tumor has invaded the submucosa.
- T2: Tumor has invaded the muscularis propria, the muscle layer of the intestine, which is approximately midway through the colon.
- T3: The tumor invades through the muscularis propria into the subserosa, or into nonperitonealized pericolic or perirectal tissues.
- T4: The tumor directly invades other organs or structures, and/or penetrates the visceral peritoneum. In T4, the term "direct invasion" includes invasion of other sections of colon or rectum by way of the serosa; for instance, invasion of the sigmoid colon by a carcinoma of the cecum.

N indicates the status of regional lymph nodes:

- NX: Regional nodes cannot be assessed.
- N0: No regional lymph nodes are invaded.

- N1: Metastasis (invasion) in one to three regional lymph nodes.

- N2: Metastasis in four or more regional lymph nodes.

M designates distant metastasis, a spreading to other organs:

- MX: Distant metastasis cannot be assessed.

- M0: No distant metastasis.

- M1: Distant metastasis, including distant lymph nodes.

Stages 0 through IV defined

The most commonly used staging system in use today is the TNM system, which can be summarized into stages 0 through IV. Staging systems are explained and correlated in Appendix D.

- Stage 0: Tis, N0, M0

- Stage I: T1, N0, M0; or T2, N0, M0

- Stage II: T3, N0, M0; or T4, N0, M0

- Stage III: Any T, N1, M0; or any T, N2, M0

- Stage IV: Any T; any N, M1

Recurrent disease

Often you'll find in the medical literature that patients who have relapsed are no longer discussed by stage, but are instead described as having recurrent disease. In some cases, recurrent disease may be the equivalent of stage I, such as is seen in the relapse of certain patients revealing local disease only. Recurrent disease in organs outside the colon, however, is more often considered to be the equivalent of stage IV.

Grading your disease

A tumor can be graded as highly aggressive or less aggressive by several measures. All colorectal cancer tumors are graded on their appearance under the microscope, known as histologic grade. Mucin-producing tumors, for example, are considered to be aggressive disease.

Assessing options

It would be wise to seek one or more second opinions about diagnosis, staging, and treatment options from a regional cancer center or university hospital. The oncologist you're already seeing may be affiliated with one of these groups, and thus may have the necessary qualifications.

Emotions at this stage

The events described above, and those that will follow over the next months or years, are very likely to take an emotional toll. There are as many reactions to cancer as there are people, and you can't always be sure how you or your loved ones will react in novel, frightening circumstances.

Although professional psychologists make fine distinctions among responses, reactions, and coping mechanisms, the emotional happenings described below are discussed not in clinical terms, but rather in terms your heart and soul will recognize.

All of the reactions mentioned below, and many others, are normal, albeit painful. You may feel that these feelings are useless or counterproductive, but like all defensive behaviors, they serve to protect your mind from harm until you can assimilate this experience and begin to build a frame of reference from the facts. Don't berate yourself if you're not feeling like the poster child for mental health week.

If weeks go by and you still feel that your reactions and responses are not serving you well, if you can't eat or sleep, if you can't stop crying, if you've lost a great deal of weight in a short time, or if you feel you are jeopardizing your source of income with suboptimal performance, see your doctor for advice. The newer sleeping pills and antidepressants are very effective in restoring sleep and appetite with minimal side effects. Objective scientific studies have shown that support groups and counseling make a profound difference in one's comfort and ability to deal with cancer. Chapter 12, *Stress and the Immune System*, and Chapter 14, *Getting Support*, describe in more detail sources of support and methods for dealing with stress and feelings.

The physical aspects of fear

If you had any hint that your symptoms might be cancer-related, you probably are already familiar with tremendous, overwhelming feelings of fear and their aftereffects. The physiology of fear is such that your body prepares you very specifically either for battle or retreat. We have evolved to note and react quickly to changing stimuli during a fearful encounter. This may explain why many people, when first diagnosed with cancer, want immediately to start a treatment—any treatment—just so they're doing something to fight back.

Unfortunately, these bodily preparations for action, such as increasing your pulse rate and redirecting blood flow from your limbs to your heart, brain, and other internal organs, are not the ideal biological events to prepare you for understanding and remembering your doctor's explanations. The moment that fear hits and adrenaline pumps, senses become heightened in preparation for life-saving action. However, that sensation that you can somehow see everything around you with remarkable clarity is not necessarily going to help you remember the doctor's description of two tests that need to be done, and a third test only if the first two are inconclusive, and where your doctor said she prefers these tests be done. Instead, you may remember exactly where you were sitting, the color of the doctor's office walls, and that stray hair of the doctor's that wouldn't stay put.

Shock and numbness

Your cancer diagnosis is very likely to seem unreal to you at first. You may awake from sleep thinking you're as you were before surgery, for example, then remember, after thirty seconds or so, that you've had extensive surgery for cancer. You might not hear people who speak to you; you may have difficulty sustaining concentration for routine normal tasks; you might feel as if you're walking underwater; you might have to remind yourself to look both ways when crossing the street. Some cancer survivors report becoming paralytic for days, unable to sleep, rise, eat, or work.

If you awake from surgery to find that you have an ostomy, you may have difficulty believing this new part of you exists, no matter how carefully and thoroughly the discussions about ostomy were conducted before surgery. You might be reluctant or horrified to look at the ostomy, or to care for it.

Shelly Weiler describes how profoundly his diagnosis affected him:

> Last year I was invincible. In one second the picture changed.

Randall, a survivor of stage II colorectal cancer, describes the shock upon his diagnosis:

> *I am a 43-year-old male from Dallas, Texas, just diagnosed yesterday. Diagnosis is so new, we don't even have staging information yet. I'm having a CT scan and more lab work this weekend to determine the extent of the cancer.*
>
> *As a result of what was first presumed to be "internal hemorrhoids" and then ulcerative colitis, I had a colonoscopy on Tuesday of this week so that the doctor could confirm the latter. Instead he found a bloody five-inch-long tumor ten inches up in my colon. They did a biopsy. Results from biopsy yesterday confirmed the new diagnosis. Looking back, and knowing what I know now, I have been having symptoms of this for two years.*
>
> *This is, obviously, quite a shocker in my house. Not just because cancer is always devastating, but because my life partner of twelve years was diagnosed with multiple myeloma, a hematologic cancer resembling leukemia, two years ago. We have been through his two bone marrow transplants, chemotherapy, radiation, the works, already. The shock comes from the reaction of "Haven't we already been through enough?" We have a dark humor about cancer, though, which has already kicked in: we've inquired about group discounts.*

Mental slowness

Many cancer patients and their loved ones, most being intelligent and competent people—even some doctors diagnosed with cancer—report not being able to remember anything of the doctor's explanation after hearing the word "cancer."

If you will be meeting the doctor in person to discuss test results and treatment choices, be prepared to have difficulty absorbing what is said. For example, you should be prepared to take notes, or take a friend or a tape recorder with you. Tell the doctor that you will be calling back with a list of questions after you have had time to absorb this information. If she expresses impatience or reluctance to help you, consider finding another doctor.

Dissociation

Many people note that upon learning of their diagnosis they were completely objective, calm and felt nothing at all, as if they were outside of their body observing this happening to someone else. This is called dissociation. Dissociation temporarily allows you to absorb information without emotional pain.

Childlike or nonsensical behavior

Some people note that they said and did things that made no sense, sometimes quite childlike things. This can be a seeking of comfort in happier times, technically called regression:

> When my husband phoned to say his CT scan showed what was almost certainly cancer, I left my office immediately. Once at home I found that, although I was 40 years old, all I wanted to do was reread my old girlhood Nancy Drew books.

Denial

Some people respond to the news of their diagnosis with the belief that there is an error in the laboratory test, or that their results have been confused with someone else's. (While laboratory errors are possible, they are not common.) This reaction, called denial, is a protective reaction to allow you to absorb an onslaught of information more slowly. Denial can be used successfully to help you forget about cancer between treatments, to return to your productive life. Denial also may be a dangerous adaptive strategy, however, if you forget medical appointments, neglect ostomy care, or become convinced that your health will improve spontaneously with no treatment.

Anger

While many people develop focused feelings of anger some time *after* their diagnosis, others may feel a generalized anger at the time of diagnosis. They may lash out at the doctor who was the bearer of bad news about the cancer diagnosis, or at loved ones, for seemingly meaningless reasons. Sometimes anger is a form of projection, a displacement of painful feelings within the self outward onto others. As such, projection serves to reduce unbearable levels of pain. At other times, the angry person may simply feel overwhelmed by having to face all of the stresses and responsibilities of normal life, plus a cancer diagnosis. Yet others feel that being angry is more socially acceptable than feeling sad. Anger can be a useful emotion if targeted properly and harmlessly, but it can also signal the beginning of depression, and can drive away the support of others that you will almost certainly need.

Sadness

Many people report that they cry or otherwise express great sadness, and that they feel better after doing so. Sadness is, of course, an entirely normal reaction to a cancer diagnosis. This change in your awareness of yourself connotes the possibilities of great losses: loss of life, loss of motility, loss of career opportunities, or loss of perceived sexual attractiveness.

> *This is so disheartening, considering I never took an aspirin for a headache and now I'm on a daily regimen of pills, pills, pills.*

Guilt

Guilt is the burden we carry for things we feel we could've handled differently. Some survivors of colorectal cancer might feel that, had they lived differently, they would not have developed cancer. This feeling haunts many survivors of many different types of cancer, but for colorectal cancer survivors, it's especially painful because the medical community in the US stresses early detection, along with prevention via dietary habits and exercise, even though some research has shown that diet and exercise are not foolproof means of avoiding colorectal cancer.

If you're feeling guilty about possibly causing your or your loved one's cancer, you need to know that no sure lifestyle-related cause of colorectal cancer has yet been found for most cases: not stress, not environmental agents, not dietary choices.

Shame

Unlike guilt, shame is the burden we carry for things we can't do anything about. Survivors of colorectal cancer may feel shame because the colon and rectum and their functions are, in some quarters, considered taboo subjects. Unlike survivors of cancers that affect an arm or the thyroid, for instance, some colorectal cancer survivors might be reluctant to discuss their condition with others, fearing their negative reaction, even if the survivor herself is comfortable with the topic.

Blame

Like anger, blame can be a form of projection. If someone has been blaming himself for his own or another's cancer, the feelings may become unbearable and he may begin looking elsewhere for an explanation. Unfortunately, some people decide that the best solution is for another person to carry this blame. Those who have been coping with stress in this way for many years sometimes skip self-blame and go directly to blaming others. If someone in your life appears to be blaming you for cancer, you might try discussing this with him. If discussion doesn't improve the relationship, it might be best to remove this person from your immediate circle of activities temporarily and deal with him only when you feel most able.

Withdrawal

Others report that they or their loved ones initially seemed detached, withdrawn or uncaring. Those who withdraw may do so for many reasons: as a habit formed during earlier stressful experiences, as a means to avoid shameful feelings about expressing emotion, in an attempt to keep emotional levels low so that others won't become upset, as an attempt to reduce exposure to painful ideas, as an effort to hide the ostomy from loved ones, and so on.

At times it's almost impossible to know what really motivates you or others, even after serious introspection, or after others tell you what they feel. Your attempts to discuss this with the withdrawn person, or others' attempts to draw you out, may make matters temporarily worse.

Reactions of loved ones

There also seems to be some difference in reaction depending on whether it's you or your loved one who is facing a cancer diagnosis. Many cancer survivors report that, in their opinion, the experience was much harder on their loved ones than on themselves. Clearly this is a topic subject to personal interpretation, as the loving caretaker isn't undergoing treatment that can cause anything from mild discomfort to serious toxicity or even death. A cancer survivor who believes that her loved ones suffered more discomfort than she did, though, may be expressing a useful feeling of immortality, a belief of being in charge of her own fate that will serve her well during treatment.

It might be useful to keep in mind that loved ones face issues that are somewhat different from those faced by the cancer survivor. They may experience guilt that they themselves remain healthy, fear that they will be deprived of the person they love most, and helplessness in the face of cancer, an erstwhile enemy by anyone's standards.

Summary

We hope that the information we've offered in this opening chapter has helped remove the edge from the fear you're feeling. Knowing that delays you may have experienced obtaining a diagnosis are common; that multiple diagnostic tests are sometimes needed; that the diagnostic process can unfold in stages with increasing levels of certainty, perhaps entailing changes in your treatment plan or your choice of doctors; that you're not alone; that what you're feeling is normal—these are the first steps of the journey.

If you attempt to compare yourself to others who appear to have the same diagnosis, bear in mind that their diagnosis may have been made using criteria that are different, perhaps in subtle ways, from those used by your own diagnosticians. This means that treatment decisions from one person to the next may differ as well.

CHAPTER 2

Finding the Right Treatment Team

*There are in fact two things, science
and opinion; the former begets
knowledge, the latter ignorance.*

—Hippocrates

CHOOSING THE RIGHT SURGEON TO PERFORM YOUR SURGERY, and the best oncologists for any additional treatment you'll need are the most important decisions you'll make during the early days of your diagnosis.

Unless you have symptoms that warrant emergency surgery, such as bowel obstruction or perforation, generally you can take a week or two to locate the best surgeon for your circumstances without compromising the outcome.

If you're pressed for time, though, or are feeling too anxious just now to pursue this issue with the necessary tenacity, you can limit your search to contacting the nearest university medical school, or to contacting the National Cancer Institute (NCI) at (800) 4-CANCER and asking for the names of several surgeons and oncologists at their institution or in your area.

In this chapter, we first look at the various types of surgeons and oncologists, and how to locate qualified candidates. Then we discuss considerations in deciding on the right surgeon and oncologists for you, including currency of medical background, affiliated treatment center, and manner of conducting practice.

Types of surgeons

There are two types of surgeons specifically trained to perform surgery when colon or rectal cancer is suspected. All candidates should be board-certified:

*   General surgeons with a secondary certification in medical oncology
*   Surgeons board-certified in colon and rectal surgery

Types of oncologists

There are several types of oncologists. Any you choose should be board-certified:

- The medical oncologist, trained in the use of chemotherapy. Colorectal cancer survivors who receive adjuvant therapy utilize the skills of this professional. The medical oncologist usually is called simply an oncologist. Board certification for this discipline is called medical oncology.

- The radiation oncologist, trained in the use of radiation therapy. Seldom is colon cancer treated with radiation therapy, but rectal cancer is, and other small areas of your body may need radiation therapy to reduce tumor bulk or to control symptoms if cancer has spread beyond the primary site. When this is the case, your radiation oncologist will usually coordinate any treatment you may need with your medical oncologist and your surgeon. Choose a radiation oncologist who is board-certified in radiation oncology.

Surgical and oncologic specialists usually are associated with university medical schools. If you cannot find a suitable specialist in your area to provide your treatment, you should plan to travel for at least one second opinion from a specialist during the course of your treatment.

General considerations

You should search carefully for a surgeon and oncologists who have a great deal of experience with your illness, and who keep informed regarding the latest breakthroughs in colorectal cancer diagnosis and treatment, because treatments are evolving with vigor. It's better to make a good choice at first rather than later, and it's especially important to find the right doctor before you make the decision to proceed with surgery and perhaps chemotherapy or radiation therapy.

If you're planning to receive adjuvant chemotherapy or radiotherapy, before deciding on a local oncologist, you should consider traveling for care and perhaps enrolling in a clinical trial. Much of the best work being done for colorectal cancer is done at university medical schools. In Chapter 20, *Clinical Trials*, and Chapter 21, *Traveling for Care,* we'll provide you with more detail, such as how clinical trials are structured and charitable groups that will pay travel and lodging costs for you.

I spoke with my gastroenterologist about surgery. He gave me the name of a few surgeons in my area. I met and spoke with one doctor who performed the surgery to create the J pouch. My disease had damaged the tissue right to the anus. He pointed out that a small amount of damaged tissue would have to be used to connect it up. It was an interesting idea. He also pointed out that there was no guarantee that it could be done on me. If the blood vessels didn't reach it was a no go. I found out later that sometimes they don't "take."

I decided to check with a research hospital, Johns Hopkins, looking for a magical mystery cure. No such luck. The GI doctor I spoke with said the diseased tissue had to come out—no ifs, ands, or buts. He had me make an appointment with the surgeon who does most of his work. The J pouch was never suggested.

I was sort of glad the traditional ostomy was the only thing discussed. I didn't like the idea of leaving precancerous cells behind, and I heard that I could get pouchitis after surgery, an inflammation of the small intestine that was used to create the pouch.

After I'd healed—about six weeks later—I saw my surgeon for a follow-up visit. He suggested I talk to an oncologist about whether chemotherapy would be necessary, because my tumor was staged as stage I. After reviewing my scans and the biopsy report, the oncologist decided additional treatment wasn't necessary.

A word about managed care: your insurance provider may have restrictions regarding whom you may consult or where you may travel for care. Check your policy carefully for such restrictions, and contact the provider before scheduling appointments that might not be covered. Some managed care providers charge only a modestly increased co-payment for out-of-plan doctors; others refuse to pay any of the doctor's fee; still others will pay most or all costs if medical necessity can be proved. If your HMO has a care coordinator, he may work with you to make special reinterpretations of the rules in your case. Often people never challenge their HMO's rules, but frequently those who do win a full settlement or a compromise.

A colon cancer survivor describes his concerns about the different opinions he's heard about treatment:

I am a 50-year-old male diagnosed by colonoscopy and CT (computed tomography) as having colon cancer. My GI doctor referred me to a surgeon at Massachusetts General Hospital who performed an extended right colectomy. After receiving the pathology report my surgeon classified the disease as Dukes stage B2.

I do not yet have an oncologist, although I have an appointment with one next week. My referring GI had originally been concerned about the possibility of imminent perforation and the initial reference had been directly to a surgeon.

My surgeon believes that there is no need for any chemotherapy. He has stated that at Massachusetts General they do not do any adjuvant therapy for a Dukes B2 diagnosis.

I have done some reading on the various chemotherapy protocols and I see that the question of chemotherapy for Dukes B2 colon cancer is controversial. From the studies that I have read, it would seem that a course of 5-FU and leucovorin would at least slightly reduce the chances of recurrence.

I don't understand a decision to not do a course of chemo if there is even a small chance of improving a prognosis. Ideally I guess I'd like the chance to talk to an oncologist on both sides of the issue.

Over the next few months, this gentleman took additional time to educate himself, sought second and even third opinions, and decided on chemotherapy.

Finding several good specialists

If you have limited time to get recommendations, you can contact the nearest university medical school or the National Cancer Institute (NCI) at (800) 4-CANCER and ask for the names of several suitable surgeons and oncologists at their institution or in your area.

In addition to these two techniques, there are several other ways to search for qualified surgeons and oncologists:

- The National Cancer Institute designates both Comprehensive Cancer Centers and Clinical Cancer Centers. The former meet rigorous standards of excellence; the latter meet less rigorous but still quite high standards. If you phone NCI's Cancer Information Service at (800) 4-CAN-CER, they can provide you with a list of these centers. Be sure to tell them if you're willing to travel for care, otherwise they are inclined to assume that you want only local references. Once you have these lists, you can phone the nearest center and ask for referrals. Note that any institution can simply include in its name the words "clinical cancer center" or "comprehensive cancer center." Be sure that the institution's title is NCI-designated. If you have a personal computer, you can access this information at NCI's web site at *http://cancernet.nci.nih.gov.*

- The American Medical Association maintains a list of all licensed doctors, AMA members or not, and can tell you if the doctor you're considering is board-certified in a surgical specialty such as colon and rectal surgery or in medical or radiologic oncology. They can also furnish information such as year of graduation from medical school and the location of residencies. The AMA's Physician Select web site is *http://www.ama-assn.org/aps/amahg.html.*

- The American Board of Medical Specialties can refer you to board-certified specialists. Visit *http://www.certifieddoctor.org* or contact them at 47 Perimeter Center East, Suite 500, Atlanta, GA 30346 or call (800) 733-2267.

- *The American Medical Directory* and *The Directory of Medical Specialists,* available at your local library, both list doctors by specialty.

- The magazine *US News and World Report,* which can be found in your local library, annually designates hospitals as Centers of Excellence. Usually this "Best Hospitals" issue is published in July. Hospitals ranked best in cancer care are listed within by cancer subcategory. With this information, you can phone several of these hospitals and ask to speak, for instance, with a surgeon who specializes in cancers of the colon and rectum. Ask this doctor for the names of several surgeons and oncologists in your area, or for a referral within her own institution if it's nearby or within your acceptable travel boundaries. You may be able to order a back issue of *US News and World Report's "Best Hospitals"* edition by calling (202) 955-2000, or by visiting their web site at *http://www.usnews.com.*

- If your family doctor or primary care physician has recommended a surgeon or oncologist, ask him why he's recommending this person. Recommendations from another doctor can range from wonderful—"Because she gets such good results"—to lukewarm.

- Phone a reputable nearby hospital, ask for the oncology floor, then ask to speak with the head oncology nurse. Explain that you'd like a recommendation for an oncologist who treats colorectal cancer, and that you'd value the nurse's opinion because she works extensively with so many oncologists.

- Likewise, phone a reputable nearby hospital, ask for the surgical floor, then ask to speak with the head surgical nurse. Explain that you'd like a recommendation for a surgeon who treats colorectal cancer.

- Use a personal computer to access the National Library of Medicine's Medline, or have a friend or relative do so for you. Search on the subjects "colon cancer treatment" or "rectal cancer treatment." Scan the last two years' worth of papers and note the authors' names. Some Medline access providers such as PaperChase show the authors' institutional affiliations; if not, phone the NCI at (800) 4-CANCER and ask where these doctors can be reached. For more information on using Medline, see Chapter 24, *Researching Your Illness*. The National Library of Medicine's free Pubmed Medline search engine is at *http://www4.ncbi.nlm.nih.gov/ PubMed/*.

- Contact the American College of Surgeons (see Appendix A, *Resources*) for the names of surgeons and oncologists who specialize in colorectal cancer.

- Your surgeon may know medical and radiologic oncologists who are well-regarded.

Choosing treatment centers

Bear in mind that when you choose a doctor, you also choose by default a treatment center. Ask the doctors on your short list to which hospitals they have admitting privileges and with which, if any, NCI-designate treatment groups they are associated.

There are several different types of treatment centers: university hospitals, cooperative colorectal cancer groups, and community clinical oncology programs.

University hospitals

In January 1999, the *New England Journal of Medicine* reported that, although patients sometimes prefer the level of emotional support provided by community hospitals, teaching hospitals provide better medical care.

University hospitals, or other research institutions funded by NCI such as Memorial Sloan-Kettering Cancer Center in New York or the Mayo Cancer Center in Rochester, Minnesota, are very likely places to find the latest advances in colorectal cancer treatment.

When regulatory agencies decide who will be allocated scarce resources or who will be given permission to provide rare services such as PET scanning, the university hospital is a likely choice because the infrastructure, such as skill levels and staffing, is already in place. In addition, the cooperative and collaborative nature of the university hospital tends to attract the most talented medical researchers. In most cases, these same researchers are also expected to provide patient care. This means that the latest treatments are likely to be offered in this setting first, that the accumulated experience level among the staff is high, and that you'll be treated by some of the most talented and knowledgeable people in the country.

University-associated hospitals and cancer centers are the institutions most likely to be designated by the NCI as either Comprehensive Cancer Centers or Clinical Cancer Centers. All NCI-designated centers are nonprofit institutions.

Some people are afraid to receive healthcare at a university or teaching hospital because they fear they will be subjected to unproven or unnecessary treatment by newly graduated medical students who may not know what they're doing. It's true that a training mission incorporated into a hospital's charter means that you may be examined or cared for by more than one doctor, but this can be an advantage as well as a disadvantage. These advantages and disadvantages differ little from having a family doctor who is a member of a large practice: while it's true that you may not always see the same doctor, it's also true that you need not go without help if she's not available. Newly graduated doctors, called interns (also called first-year residents, or postgraduate year-one students) are seldom charged with care or decision-making in the absence of your attending doctor or an oncology resident. You're always free to say that you prefer that a procedure or exam be done by someone with more experience.

In the US, unproven treatments are never performed without clear written informed consent if your hospital receives any federal funds or is governed by local laws regarding informed consent. If you are approached to take part in a study of an unproven treatment, called a clinical trial, you always have the right to refuse, and if you do decide to enroll, you always have the right to withdraw later.

A most important fact of which all cancer survivors and their loved ones should be aware is that, for cancer treatment, a placebo is virtually never used. The new, unproven treatment is offered either in clinical trials that compare the new treatment to standard, approved treatment or that offer the new treatment only—for cancer, new treatments are never compared to an inactive sugar pill as are drugs in other kinds of (noncancer) clinical trials. When there is no standard treatment to which the new treatment can be jux-taposed, such as the very first bone marrow purging procedures in the early days of bone marrow transplantation, this lack is clearly communicated by those attempting to ensure that consent is indeed informed consent.

Note that a community teaching hospital is not the same as a medical school training hospital, although the community hospital may have residency programs that accommodate certain university medical school training needs such as emergency room rotations.

Cooperative groups

Cooperative groups comprise university hospitals and cancer treatment centers that take part in administering very large multi-center trials of new treatments. There are about 13 clinical trial cooperative groups in the US. A list of the centers in these groups can be obtained by phoning the NCI's Cancer Information Service at (800) 4-CANCER.

Community clinical oncology programs

This program links community doctors with the clinical trial cooperative groups described directly above in the section called "Cooperative groups." For a list of groups in your area, phone the NCI at (800) 4-CANCER.

Treatment at no charge

The National Cancer Institute provides free cancer care to those who qualify, but only within clinical trials. A referral from your local oncologist is necessary for entry into a trial. Non-US citizens as well may be admitted at the discretion of the principal investigator of the trial.

St. Jude Children's Research Hospital in Memphis, Tennessee, provides free treatment for children.

Some university and community hospitals have a policy guaranteeing that they will provide medical care for local residents who cannot pay.

Checking credentials of candidates

If a check on credentials wasn't part of the process you used to come up with a list of candidate surgeons and oncologists, you can check credentials now. Any doctors recommended by NCI or from a clinical center have undoubtedly already had a thorough check of their backgrounds and qualifications, however you might want to see these credentials for yourself.

You can check doctors' professional qualifications in some of the same publications listed as aids to locating qualified surgeons and oncologists:

- The *AMA Directory of Physicians* lists the doctor's name, medical school attended, year licensed, primary and secondary specialty, type of practice, board certification, and physician recognition awards. (Available in libraries or at *http://www.ama-assn.org*.)

- The official *ABMS Directory of Board Certified Medical Specialties* includes specialty, when certified, medical school and year of degree, place and dates of internship, place and dates of residency, fellowship training, academic and hospital appointments, professional association memberships, type of practice, and current address, telephone, and fax. (Available in libraries, at *http://www.abms.org*, or at (800) 776-CERT.)

- Your state medical licensing board should be able to tell you the status of your doctor's license, when the doctor was first licensed by the state, and the status of any misconduct charges or disciplinary actions.

- An easy way to check on your doctor's credentials is to call Medi-Net, a consumer information service that provides healthcare consumers with a background check on any doctor who is licensed to practice in the United States, including credentials, degrees, training, board certifications, as well as any disciplinary actions or sanctions taken against the doctor. Each complete Medi-Net physician profile costs $15.00 per doctor (less for subsequent profiles ordered at the same time). Preliminary information is provided on the telephone, with detailed reports mailed or faxed to callers usually the same day. To order a report, call toll-free (888) ASK-MEDI (275-6334) or (800) 972-MEDI (972-6334), or on the Internet at *http://www.askmedi.com.*

Another way to reassure yourself about the currency of the candidate doctor's knowledge is to see what he has published.

- Again, use a personal computer to access Medline, or have a friend or relative do so for you, this time searching by the doctor's last name and first initial to see what she has published. Note that the US National Library of Medicine offers a free Medline search engine at *http://www4. ncbi.nlm.nih.gov/PubMed/.* (If you don't have a PC, try your local library. Many have computers for public use.) In general, if the doctor you're considering has published two or more papers in the last five years on topics that you feel pertain to your condition, she's worth a visit. Keep in mind, though, that many excellent oncologists are involved in research during their training years, then move into private practice and cease publishing. Lack of published material does not mean a doctor is inadequate, nor does the existence of many publications guarantee that she will be a good, caring practitioner. Published papers are just one of many gauges of a doctor's ability.

Choosing the best from a short list

Once you have found one or more board-certified surgeons and oncologists who seem excellent, you can interview them to make sure they're good candidates. This is especially important for choosing a medical or radiation oncologist. No matter how many recommendations you receive or sterling credentials you have uncovered, until you have a candid conversation with the human behind the stethoscope, you won't know if this is a person with whom you'll feel comfortable for a series of treatments that may last many months.

Schedule a meeting to ask any questions that you have about medical background and about the doctor's attitudes and office policies, such as:

- How many surgeries for suspected colorectal cancer has the surgeon performed? If interviewing a medical or radiation oncologist, how many patients with your type of colon or rectal cancer has he treated?
- To what hospitals does he have admitting privileges?

- With which clinical trials is he familiar? It's important to have medical and radiation oncologists familiar with the latest research in colorectal cancer.

- With which institutions is he affiliated? For instance, has he a faculty appointment at a medical school in addition to a private surgical or oncology practice?

- What surgery or treatment does he recommend? After the appointment, evaluate how this recommendation compares with what your reading has taught you.

- What is his policy for handling emergency calls during non-business hours?

- How will test results be communicated? Will ancillary doctors be given permission to communicate directly with you, the patient? Does the doctor object to leaving information on your answering or fax machines, if that's a method you prefer?

- Are family members welcome to call with questions? Some doctors prefer communicating only with the patient.

- Does the doctor's philosophy about health and life mesh well with your own? For example, does he espouse treatment at all costs over quality of life?

- Use some of this interview time to describe yourself and your expectations, such as how much participation you would like to have in health-care decisions.

Overall, you want to make sure that the surgeon and oncologists you choose have excellent medical credentials, extensive experience with colorectal cancer, and are affiliated with treatment centers that offer up-to-date resources. You'll want to weigh in other considerations such as communication skills, personal style, and office location.

Summary

Now that you have information regarding the differences among oncologists and surgeons, the wisdom of utilizing a board-certified specialist, and the advantages of care at a well-regarded cancer center or large cooperative colorectal cancer group, you are equipped to find a good doctor and turn your attention to such issues as the details of your treatment and finding the emotional and instrumental support you will need.

CHAPTER 3

What Is Colorectal Cancer?

Physicians think they do a lot for a patient
when they give his disease a name.

—Immanuel Kant

IN THIS CHAPTER, WE WILL ATTEMPT TO CATEGORIZE INFORMATION about colorectal cancer so that you can begin to build a frame of reference for understanding your disease. First, we will discuss colorectal cancers in the broader context of all cancers. Then we will look at variations in colorectal cancer by age, gender, race, geographics, and other characteristics. Finally, we'll look at what is known about the possible causes of colorectal cancer.

What are the colon and rectum?

The colon, or large intestine, comprises the last six feet of the intestine, which is about twenty-six feet long. It begins just past the ileum, which is part of the small intestine. The colon changes to rectal tissue in its last six inches, but the boundary between the colon and rectum is not clearly delineated. For this reason, colon and rectal cancers are sometimes grouped together as colorectal cancer. See Figures 3-1 and 3-2.

The colon is responsible for absorbing water from what we eat, and for collecting food waste until we are able to expel it from the body.

As the colon loops through the abdomen in the shape of an upside-down "U," it passes near many other critical organs: the spleen, liver, pancreas, male and female sexual organs, and so on. Each of these can be affected by the spread of colorectal cancer beyond the colon.

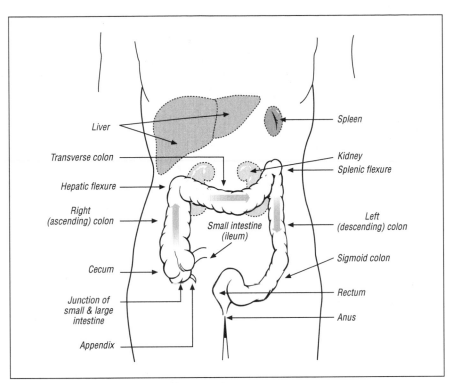

Figure 3-1. The path of the colon (front view)

Colorectal cancer

Colorectal cancer begins as the uncontrolled growth of cells that line the innermost surface of the large intestine and rectum.

As with other cancers, the wayward cells that characterize colorectal cancer do not always die as normal cells do, nor do they honor the cycles of orderly cell division as normal cells do: many have no resting phase, instead dividing continuously. What's worse, they divide before they are fully mature, which makes them unable to function as normal cells of the colon do. This means that our bodies accumulate nonfunctional colon cells that, by dividing rapidly or by not undergoing normal cell death (apoptosis), crowd out other functioning colon cells and other nearby normal cells within affected organs.

For some forms of cancer such as leukemia, this overgrowth and crowding out of normal cells in the bloodstream is enough to cause serious health problems and eventually death. But for most solid tumors, an additional step

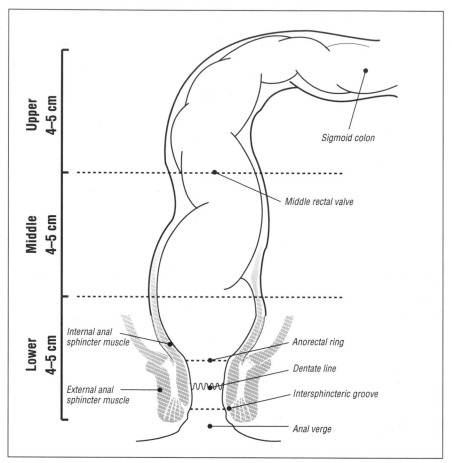

Upper 4–5 cm

Middle 4–5 cm

Lower 4–5 cm

Sigmoid colon

Middle rectal valve

Internal anal sphincter muscle

External anal sphincter muscle

Anorectal ring

Dentate line

Intersphincteric groove

Anal verge

Figure 3-2. The rectum and anus (front view)

must occur: the abnormally proliferating cells must develop the ability to invade other organs. This invasiveness distinguishes benign tumors from cancerous tumors.

Many studies have shown that most cases of colon cancer begin with noncancerous growths called polyps. Polyps usually are pedunculated—that is, extending from the surface of the colon much like a tiny balloon. Some, however, lie flat against the surface of the intestine—sessile polyps—and may be hard to detect with the diagnostic tools in use today.

Polyps are known to progress gradually through stages of change from harmless to cancerous. For most people, polyp removal in the precancerous adenomatous stage is sufficient to keep the patient free of colon cancer, and general screening guidelines are aimed at detecting colon cancer at this stage. Exceptions are those people who inherit genes that predispose them to a form of polyp growth that results in hundreds or thousands of polyps that are too numerous to be removed with a colonoscope (and are very likely to regrow), or those who inherit a familial syndrome that causes polyps to form at such a young age that, unless the family history were known, relatively late screening at age 50 would be too late.

The following sections discuss the unique aspects of colorectal cancers.

Types of colorectal cancers

There are several subcategories of colorectal cancers. Subtypes of colorectal cancer, as defined by the National Cancer Institute, include:

- Adenocarcinoma, which accounts for the majority of cases

- Mucinous (colloid) adenocarcinoma

- Signet ring adenocarcinoma

- Neuroendocrine scirrhous tumors

If you attempt to compare yourself to others who appear to have the same diagnosis, bear in mind that their diagnosis may have been made using criteria that are different, perhaps in subtle ways, from those used by your own diagnosticians. This means that treatment decisions from one person to the next may differ as well.

Metastasis

The spread of a primary tumor into other organs as independent secondary tumors is called metastasis. The secondary tumors that appear within these other organs are called metastases.

A mechanistic theory that explains the spread of many (but not all) cancers appears to be the best explanation for the spread of colorectal cancer: the transport of cancer cells via the bloodstream or via lymphatic fluid.

Colorectal cancer tends to spread to nearby sites, such as the lining of the abdomen, called the peritoneum, and to the nearest lymph nodes (there are many lymph nodes throughout the abdomen, especially near the intestine). It also spreads preferentially to certain organs such as the lung, liver, and brain. The liver is a common site of metastasis for colorectal cancer because the return flow of blood from the intestine to the heart is unique in first passing through the liver.

Incidence and trends

Using Surveillance, Epidemiology, and End Results (SEER) statistics from 1995, the American Cancer Society projects that new cases of colorectal cancer in 1999 will number 129,400, a decrease to fourth most common cancer in the US, following prostate, breast, and lung cancers in incidence.

However, ACS estimates that colorectal cancer will remain the second most common cause of cancer deaths. About 56,600 people are expected to die from colorectal cancer in the US in 1999.

These numbers represent a decrease of 9.1 percent in new cases from 1973 to 1996: a 7.1 decrease in incidence among males; a 12.0 percent decrease among females. Incidence rates rose until 1986, and have been dropping since.[1]

A decrease of 22.6 percent in deaths in the same time period has occurred: a 17.9 percent decrease among males; a 27.6 percent decrease among females.

Detailed incidence and mortality rates for colon and rectal cancers differ, though.

Colon cancer

According to 1996 SEER statistics, from 1973 to 1996 colon cancer incidence in the US decreased 5.1 percent, with a 1.5 percent decrease among males and a 9.5 percent decrease among females. Differences in these incidence numbers by gender are discussed in the section "Who gets colorectal cancer?".

Rectal cancer

According to 1996 SEER statistics, rectal cancer incidence from 1973 to 1996 decreased 17.6 percent: 17.5 percent in males and 18.6 percent in females.

Who gets colorectal cancer?

You would be a most unusual person if you didn't wonder why you developed cancer, and where you are in the spectrum of others with the same disease.

Geographic latitude

There is a striking pattern of steady increase in colon cancer among those living increasingly far from the equator. Colon cancer among those living within ten degrees of the equator, for instance, is virtually unknown. This geographic pattern of disease transcends all other lifestyle and environmental risk factors, including gender, diet, exercise, national industrialization, and socioeconomic class.

Researchers have tentatively attributed this pattern of increasing incidence to decreasing amounts of vitamin D in skin as a result of lessened exposure to sun, and to its corresponding lowered effect on calcium metabolism.

Gender

Males of all ages are diagnosed more frequently with colorectal cancer than are females. According to 1996 SEER statistics, the age-adjusted incidence rate among males is 51.1 per 100,000, and the age-adjusted rate for females is 36.2 per 100,000. Natural estrogen, oral contraceptives, and estrogen-replacement drugs appear to protect females from colon cancer, perhaps owing to their effect on calcium and vitamin D metabolism.

Race

According to 1996 SEER statistics, white Americans are diagnosed with invasive colorectal cancer less often than black Americans: 43.0 per 100,000 versus 50.4 per 100,000. Blacks with colorectal cancer are diagnosed in later stages, at an earlier age, and survive for shorter periods of time. This difference is thought by some to be attributable to differences in access to health-care among socioeconomic classes in the US.

For other US ethnic groups, rates of incidence per 100,000 are:

- Hispanic: 29.0
- American Indian: 16.4
- Asian/Pacific Islander: 38.6

Age

Colorectal cancer is clearly a disease correlated to increasing age. Incidence for those aged 50 to 54 is 48.1 per 100,000 people; for those aged 75 to 79, however, the incidence is 347.3 per 100,000.

Although primarily a disease of older adults, colorectal cancer is not unknown among those aged 40 and younger, who account for 2 to 6 percent of colorectal cancer cases.

Socioeconomic class

In the US, incidence of colorectal cancer is evenly distributed among the socioeconomic classes. In certain other countries, however, particularly in the less industrialized countries, higher socioeconomic classes have a higher incidence of colorectal cancer, a phenomenon that some researchers say correlates to the presence of more red meat in the diets of the upper classes.

What causes cancer?

Before a clear discussion of the causes of colorectal cancer can ensue, you need to know a bit about what causes cancers in general.

Human DNA is stored on 46 paired chromosomes. With a couple of exceptions, each cell in our bodies has one copy of all 46 chromosomes, coiled tightly in a ball, stored in the cell nucleus. Each chromosome is composed of two long strings of genes held together like a ladder, with rungs consisting of electrochemical bonds.

All instances of cancer are accompanied by changes in the tumor cell's DNA. At times, one or more genes are entirely missing, or have been altered by viruses that insert their genes into ours, or have been half-spliced with another gene after DNA strands from two entirely different chromosomes accidentally overlap, break apart, and rejoin. Such chromosomal changes are well known among colorectal cancers and other cancers. In some cases, an entire chromosome may be missing.

These changes become potentially harmful when genes are engaged to manufacture proteins. All of the body's work is accomplished using proteins. Our bodies build proteins from genes by reading the base pairs of DNA in groups of three, until special repeating sequences recognized as terminators are encountered. Each triplet encodes for one amino acid, and the complete string of amino acids comprise a protein. The string of amino acids that accumulates—that is, the protein built as the DNA is transcribed—is unique to that gene.

If the gene is damaged by the crossing-over of two chromosomes, a protein built from it will be based half on one gene and half on another, and most likely will be completely nonfunctional, or even toxic. If one base pair is deleted from DNA, the transcription of the three base pairs into one amino acid is shifted off by one, almost exactly like placing one's fingers on a piano or computer keyboard in the wrong starting position: every subsequent movement up and down the keyboard will produce wrong notes or wrong letters when the starting point is wrong. Thus, when one or more base pairs are missing, the resulting protein will be entirely different from that which the body is expecting to accomplish some metabolic task.

Often these mutations are harmless, but when a great many accumulate, and especially when these changes occur in or very near genes that regulate cell growth, orderly cell death called apoptosis (as does the p53 gene), or maturation of cell division and reproduction, uncontrolled growth, either benign or cancerous, may result.

Cancerous growths are distinguished from benign growths by their ability to invade other tissues and, in colon cancer, can arise from longstanding precancerous polyps.

Often, the higher the number of damaged genes the more likely cancer is to result, as more and more cellular functions become affected by nonfunctioning proteins. Some cancers, though, such as acute promyelocytic leukemia, can result from damage to just two genes.[2]

What causes colorectal cancer?

Many people try to determine what gave cancer a foothold, sometimes from intellectual curiosity, and sometimes from a determination not to suffer a relapse.

With one exception—the familial cancer syndromes—no sure cause of colorectal cancer has been found, but several highly suspicious circumstances or substances may explain the development of some colorectal cancers. It's probable that you'll never know the exact cause of your illness, but the following discussion can offer possible explanations.

Genetics

Many people diagnosed with colorectal cancer become concerned that their siblings or children also may face an increased risk of developing this disease.

Attempts to understand any increased risk among family members may be difficult if the way that many research studies use the word *genetic* is not understood. We who are not involved in research tend to use the word *genetic* interchangeably with *heritable or inherited*, but the study of genetics encompasses a broader meaning, and researchers sometimes are not referring to genetics in the heritable sense when they use the word genetics. Many genetic changes occur within cancerous cells, but only genetic changes or errors that arise and persist in sperm or ova can be inherited.

Nonetheless, several inherited forms of colorectal cancer have been identified:

- Hereditary nonpolyposis colorectal cancer (HNPCC), characterized by development of about the same number of adenomatous polyps seen in the general population, and by development of colon cancer in three first-degree family members within two generations, at least one of whom is younger than 50:

    - Lynch syndrome I manifests as multiple episodes of early onset colon cancer in the same family, often occurring on the right side of the colon or prior to the splenic flexure (see Figure 3-1).

    - Lynch syndrome II manifests as multiple cases of cancer in the family, including colorectal cancers, gastric cancers (stomach, biliary tract, small intestine), ovarian, urinary tract, and endometrial cancers.

    - Muir-Torre syndrome, exhibiting multiple cutaneous sebaceous tumors and, frequently, internal tumors, of which colon cancer is the most common.

- Familial adenomatous polyposis (FAP), characterized by the presence of hundreds or thousands of polyps in the colon that almost always progress to full-blown colon cancer if the colon is not surgically removed.

- Gardner's syndrome, a subtype of FAP, includes families having adenomatous polyps of the colon, soft tissue tumors (sebaceous cysts and fibromas, also called desmoid tumors), bony tumors, osteomas, and hyperpigmented lesions of the retina.

- Attenuated familial adenomatous polyposis (AFAP) is now considered a subtype of FAP, and is characterized by the presence of less than 100 polyps as well as a later age of onset of polyps and of colorectal cancer.

• Peutz-Jegher's syndrome, exhibiting pigmented skin patches around the mouth, hands, or anus; and hamartomatous polyps—polyps that are benign, but may eventually develop into cancers of the small bowel, stomach, or colon. Breast or ovarian cancers in females are sometimes linked to this disorder, as is pancreatic cancer in males and females.

• Juvenile polyposis syndrome, exhibiting hamartomatous (benign) polyps that may eventually develop into gastrointestinal cancer.

• Cowden's disease, characterized by hamartomatous (benign) polyps and related growths on the face, mouth, and hands, and associated with malignancies such as colon, breast, uterus, bladder, lung, and thyroid cancers, as well as melanoma and liposarcoma, tumors of the central nervous system, and squamous cell carcinoma of the skin.

• Intestinal ganglioneuromatosis, an overgrowth of nervous system cells in the intestine that is associated with intestinal polyps that can transform to gastrointestinal cancer. This syndrome also is linked to multiple endocrine neoplasia type IIB (MEN IIB), which gives rise to thyroid cancer and pheochromocytomas.

Known inherited forms of colorectal cancer account for only about 10 percent of diagnoses, but in general, the risk of getting colon cancer is about 6 to 12 percent higher than the general population's if you have a first-order relative (father, mother, or sibling) with colon cancer. Many researchers have noted that those with so-called "sporadic" colon cancers—cancers thought not to be inherited—also have a number of family members with colon cancer, or with breast, ovarian, or endometrial cancers. This suggests that unknown heritable factors are in play, and that perhaps environmental factors that families share, such as diet or water supply, can trigger an otherwise not very strong predisposition to colon cancer.

Copious information about inheritance of a predisposition to colon cancer is available in Alfred Cohen's 1995 text, *Cancers of the Colon, Rectum, and Anus*, and in current medical journals, the abstracts of which are made available free of charge by the US National Cancer Institute. They are accessible using a computer and Internet browser software; see Chapter 24, *Researching Your Illness*.

Anyone with a first-order relative (mother, father, sibling, child) diagnosed with colon cancer should consider genetic counseling to assess their risk, and should have screening tests earlier in life, and more often, than those in the general population.

Anyone with a known familial colorectal cancer syndrome such as hereditary nonpolyposis colon cancer (HNPCC) or familial adenomatous polyps (FAP) should consult a physician regularly about screening. Depending on your family history, your doctor might recommend screening as early as age 20, or even in childhood.

Additional screening information can be found in the back of this book, on the page titled "Colorectal Cancer Screening." You might wish to share copies of that page with your family and friends.

Autoimmune diseases

Certain autoimmune illnesses, such as diabetes and the inflammatory bowel diseases ulcerative colitis and Crohn's disease, predispose one to developing colorectal cancer. For example, in three European populations followed for 17 to 38 years, the risk of developing colon cancer among those who had extensive ulcerative colitis was 20 times higher than the risk faced by the general population.[3] The risk among those with Crohn's disease is higher than that of the general population—about fourfold—but not as pronounced as that faced by those with extensive ulcerative colitis of long standing.

Foods

Not surprisingly, diet and its effect on colorectal cancer have received much scrutiny, as foods and the contaminants they may contain come in direct contact with the gastrointestinal tract and spend from 26 to 40 hours therein.

High consumption of red meat has been linked in some studies to an increased risk of colorectal cancer, but other studies show no connection.

Some studies, but not others, show that an increased amount of fat in the diet correlates to an increased risk of developing colorectal cancer. Dissenting studies have found that obesity, rather than fat in the diet, accounts for this increased risk. Still other studies have found that the source of fat is more important than total fat in the diet, with vegetable sources being safer than animal sources.

In several studies, diets low in calcium, vitamin D, selenium, and folate correlate to higher rates of colorectal cancer. This is consistent with recent evidence that those who take multivitamins containing folate for many years sustain lower rates of colorectal cancer, and with evidence that many populations living farthest from the equator—and thus experiencing the lowest amount of sun exposure and subsequent lack of vitamin D formation in skin—sustain the highest rates of colorectal cancer.

Vegetables, especially cruciferous vegetables such as broccoli, cabbage, and cauliflower, appear to confer a protective effect against colon cancer. Fruits have a beneficial effect as well, but do not have as pronounced an effect as do vegetables.

In some but not all studies, diets high in fiber and roughage appear to protect against development of colon cancer. Other studies have shown confoundingly low rates of colorectal cancer in countries such as Japan, where fiber is not a significant part of the daily diet. The Japanese consume higher quantities of soy than other populations do, however; the properties of soy that resemble estrogens may protect the Japanese from colorectal cancer in spite of a lower level of fiber in the typical Japanese diet. Results of studies on fiber can be difficult to compare, as some, for example, examine vegetable fiber while others examine fiber in whole grains. A recent large study of 88,000 women found no association between low dietary fiber and an excess risk of colon cancer.[4]

Alcohol consumption has been correlated to an increased risk of developing colorectal cancer, and especially rectal cancer, in some studies; however, other researchers feel this association is, at best, small.

Exercise

A recent review of many studies on physical activity and colorectal cancer has shown that those who exercise regularly may experience lower rates of colon cancer.[5] Another study shows a protective effect for men, but not women.[6] A third shows protective effect against colon cancer but not rectal cancer.[7]

Although the exact protective effect of exercise and its true impact on risk is not known, exercise is known to quicken the digestive process to approximately two-thirds of that found in sedentary people, and to induce bowel movements. This relatively rapid passage of food byproducts through the colon may minimize exposure to potential carcinogens, substances that cause cancer.

Medications

One study has found a significant association between constipation, the use of laxatives and an increased risk of developing colon cancer.

Many studies have found that a protective effect against colorectal cancer is conferred by use of aspirin and other nonsteroidal anti-inflammatory drugs (NSAIDs) such as ibuprofen. NSAIDs inhibit the production of prostaglandins, body products that play a role in inflammation and that may play a role in the development of colorectal cancer. Consult your doctor before using NSAIDs, however, as serious side effects might occur in some people.

Estrogen exposure

The use of estrogen-containing medications, an increasing number of pregnancies, and lower age at first menstruation are associated with lower rates of colorectal cancer. Researchers speculate that estrogen's beneficial effect on calcium and vitamin D metabolism may contribute to this lowered risk.

Divergence in rates of colorectal cancer among men and women in the last 25 years has been attributed by some researchers to the increased use of oral contraceptives and estrogen replacement therapy by females in the fourth quarter of the twentieth century.

Tobacco use

Smoking cigarettes is known to be associated with development of adenomatous polyps, a precancerous colon condition, and with increased rates of rectal cancer.

Moreover, recent studies that contradict earlier studies have shown that those who smoke a pack or more of cigarettes a day have an increased risk for developing colon cancer, a risk that persists even years after cessation of smoking. This risk appears not to extend to those who smoke cigars or pipes. The risk is greater for overweight females who smoke more than 20 cigarettes a day.

Risk associated with other cancers

Those previously diagnosed with ovarian, endometrial, or breast cancer face an increased risk of developing colorectal cancer.

Obesity

For men, excessive weight predicts an increased risk of colorectal cancer; in women, abdominal obesity—a high waist-to-hip ratio—is a more reliable risk indicator.

Parasites or pathogens

Asians living in Asia seldom develop colorectal cancer, except for Chinese living along riverbanks. This has caused some researchers to speculate that certain pathogens, perhaps only those specific to the Asian subcontinent, might release toxins, or induce bodily responses, that culminate in colorectal cancer.

The aging immune system

Some researchers feel that the greatly increased rate not only of colorectal cancer, but also of most other cancers among those over age 65, hints at a general weakening of the immune system with age. Others feel that this more likely may be an artifact of the modern, industrialized world we live in: that genetic damage from substances in an industrialized environment accumulates over time, and first becomes apparent among the oldest.

Summary

The preceding pages have attempted to categorize information about colorectal cancer so that you may begin to build a frame of reference for understanding this disease.

Key points to remember:

- About 10 percent of colorectal cancers are attributable to inherited disorders.

- Lifestyle choices such as diet, exercise, and calcium/vitamin D metabolism appear to play roles in the risk of developing colorectal cancer.

- Increasing age is a prominent risk factor for colorectal cancer.

CHAPTER 4

Prognosis

To lose one's health renders science null,
art inglorious, strength unavailing,
wealth useless, and eloquence powerless.

—Herophilus

ALMOST EVERYONE WANTS TO KNOW HOW SERIOUS THEIR CANCER IS, and what their prospects are for survival. This questioning is completely normal.

In this chapter, we first review factors that limit the ability of this book—or any printed resource—to predict outcomes for colorectal cancer. The last half of the chapter describes what prognostic factors have been studied, and what factors matter the least and the most. It is important to grasp that several poorly understood circumstances limit one's ability to say that events will happen in a certain way for a person diagnosed with colorectal cancer. It's also important to know that many, but not all, prognostic factors for colon cancer also pertain to rectal cancer, as the border between these two diseases is quite literally obscured as colon tissue blends into rectal tissue.

When you've finished this chapter, you won't have an absolute, unchanging answer about your prognosis. However, you'll have an idea of factors that might influence your prognosis, a respect for the complexity of the topic, and an awareness of the dangers of predictions.

Limitations on accurate prognosis

The limitations on the ability to predict the course of colorectal cancer include the general limitations of all medical studies and statistics; that is, there are still many unknowns, and not all unknowns can be predicted from what we do know. There are also limitations specific to colorectal cancer, such as improvements in treatment, the differences between various cancers, and differences in patients and in colorectal cancer types. The following are factors to keep in mind when reading any discussion of prognosis for colorectal cancer, no matter how recent.

Improving treatments

First, owing to intense research, information regarding prognoses stated unequivocally today might be obsolete tomorrow. The increasing use of adjuvant therapies and the tremendous gains made in supportive care, such as new antifungals and antinausea drugs, are examples. As always, your doctor, a well-trained and skilled person who most likely you chose carefully as outlined in Chapter 2, *Finding the Right Treatment Team*, is your best resource for the most current information. You might also choose to follow the progress of new treatments on your own. Ways to do this are discussed in Chapter 24, *Researching Your Illness*.

Difficult classifications

The four generalized classifications of colorectal cancer make discussing research results complex. Chapter 3, *What Is Colorectal Cancer?* and Appendix D, *Staging System Equivalents*, discuss and delineate the systems used to categorize the spread of colorectal cancer, and the problems and complexities encountered in doing so. For instance, all of these factors amount to subclassifications that may affect outcome:

- Left-colon disease may exhibit different behavior from right-colon disease.

- The location and contiguity of affected lymph nodes further refines the TNM classification.

- The rate at which tumor cells are dividing and the amount of damage to the DNA in tumor cells may affect response to therapy.

- The pattern of movement of cancer cells into the intestinal wall may affect outcome.

- The absence of mucin-producing cells might yield a better outcome.

This means that multiple studies from different institutions, which yield conflicting results from the same treatment regimen, may not compare readily to each other, and, most importantly, may not apply to you and your specific circumstances.

Limitations of statistics

Survival statistics are developed using groups of people, many of whom are not very much like you, even if they appear to have the same disease, categorized using the same system or by a single research center. Your chances may be considerably better, for instance, than those of someone who has several chronic illnesses such as heart disease, diabetes, or lupus along with colorectal cancer. In addition, many of those whose cases find their way into medical journals, and who become the basis for statistics regarding the success of one technique versus another, are those who have had many different treatments and who may have one or more organ systems compromised owing to repeated toxic treatments. More is said about this later.

Those of you who studied statistics in school are aware that many different statistical methods exist to manipulate data, any two of which may in some cases give differing results. Statistical analysis is really just a method for making sense of large amounts of otherwise incomprehensible data. Consequently, sometimes the statistical model chosen represents only science's closest guess regarding how to analyze the outcome of treatment. Some statistical models chosen may not be a good fit for some collections of data. In spite of the best faith on the part of researchers and statisticians, these inconsistencies may creep into research papers. For more information on this topic, see Steven Jay Gould's essay, "The Median Isn't the Message." Steven Jay Gould is a popular evolutionary biologist, and a survivor of a rare form of cancer called abdominal mesothelioma. His essay can be found at:

- Cancerguide: *http://www.cancerguide.org/median_not_msg.html*
- Dartmouth College: *http://www.dartmouth.edu/~chance/teaching_aids/median.html*
- The June 1985 issue of *Discover* magazine

Correlation is not causation

Just because a characteristic applies to people who have something in common does not mean that the characteristic causes that commonality. For example, say that everyone who has ever entered a college registration office has had a nose. You could say that there is a correlation between being able to walk into that office and having a nose, but you cannot say that having a nose causes a person to walk into that office, or that walking into the office causes a nose to grow.

Beware of correlations. They are not necessarily causative.

Complexity of the immune response

Humans and their capacity to withstand stressors are, thank goodness, always confounding medical theory. Everyone knows of someone who was told he had only three months to live, but is still alive long after. People can argue that these cases represent misdiagnoses, but this explanation is not likely to cover all such instances, and gives no credit for variables such as the many immune-system factors that are still unknown.

We have a great deal to learn about the immune system and are learning great amounts quickly owing to well-financed cancer research and the sharing of knowledge across scientific disciplines.

How colorectal cancer is not like other cancers

Some of the facts that apply to other cancers do not apply to colorectal cancer. For example, some other cancers are not treated as successfully with surgery as colorectal cancer can be.

Another difference can be found in the spread (metastasis) of colorectal cancers to other sites within the body. Although at the time of this writing heavy involvement of distant organs outside the colon does imply a worse outcome, it is not universally true that *any* spreading of colorectal cancer to another organ is necessarily predictive of a poor outcome:

- In carefully selected patients, spread to the liver can be addressed with surgery or certain other techniques (see Chapter 6, *Modes of Treatment*). Twenty to thirty percent of those with liver metastasis who are deemed eligible for surgery might be cured if a solitary liver lesion is successfully removed.

- Spread of a solitary lesion to the lung can, in some instances, be cured with surgery.

- Spread to nearby lymph nodes may entail a better prognosis if the spread skips the node(s) nearest the tumor instead of affecting consecutive nodes.

- Spread of colorectal cancer to the most adjacent organs such as the ovary, bladder, or prostate often can be totally removed by the surgeon.

Thus, general statements that are true for other cancers that have spread might not apply to colorectal cancer.

Physical characteristics of patients in studies

Many colorectal cancer patients who enter clinical trials, especially phase I and phase II clinical trials, have had previous treatment that has failed. This means that the percentages of survival found in phase I and phase II studies of new substances or techniques, using pretreated patients, may be lower than the survival rates that will be found as the treatment moves into phase III trials, and then general use as first-line therapy.

The same treatments used on any one person may produce better results than those recorded in trials; the same treatment used on the general population of colorectal cancer patients may produce better results than were seen in clinical trials with pretreated patients.

The progress of research

For all cancers, very few characteristics of tumors or of disease have meaning in the absence of a discussion about treatment. In other words, as new and better treatments emerge, they tend to dilute the effects of tumor traits that once were considered deadly.

At the time this book was being written, there were about 185 clinical trials underway for colorectal cancer funded by the National Cancer Institute, and this number does not include trials funded solely by pharmaceutical companies. For a better understanding of what this may mean for those who are diagnosed today, consider that ten years ago we did not have:

- Granulocyte colony stimulating factor, G-CSF (Neupogen), approved in 1991 for growing new white blood cells to prevent you from catching infections if chemotherapy wipes out your white blood cells, and to help you recover more quickly if you do catch an infection.

- Erythropoietin, Epoetin (Epogen, Procrit), for growing new red blood cells when bone marrow has been suppressed by chemotherapy or radiation therapy.

- Monoclonal antibodies, proteins produced by white blood cells that are grown outside the body and "taught" to travel to and preferentially attack tumors. They are almost unique in their ability to avoid damaging most healthy tissue, and thus are less likely to cause serious side effects.

- Stem-cell support for reconstituting bone marrow after high-dose therapy. Stem cell support following chemotherapy for colorectal cancer is now in clinical trials.

- Magnetic resonance imaging (MRI) for finding very small tumors that had spread to the brain and spine was not readily available until about eleven years ago.

- Positron emission tomography (PET) for distinguishing benign lesions from cancerous lesions by detecting differences in glucose metabolism.

- Imaging compounds that permit the surgeon to detect and remove the smallest of cancerous lesions.

- Floxuridine (FUDR), a prodrug of 5-fluorouracil. FUDR is harmless to cells until transported within a cancerous cell, where it is converted to 5-FU. This drug is used for chemotherapy specifically directed into the liver.

- Capecitabine (Xeloda), a prodrug of 5-FU that is administered orally and sometimes causes tumor shrinkage in those who have failed first-line therapy with 5-FU. A similar drug, tegafur-uracil (Orzel), is still in clinical trials.[1]

- Irinotecan (Camptosar, CPT-11) was approved by the FDA in 1996 for use in colorectal cancer patients who fail to respond to 5-FU. Studies are now underway to assess the value of combining irinotecan with 5-FU as first-line therapy.

- Oxaliplatin, a platinum-based anticancer drug, is in late-stage clinical trials for colorectal cancer at the time of this writing. Many researchers expect that it soon will be approved by the FDA for this use. Oxaliplatin is the first of the platinum-based drugs to prove effective against colorectal cancer. Because it is in a different biochemical class from 5-FU, it might be effective against tumors in cases when 5-FU has ceased to work.

- Various promising therapies directed specifically to the liver, a common site for metastasis. At the time of this writing, these therapies include cryosurgery, hepatic arterial infusion, radiofrequency ablation, and tumor embolization. For details on these therapies, see Chapter 6 and Chapter 23, *The Future of Therapy*.

Thus, bear in mind that the not too distant future holds great promise.

The aging of printed material

Owing to the amount of time it takes to enroll patients into trials, perform research, analyze results, write the research paper, peer-review the research paper, print the results in a medical journal, and summarize many such papers in a textbook, there can be a lag of at least one year, and usually many more, between the completion of research and the results being disseminated among doctors and the concerned public. During this interval, research has continued and better information may have become available. For this reason, we encourage you to become familiar with medical journals that report progress in the treatment of colorectal cancer. Methods for finding and understanding the basics of research papers are discussed in Chapter 24.

Remember that what you read about survival and treatment success here, and in all but the newest texts, will never be as current as the information you can receive from a well-trained oncologist active in his specialty who has access to medical journals and to other researchers.

The following passage, written by a colorectal cancer survivor, illustrates his keen understanding of the factors discussed above:

> *A problem with a quantitative response is that they will most likely cite the median survival rate and median survival time. You also need a course in probability statistics and an understanding of the distribution curve to really understand the answer. Also, the answer does not go into the options for influencing the outcome. The statistics are probably based on clinical trials started years ago and do not reflect the current optimization of adjuvant chemotherapy; the influence of CPT-11 or Xeloda, which only recently received FDA approval; Oxaliplatin, which has not yet been approved by the FDA; nor a variety of techniques, such as RFA for controlling metastases.*
>
> *Then there are the clinical trials and drugs in the pipeline that need to be factored in as to their influence on achieving cure and extending life.*
>
> *I had considered taking the disease-free survival curve from the relevant clinical trial for me, enlarging it, framing it, and hanging it on the wall in front of my desk as a defiant gesture. Right now I am hell bent on defying those statistics.*

Which factors matter least and most

With all of the above in mind, please see the summary below of the features of colon or rectal cancer, and of the patients who have colorectal cancer, that seem to matter or not, regarding outcome of treatment. This summary was prepared using the US National Cancer Institute's PDQ *State-of-the-Art Physicians' Treatment Statements* for colon and rectal cancers, and the text *Cancer of the Colon, Rectum, and Anus,* edited by Alfred M. Cohen. Many additional Medline and journal references from 1992 through 1999 were used to revisit the issue for the most recent prognostic factors.

Even with the following list of risk factors, nobody will be able to speak in absolute terms about your overall prognosis. You may have at least one risk factor for a poorer prognosis; and you will undoubtedly have several factors that point to a better prognosis.

The most important point to remember about your prognosis is that what are used today as reliable prognostic indicators may become meaningless when new treatments that surmount old difficulties are engaged. You might find it encouraging to read Chapter 23 after you have read this chapter.

The order of the sections that follow does not imply a greater or lesser effect on outcome.

Stage

At the time of this writing, the National Cancer Institute states that the most important factor contributing to long-term survival following curative surgery for colon or rectal cancer is the stage, or spread, of cancer found at the time of surgery. Stage, or more correctly, pathologic stage, is determined after surgery gives access to colon, rectum, liver, and lymph node tissue that can be biopsied, and direct visual or assisted imaging assessment of other abdominal organs.

There are several staging systems, including the TNM, Dukes, the Modified Astler-Coller (MAC) staging schemas, and a separate staging system used just for analyzing CT scans prior to, or in the absence of, surgical surveillance. Many cancer centers have abandoned the older staging systems in favor of the TNM system. All are based on the invasiveness and spread of disease. These systems are detailed in Appendix D.

Some aspects of disease spread that contribute to prognosis are:

- The degree of penetration of the tumor through the bowel wall correlates to a worse prognosis. In Chapter 18 of Cohen's 1995 text, *Cancer of the Colon, Rectum, and Anus*, Hamilton writes: "Infiltration through the muscularis mucosae is virtually required for risk of metastasis in colorectal carcinoma...As a consequence, 'in situ' and 'intramucosal' adenocarcinomas of the large bowel...pose virtually no threat to the patient."

- The spread to other organs. The tumor burden the body is carrying is directly related to outcome, with higher tumor burden within many organs related to poorer outcome than disease spread only to one organ.

- Presence of bowel obstruction.

- Presence of disease in lymph nodes. An increasing number of nodal sites involved correlates to a poorer prognosis. Patients with less than four involved lymph nodes have significantly better survival odds than those with four or more involved nodes.

- Malignant ascites, a collection of tumor-cell bearing fluid in the abdomen, is associated with a poorer outcome.

- The existence of just one lesion predicts a good outcome. Primary tumors that develop together (synchronous) yield a prognosis that matches the behavior and stage of the most serious tumor. Multiple primary tumors are more easily eliminated than multiple or large metastases from one primary.

- Metastases to liver, lung, abdomen, or pelvis can in some cases be treated with surgery and chemotherapy, and may result in long-term survival for up to 30 percent of patients deemed eligible for a second surgery.

For rectal tumors, the National Cancer Institute states that these prognostic factors, in addition to those listed above, bear on outcome:

- Size, with primary tumors smaller than two centimeters in the largest dimension having a better prognosis.

- Well-differentiated tumors that resemble mature, normal cells are more successfully treated than poorly differentiated tumors. Often, poorly differentiated tumors are more aggressive than well-differentiated tumors.

- Infiltrating rectal tumors have a worse prognosis than those of the expanding type.

Individualized prognostic factors

Many other measures of tumor burden or tumor behavior have been sought and studied as means to predict outcome, but as of now, none is as important as the pathologic stage. Many individual features of the patient and of the tumor may come into play, however. The remainder of this chapter discusses these factors.

Site of disease

The location of tumors may in part affect your survival:

- Peritoneal carcinomatosis, the implanting of numerous tumors on the inside lining of the abdomen and the pelvis, is considered a bad sign if many large tumors are found at surgery and cannot be completely removed. One study quantifies large tumors to be those greater than 5 centimeters; one medical reviewer specifies greater than 5 millimeters. Involvement of only one or two of the five abdominopelvic regions is considered a good sign.[2]

- The portion of the intestine in which the tumor develops is thought to contribute to outcome: tumors arising in the appendix have better outcome than those arising in other parts of the colon;[3] right-side disease (excepting that in the appendix) may, in some patients, have a worse prognosis than left-side disease. Left-side disease expressed the desirable p53 gene more often (see "Genetic characteristics," later in this chapter).

- In females, the spread of large secondary tumors to the ovary is correlated to worse prognosis.

- Bone marrow involvement confers a worse prognosis.

- Tumors that adhere to adjacent structures are thought to be more likely to recur.

- If the spine is involved, the preoperative neurological status and the number of vertebrae affected correlates to a worsening prognosis.

Tumor aggressiveness (tumor grade)

Many researchers believe that an aggressive tumor correlates to a bad prognosis:

- Histologic grade and the number of tumor cells actively dividing (percentage of S phase content) are thought to contribute to recurrence of disease.

- An unusually high number of blood vessels in a tumor, a sign of robust tumor growth, is thought to predict recurrence, even in node-negative disease. A tumor must grow beyond 2 millimeters in order to break apart and spread (metastasize). Tumors cannot grow beyond a few millimeters without an increased blood supply.[4]

- Poorly differentiated tumor cells, an indicator of rapid cell division, are correlated to higher tumor grade and greater aggressiveness. Poorly differentiated tumors connote a worse prognosis than well-differentiated tumors diagnosed at the same stage.

Histology

Many studies of the tumor's appearance under the microscope have been done in an attempt to correlate the cell's appearance to prognosis. The results can be difficult to interpret because almost every histologic characteristic has been correlated in some way to prognosis. Here are several characteristics that appear consistently in the medical literature:

- Mucinous adenocarcinoma has been shown in some studies to be a poor risk factor, but not in other studies.[5]

- Signet-ring cell carcinomas appear to have a worse prognosis than ordinary colon adenocarcinoma.[6] This correlation might be attributable to the more common presence of signet-ring carcinoma in those under age 40 and the fact that younger people often are diagnosed at a later stage. Another study notes that those with signet-ring histology are not diagnosed until disease is advanced.[7]

- Poorly differentiated tumors connote a worse prognosis than well-differentiated tumor when stages are equal.

Immunophenotype

Immunophenotyping is a way of identifying how certain genes within a tumor exhibit themselves in the tumor's appearance or behavior. The tumor cell's genotype is its collection of genes; its phenotype is the collection of physical characteristics that result from having one set of genes versus another. For example, if you have brown eyes, your gene for brown eyes is part of your genotype; the brown of your eyes is the phenotype.

The science of immunophenotyping, or immunotyping, is a rapidly advancing subfield of cancer research. Some researchers say that advances in this method of analyzing tumor cells will provide us with the most meaningful information possible for designing patient- and tumor-specific anticancer products.

Thus far, immunophenotyping has concentrated mainly on identifying cell surface antigens—that is, proteins that protrude from the cell's surface and act as identifying signals and attractants to other cells and to other molecules. All cells have these surface antigens, which are proteins and which cancer cells produce in greater abundance or in different quality from normal cells. This allows cancerous cells to be sensed, measured, or treated, separately from healthy cells, using new tools being developed. Some can be detected in blood; others can be detected only in tumor tissue that has been biopsied.

Your doctor can look for certain antigens in your blood to let him know if you might be experiencing a recurrence of disease. For example, your doctor might ask for blood tests every three, six, or twelve months, looking for one of more of these substances.

At this time, CEA (carcinoembryonic antigen) is the most commonly followed blood antigen for detecting disease recurrence, as a majority of colorectal cancer survivors show elevated CEA levels upon recurrence of disease. The routine use of antigen detection alone for monitoring response to treatment and continued absence of disease, however, is not recommended. A single blood test showing an increase in CEA is not considered a reliable indicator of recurrence in the absence of other findings. CEA can become elevated as a result of other bodily or disease processes, or as a result of changes in smoking or alcohol consumption habits. Tumors that are either highly or poorly differentiated are less likely than moderately well-differentiated tumors to produce abnormally high levels of CEA; mucinous tumors or tumors that are localized are less likely to elevate blood levels of CEA. One study has shown that liver metastases are more likely to elevate CEA than tumors in other locations.[8] Some clinicians find that CEA might not become elevated upon recurrence, even when gross metastatic disease is present, and that changes from initial test values often are meaningful, even if the patient's CEA level remains within normal laboratory ranges. Different laboratories sometimes use different manufacturers' assays to measure CEA levels, and their results cannot always be compared with accuracy. Thus, some clinicians say that at least two consecutive increases in CEA must be found before recurrence is likely. In summary, tests such as colonoscopies, chest x-rays, and magnetic resonance imaging (MRI) along with CEA blood testing all contribute to the total picture either of continuing health or of a recurrence of disease.

Radioimmunoguided surgery (RIGS) is a combination of imaging and surgical technique. One study has shown that five-year survival of those who were treated with RIGS was 60 percent; a matched group treated without RIGS experienced 0 percent survival after five years. Additional studies are needed to replicate these results. RIGS is based on the fact that an antigen called TAG72 on the surface of cancer cells can be detected with monoclonal antibodies. Antigens are unique protein tags that extend from the cell's surface; monoclonal antibodies are manmade proteins that are identical to those our bodies make, and are manufactured to target preferentially tumor cells by recognizing their cell surface antigens. These antibodies, which have a safe radioactive isotope attached to them, are injected a few weeks before surgery and subsequently attach to TAG72 on tumor cells. During surgery, a hand-held gamma counter is used by the surgeon to spot otherwise invisible sites of disease.

Other examples of experimental cell surface antigens that appear to correlate to tumor activity for colorectal cancer follow. Please note that, because new tumor markers are discovered regularly, this list is not exhaustive. Moreover, to date, none has been shown to be more accurate than CEA in tracking tumor activity. Some have been reported as the result of just one or two research studies, and need further scrutiny before becoming useful in the clinic. Nonetheless, you may see some of these biochemical markers on pathology reports in the future:

- Antigen CO17-1A is detectable with monoclonal antibodies when colorectal cancer is present. This antigen, also the target of treatment involving a monoclonal antibody that is now in clinical trials (see Chapter 6), can be used to highlight cancer cells in imaging studies using a scintigraphic agent connected to a monoclonal antibody that attaches to this antigen.

- Variants of CD44, an antigen on the surface of white blood cells, are higher in patients with active colorectal cancer. Variants 8 and 10 are higher in all patients; variant 6 is higher in primary tumors, but not in liver metastases.

- SLX (sialyl Lewis X antigen) rises with tumor activity. Patients with tumors that are negative for SLX have the best prognosis. In one study, increasing SLX levels correlate to disease recurrence and depth of tumor invasion.

- Lower levels of alfa-catenin are linked to poorly differentiated tumors with a higher potential to spread, and a worse prognosis.

- Lower levels of P-selectin correlate to lower tumor growth and fewer metastases.

- Increased levels of the ICAM-1 antigen in blood are linked to higher stages of colorectal cancer. Blood levels of ICAM-1 were higher in patients with liver metastases.

- Levels of ELAM-1 were higher in those with lung metastases.

- Tumors that do not express the MRP1/CD9 antigen have a significantly higher frequency of blood-vessel penetration of the tumor, and of liver metastasis. These findings were independent of the presence or absence of disease in lymph nodes.

Genetic characteristics

An examination of the genetic material—the DNA and chromosomes—of tumor cells often reveals differences between cancerous and noncancerous cells. Some of these differences correlate to survival; some are expected to become the basis for newer, more targeted treatments.

Colorectal tumors are often, but not always, tested for genetic abnormalities. Some genetic abnormalities may be present in all tumor samples from the same patient; some present in one sample but not in others; some are present at diagnosis but others accumulate as time progresses.

There have been many studies for many cancers that indicate a statistical correlation between certain kinds of genetic damage and outcome. The prognostic significance of some genetic aberrations is not entirely clear. Some have been detected in only one study and need to be confirmed with further research. Moreover, a correlation alone is never strong enough evidence to prove causality:

- Damage to one of the cell-death genes, p53, which resides on chromosome 17, appears to affect negatively the outcome of many cancers, including colorectal cancer, but at least one study has found that it does not affect prognosis in colorectal cancer.

- Absence of DCC, the "deleted in colon cancer" gene protein, appears to have a negative effect on survival.

- Extra copies of chromosomes 7, 13, or 20 have been correlated with a worse prognosis for colorectal cancer survivors.

- Loss of one copy of chromosome 11 is correlated with a lower incidence of spread of colorectal cancer to lymph nodes.

- Losses of chromosomes 8 or 18, or of the long arm of chromosome 18 (18q), have been correlated with a worse prognosis for colorectal cancer.

- Loss of genes at positions (loci) 32 or 36 on the short arm of chromosome 1 (indicated as 1p32, 1p36) are linked to a worse prognosis for colorectal cancer survivors.

- Loss of the gene at position 13 on chromosome 17, indicated as 17p13.3, was found in one half of colorectal cancer tumors biopsied by one group of researchers.

- Rearrangements of genes on chromosome 8 are found in some precancerous polyps. This implies that chromosome 8 plays a part in the development of colorectal cancer.

- Those with hereditary nonpolyposis colon cancer are less likely to have extra copies of chromosomes, or missing copies of chromosomes, than those with sporadic colorectal cancer.

- Tumors that are positive for the RER gene have a better prognosis.

- Mutations of the K-ras gene are linked to a worse prognosis, as these tumors tend to be nonresponsive to the chemotherapy drug CPT-11 (irinotecan).

- An increase in the expression of the c-myc gene is accompanied by a failure to respond to the chemotherapy drugs 5-fluorouracil and leucovorin.

Byproducts of tumor metabolism

Increasingly fine biochemical tools provide a means to assess tumor progression or the success of treatment. Many of these tools, such as polymerase chain reaction (PCR), flow cytometry, and in situ hybridization (ISH) can detect substances in blood or in other tissue that reflect tumor activity.

Some of the substances described below have been detected only in one study. More research is needed to strengthen their meaning regarding prognosis; a correlation alone is never strong enough evidence to prove causality:

- P-glycoprotein (P-gp) which is expressed by tumors that have become resistant to many chemotherapy drugs (multiple drug resistance or MDR) is correlated to a higher risk of recurrence in those staged at Dukes B2.[9]

- Cytokeratin-producing cells that are found in the bone marrow when no signs of metastases exist upon physical examination have been linked to higher risk of recurrence of disease in the liver and in the lungs.[10]

- One form of the growth factor VEGF, type 3, increases when liver metastases are present. VEGF type 3 is found in the presence of new blood vessels in growth; tumor growth is accompanied by the growth of new blood vessels to feed the tumor.

- A substance known as guanylyl C cyclase is found in lymph nodes when colorectal cancer cells exist in extraintestinal tissue.

- When increasing levels of soluble urokinase receptor (suPAR) can be detected in blood, a recurrence of colorectal cancer may be unfolding.

- The substance tenascin (TN) is associated with thick bands around well-differentiated tumors, but only with interstitial bands in poorly differentiated tumors. The pattern of tenascin might be useful in distinguishing less aggressive from highly aggressive tumors. In general, aggressive tumors correlate to a worse prognosis.

- Increased amounts of matrix metalloproteinase-1 (MMP-1) appear to correlate to a worse prognosis, independent of Dukes staging. Matrix metalloproteinase-1 is part of the process by which tumors spread and attach to new areas.

- Decreasing levels of C-adherin have been linked in some studies, but not others, to spread of disease. C-adherin is a component of the cellular glue that keeps an organ intact. When tumor cells begin to spread (metastasize), this glue breaks down.

- Serum levels of hepatocyte growth factor (HGF) increase when liver or lymph node metastases are present, and as tumor size increases.

Patient characteristics

Many cancer survivors wonder if their ethnic background or gender, for example, have a bearing on successfully fighting the disease. These are the factors that appear to matter most for colorectal cancer.

Age

Age greater than 70 is not a predictor of bad outcome unless emergency surgery is necessary at first diagnosis to control severe symptoms of disease, such as bowel obstruction or perforation. Several studies indicate that general health status or tumor bulk is more important than age in predicting the success of treatment. Older patients in good health who can withstand full surgery or a full chemotherapy or radiotherapy regimen, with few delays, do better than those who must repeatedly postpone treatment owing to side effects or other illnesses.

Many studies have shown that younger patients, those under age 40, are more likely to experience a recurrence of disease after curative surgery than those over age 40. Reasons proposed for this include:

- A more deadly form of the disease, with or without a family history of colon disease
- Later diagnosis, owing to neither young people nor their physicians suspecting colorectal cancer as the cause of symptoms

The tendency for those under age 40 to experience a recurrence of disease is still being investigated.

Race

Survival statistics for black Americans are lower than for white Americans in the earlier stages of colorectal cancer, even after other factors such as socioeconomic class are taken into consideration. This difference in survival holds even ten years after treatment.

Weight

One study found that, in females only, obesity at time of diagnosis signals a worse prognosis. Obesity is defined as weight greater than 20 percent above one's ideal weight. Although several studies have found a correlation in both men and women between obesity and risk of developing colorectal cancer, or waist-hip ratio (WHR) and risk of developing colorectal cancer, few studies have examined the effect of weight on prognosis.

Physical ability

Performance status (Karnovsky or ECOG scales) measures the patient's ability to do everyday things. The lower the performance status at diagnosis, the poorer the outcome. This measure does not apply to temporary setbacks while coping with the side effects of treatment or recovering from surgery.

Pregnancy

Pregnancy corresponding with colorectal cancer—usually rectal cancer—correlates with poor prognosis only if the symptoms of colorectal cancer are mistaken for those of pregnancy and result in a delayed diagnosis. Diagnosis sometimes can be delayed owing to risks to the fetus associated with testing for colorectal cancer.

Other patient characteristics

- Presence of adhesions after curative surgery is thought to contribute to recurrence.[11]

- Reduced levels (reduced expression) of HLA class I antigens—antigens detectable on white blood cells during an immune-system response—correlate to increased aggressiveness, higher grade, and passage of the tumor through the intestinal wall. In other words, a reduced immune system response to tumor appears to be linked to tumor aggressiveness and spread.[12]

- Increased levels of HLA II antigen HLA-DR—another white blood cell antigen detectable during an immune response—along with relatively low PCNA-LI levels, occur in patients with the best prognosis.

- Untreated anemia and resulting low hemoglobin levels are correlated with a worse prognosis.

Blood transfusions

Several studies have examined the difference blood transfusions during and just after surgery may make on the recurrence of disease. Initially, it was thought that blood donations from another were responsible in some way for the increased risk of recurrence among colorectal cancer patients treated with curative surgery. Subsequent studies revealed, however, that even using one's own blood that had been stored prior to surgery can increase the likelihood of recurrence. The conclusion appears to be that those who bleed less during surgery are less likely to experience a recurrence of disease. Many factors, such as the involvement of multiple organs with colorectal cancer, the overall status of the patient's health, and surgical technique, contribute to bleeding during surgery. At this time, it's not clear which of these factors is most important.

Emotional responses

Although there are often similarities in how people with colorectal cancer feel about the effect of their disease on the future, and in how they choose to adapt to it, differences exist as well. Each person tends to find his or her own way along the path.

Sue Browne describes her peace of mind about what she and her husband might face:

> At the end of May he gets another CT scan to see if his new treatment is working. We have had a few dress rehearsals of "what-ifs" and "what to dos," so we have some plan in the event of bad news. I continue to be optimistic, yet realistic. It has been six months since his diagnosis, but it seems like a lifetime ago that we thought cancer only happened to other people.
>
> There are so many positives that have come out of this life experience. Steve and I have always considered ourselves as soulmates, but that is nothing compared to what we are now. I don't know how I could love him more than I do, but each day that passes it is even better. We appreciate each precious moment of togetherness and finding new avenues to explore in each other's lives. For all this, I consider this cancer a gift.

Denial

Some people prefer not to think about the possibility that colorectal cancer may shorten their lives. Denial about prognosis can be a very healthy way to live, as long as it doesn't cause you to miss doctor appointments or bypass valuable treatment.

Randall discusses why he really doesn't want to know too much about the future:

> For about a day, my oncologist pondered doing a rare test on me for a particular genetic abnormality which some recent literature in JAMA suggests might increase the odds of recurrence among folks with stage II colon cancer. In fact, we drew the blood for it but had a hard time finding a local lab that could do the test. Then my doctor changed his mind. I was glad in hindsight. I suppose there are all kinds of genetic signposts to the future, which, if discovered now, would only be a source of "oh my god when is that going to happen to me?" anxiety. I'll wait and see what tigers or angels are around corners as I turn them, thank you very much!

Anger

Anger about the possibility of premature death is normal and expected. Moreover, as colorectal cancer is one of the cancers that some researchers believe might correlate to some lifestyle choices, some survivors who "followed all the rules" may feel angry that their prognosis is not good in spite of their having lived a healthy lifestyle.

Bargaining

When confronted with news about the possible outcome of your disease, it's possible that your first reaction will be to seek information about better treatments and better outcome. This can be a very fruitful reaction: many cancer survivors have found better treatment within a clinical trial owing to this tenacious reaction.

For some survivors of colorectal cancer, bargaining takes other forms. Some diagnosed as stage IV for which curative treatments might not succeed may bargain to live until their next birthday or until Christmas, for instance. They may bargain with themselves and their caretakers for a pain-free death, and plan accordingly.

Depression

Depression about the uncertainty of the future after being diagnosed with colorectal cancer is entirely normal. In fact, depression is recognized as a major emotional consequence of those being treated for any cancer. The likelihood that one's prognosis might not be good is very likely to make depression worse.

Acceptance

Some survivors feel that they can face whatever the future holds. A conviction may develop that life is worth living and enjoying to its fullest, in spite of a possible decrease in the amount of time that remains.

> *Our two worst enemies are helplessness and hopelessness.*

> *You can help yourself to make every day of your life—whether 1, 3, 456, or 2,223 days remain—as full as possible. You can help control side effects of medication, pain, anxiety, and depression. You can help find the best medical treatment.*

> *You can hope for remission, more time, quality of life, sunshine on maple trees, spending time with your family, having fun, and, if it happens, dying comfortably and with loved ones near. If you are religious, you can hope for life that continues [after death] and seeing loved ones again.*

> *Cram your life full of fun, beauty, and the things you love.*

Summary

This chapter has reviewed many of the known factors that might influence the outcome of colorectal cancer and its treatment. As stated at the beginning of this chapter, however, these factors are only relevant with respect to treatments in use at the time this book was written. Newer treatments may rise above current limitations such as genetic damage or tumor burden. Your doctor is always your best source of up-to-date information.

Prognosis most often is influenced by these circumstances:

- Complete removal of all precancerous polyps.
- Stage at diagnosis. In general, advanced stage is linked to a worse prognosis. Some components of stage are:
  - Degree of penetration through the bowel wall
  - Spread of disease to other organs
  - Presence of disease in lymph nodes—with important exceptions described in this chapter

- Presence of bowel obstruction.

- Presence of malignant ascites, a collection of tumor-cell bearing fluid in the abdomen.

It's most important, though, to realize that seldom is the prognosis of any one person clear-cut. Many factors contribute to survival; this chapter touched on these sometimes complicated factors.

CHAPTER 5

Tests and Procedures

*X-rays: their moral is this—that a
right way of looking at things will
see through almost anything.*

—Samuel Butler

WHEN YOUR DOCTOR SUSPECTS THAT YOU MAY HAVE COLORECTAL CANCER, she will order one or more tests in an effort to arrive at a firm diagnosis. After diagnosis, several of these tests may be repeated throughout your treatment in order to gauge how well you are responding to treatment, and several will be performed after your treatment to confirm that you are still in remission.

This chapter begins with a description of general preparations to keep in mind for all procedures, then we list tests and procedures alphabetically. For each test, we state whether it is inpatient or outpatient, describe what the test or procedure accomplishes, tell how to prepare for the test, detail how it is administered, relay how most people rank the test regarding pain, discuss recovery issues, and outline any risks.

The tests that are described here are those most commonly used for colorectal cancers, but your doctor may order additional tests not described below. An excellent resource for finding information about other tests is *Everything You Need to Know About Medical Tests*, published by Springhouse and written by more than 70 medical experts. This 690-page book has descriptions of more than 400 tests. See the bibliography for other recommendations.

General information

Some of the tests described here are necessary to determine whether surgery is really necessary or if instead you are suffering from a benign condition. An almost certain knowledge that cancer is present is important before surgery or adjuvant therapy.

Other tests described here are used during or after treatment to determine that disease has not returned or that side effects and late effects have not arisen.

Pain control

It's not unusual to feel nervous about tests. You have the right to ask for and receive pain medication before any potentially painful test is administered. If you are an adult patient, you may already have some idea of your ability to tolerate pain, but if you have any doubts, ask in advance about options for controlling pain. Various pain-controlling medications can be requested, such as the injected sedative Demerol; the sedative and brief amnesiac Versed, also injected; the topical cream EMLA, which contains the drug Xylocaine, familiar to us from dental care; or the short-acting anti-anxiety tablet Ativan.

Pediatric colon cancer is rare. Nonetheless, if you are the caretaker of a child with colorectal cancer, pay special attention to the control of pain. Lobby for pain relievers, and become informed about less invasive procedures. Communicate as honestly as possible with your child about the details of upcoming tests. Nancy Keene's book, *Your Child in the Hospital* (O'Reilly & Associates, 1999), does an excellent job of describing ways to help children cope by explaining tests in advance, play-acting with toys, and using pain-killing medications such as EMLA. One point she makes most clearly is that communicating the details to children is mandatory because the child's anxiety decreases and trust increases when he knows what to expect.

Make comfort a priority. Many of the tests done today require that you lie on a table for extended periods while cameras and x-ray machines do imaging. Get comfortable for this opportunity to nap by asking for extra blankets and finding a position that you can maintain pain-free for long periods. Ask for pillows to support your back and knees if you suffer from back pain.

Unnecessary testing

Become aware of alternatives to testing. For tests about which you feel unaware or uneasy, ask the following:

- Why is this procedure or test necessary? Will it change my treatment plan?

- Is there a safer or more comfortable alternative?

- What are the risks and side effects?

- How will pain be controlled?

- Please explain this procedure to me, or provide me with literature that describes it thoroughly.

- How experienced is the technician or doctor performing this procedure?

Inform and be informed

Never assume that the hospital staff administering the tests are fully aware of your circumstances. Always tell the technicians doing tests that you are a colorectal cancer survivor. Tell them of any other health problems or allergies you have, such as previous allergic reactions to the iodine in shrimp; of any prescribed or over-the-counter medications you are taking; of your previous surgeries, particularly if most or all of your large intestine was removed.

If you are an ileostomate, instructions may differ for premedication, or for cleansing the small intestine before an imaging procedure such as CT scanning. Always tell the medical staff that you have had a total colectomy. Verify in advance with your surgeon or oncologist any instructions regarding use of laxatives.

One ostomate describes a frustrating experiences that he and a friend, a fellow ileostomate, had with their doctors:

> One of the people in my ostomy group went in to have some things checked on, and to have some surgery. One of the first things the medical staff said was, "You need to have an enema or take a laxative to clean out your system." She said, "No, I don't think so." The doctor was really irate that she wouldn't take a laxative. She said, "Why would I do that?" "Because that's the procedure." "You don't understand. I have an ileostomy. I don't have a large intestine to clean out." "We always do a laxative before we do this procedure." "I'm not doing it. You can rant and rave as much as you want." Here's somebody in the hospital that you'd think knew these things talking to someone who's had an ileostomy for twenty years.

> When you see a doctor, you need to tell them if they're not aware that you've got an ileostomy. You need to have some idea of what does and doesn't work. There's no reason to take an enema if you have an ileostomy.

I can get the same effect by drinking clear liquids for one day. Six to eight hours is a long time for anything to remain in your small intestine.

Whenever a doctor prescribes something for me, I need to question whether it's a long-acting, extended release drug—any kind of thing that's supposed to reside in the large intestine to finish letting out its medication.

Timely results

To spare yourself agonized waiting, you should discuss in advance with your treatment team how test results will be relayed to you. Some patients mistakenly assume that their doctors will take the initiative and contact them when in fact it may be the doctor's policy that the patient should take the initiative and call for results. If you know that your best method of coping includes acquiring as much information as possible as quickly as possible, tell your surgeon or oncologist that you appreciate timely communication, and offer to expedite communication by making yourself available at the appropriate time. Be aware that some physicians are reluctant to leave test results on an answering machine without assurance from you that this is not a violation of your privacy. In addition, many ancillary doctors involved in your testing may choose for ethical reasons to communicate only with your primary oncologist or surgeon unless otherwise instructed. Discussing these issues in advance with your doctors is wise.

Steve's story

Sue Browne, author of a book of cancer survivor success stories, tells of her husband's diagnostic tests:

When Steve's stomach pains started, we just thought this must be new-job stress or a flu bug. It began as just slight abdominal pains, and soon turned into one of those dreams that jerks you awake. We could not understand what was going on, and why our lives had taken this turn.

Since Steve was 52 at the time and was due for a physical anyway, he went to a doctor recommended by a neighbor. They did a routine FOBT (fecal occult blood test) to check for blood in the stool and it came up positive. They did another test, and again, positive. So now we had stomach pains and blood in the stool. A colonoscopy appointment was set up, but it was a month away. Meanwhile, the stomach pains were getting

*too hard to ignore, so back to the doctor we went. X-rays were then
ordered and a vague mass was found in the large intestine, warranting
further analysis by doing a barium enema to be able to see this mass
more clearly. After they did the barium enema, the surgeon had the news
for us that there was a three-inch tumor that needed to be surgically
removed and a biopsy done.*

Surveillance for recurrent disease

All patients treated for colon or rectal cancer need follow-up surveillance for
recurrent disease or the development of second cancers. Ask your doctor
about the timing of these tests, which vary depending on individual factors.

In Chapter 6 of the 1997 text *Surgery for Gastrointestinal Cancer*, Paul Sugarbaker, MD, recommends these tests after treatment for colorectal cancer:

- Physical examination and assessment of symptoms
- CEA and CA19-9 blood tests
- Colonoscopy or barium enema (contrast radiographic studies)
- Laboratory tests for blood counts, liver, and kidney function
- Chest radiographic studies (x-rays)
- CT of the abdomen and pelvis, if specific symptoms warrant
- PSA blood test
- Rectal examination
- Mammogram and breast check
- Pelvic examination and cervical cytology (pap smear)
- Radioimmunoscintigraphy (OncoScint is a commonly used agent)

In the 1995 text *Cancer of the Colon, Rectum, and Anus*, Drs. Parikh and
Attiyeh suggest the following tests:

- Physical examination and assessment of history and symptoms
- Examination of pelvis and groin
- Occult fecal blood test
- CEA blood tests
- Colonoscopy or barium enema (contrast radiographic studies)

- Chest radiographic studies (x-rays)
- CT, MRI, or ultrasound, if specific symptoms warrant
- Rectal examination

Descriptions of tests

The following information provides the specific details of experiencing various tests. This information will help you relax, and will prepare you to ask questions or request pain medicine if necessary.

Abdominal surgery (laparotomy)

Laparotomy is the medical name for any incision into the abdomen. Laparotomies are routinely performed for diagnosing and curing colorectal cancer, and are discussed in detail in Chapter 6, *Modes of Treatment,* and Chapter 7, *Experiencing Hospitalization.*

Anorectal function examination

This outpatient examination usually involves more than one test, perhaps including anorectal manometry (ARM), electromyelography (EMG), endo-anal echogram, and others.

See also Sonography.

Preparation: For some tests, you may be asked to stop taking aspirin or other non-steroidal anti-inflammatory drugs (NSAIDs) a few days beforehand, and blood may be drawn to check for various conditions. At the time of testing, you'll be asked to undress from the waist down and lie either on your back or side.

Method: For some such tests, a small balloon or a tube the diameter of a straw is inserted past the anal sphincter. For others, a fine needle is inserted into the sphincter muscle. You'll be asked to exert both modest and strong pressure using your anal sphincter, and you may be asked to report if you feel as if moving your bowels is necessary.

Pain: No pain is associated with insertion of a balloon or tube. A small amount of pain is reported when a fine needle is used to measure electromuscular activity of the anal sphincter.

Recovery: No special recovery precautions are necessary.

Risks: There is a small risk of bleeding or infection at the insertion site if a fine needle is used to measure electromuscular activity of the anal sphincter.

Barium enema (single- or double-contrast)

See X-rays.

Blood product transfusion

This outpatient procedure is a means of replenishing your red blood cell and platelet blood supply if surgery, chemotherapy, or radiation therapy have significantly lowered your red blood cell and platelet supply, or have limited your bone marrow's ability to produce new blood cells.

Preparation: You should check the blood product brought to you for infusion to be sure it matches your blood type. Platelet matching may also become necessary after many platelet transfusions, as the body gradually becomes sensitized to and attacks donated platelets. Be sure to tell the nursing staff if you have ever had an allergic reaction to donor platelets.

Method: An intravenous (IV) line is inserted into a vein in your forearm, or into your central catheter if you have one that can be used for transfusions. The blood product to be transfused is hung from an IV pole and is dripped into you over a period of about four hours. If you have chills, fever, or difficulty breathing during a transfusion, notify the nursing staff immediately. This may be the beginning of an allergic reaction.

Pain: If you have no catheter and an IV line is inserted into your vein, you may feel mild pain during its insertion.

Recovery: There are no recovery issues following transfusion. On the contrary, you can expect to feel much less tired almost immediately after red blood cells are infused.

Risks: There is a risk of serious allergic reaction if donated blood products are not properly matched to yours. There is a slight risk of infection at the site of IV insertion.

Blood tests

Various blood tests detect various conditions. Each blood test's purpose is discussed following the name of the test. All are outpatient procedures.

Preparation: Most blood tests require no preparation; however, some may require an overnight fasting diet or the cessation of certain medications for a few days. Always tell your doctor and the staff administering the test of any drugs, prescription or over-the-counter, that you are taking. Zantac (Ranitidine), for example, can suppress platelet production and could cause an inaccurate result in a complete blood count.

Method: Most blood tests are performed by drawing blood into a syringe from the vein just inside the elbow. If your veins have been damaged by chemotherapy, if they are hard to find, or if they roll—more common in muscular people—the technician (phlebotomist) may use a vein on the back of the hand or on the back of the lower forearm. Some implanted catheters (see "Catheter insertion," later in this chapter) can be used for blood draws.

You can make your veins easier to access by doing the following:

- Lay a wet, warm cloth on the vein just before blood is drawn, or ask to use a restroom to soak the forearm in warm water.

- Vigorously pump the muscles in that arm just before the draw.

- Hang the arm lower than the rest of the body for a few minutes just before the draw.

- Drink lots of fluids starting four hours before blood is to be drawn.

Once a vein is accessed successfully, a blood draw takes under three minutes.

Pain: Most people report minor pain or no pain during a blood draw. If, however, you are afraid of needles, of the pain of needles, or the sight of blood, you are not alone. Here are a few tips for reducing fear and pain during a blood draw:

- Slap or rub the injection site just before the draw so that you will be less likely to feel the insertion.

- Ask for EMLA cream to use two hours before your appointment. Keep the site covered with an airtight bandage until your draw.

- Ask the phlebotomist, most of whom are quite skilled at reducing pain, to stretch the skin at the injection site.

- Look away while the blood is drawn.

- Think of someone who delights you and makes you smile.

- Ask the phlebotomist about his or her life, photos, liking for the job and so on.

For some children, blood draws can be a difficult ordeal. It might be possible for the technician to use a finger-prick or the earlobe if only a small amount of the child's blood is needed, after the area has been numbed with EMLA cream.

Recovery: Most blood draws entail no recovery, but you may have slight, painless bruising at the injection site the following day. Stretching the skin to make the blood draw less painful may increase this chance of bruising. Steady pressure on the injection site for 60 seconds or more directly after the needle is withdrawn facilitates clotting and can reduce the chance of bruising.

Risks: Unless you have blood that won't clot normally, there are only minor risks associated with a blood draw, such as the possibility of painless bruising.

Specific blood tests: Blood tests are listed alphabetically. Normal values for these blood tests are described in Appendix B.

Alkaline phosphatase
   This product's value may be abnormal if liver function is affected by the tumor, or if bone is being dissolved, for example, when calcium levels are out of balance.

Bilirubin
   As with other liver products, the level of this substance is a reflection of the tumor's effect on liver function.

Carcinoembryonic antigen (CEA)
   This product of tumor metabolism rises in the presence of certain types of colorectal cancer. It is not always accurate enough to use alone to track the progression or regression of cancer, but it is meaningful in concert with other findings and in the presence of certain symptoms. It is most reliable for signaling the presence of liver metastases.

CA19-9
   Like CEA, this product of tumor metabolism rises in the presence of certain types of colorectal cancer. It is not accurate enough to use alone to

track the progression or regression of cancer, but it is meaningful in concert with other findings and in the presence of certain symptoms. As of July 1999, its use is still experimental.

Complete blood count (CBC)

This test measures the three blood cell types and reports on their proportions, age, and other important parameters. During chemotherapy and radiation therapy, white counts in particular can drop and make the patient susceptible to infections. See Appendix B for more detail on complete blood counts.

Creatinine (serum creatinine)

This substance is an indication of how well your kidneys are working. Colorectal cancer can press on the ureter—the tube leading from kidney to bladder—and can impair kidney function. Creatinine may also reflect the amount of dangerous toxins being released by the tumor as it breaks down, called tumor lysis syndrome.

Electrolytes

Levels of various minerals in the blood are sometimes a reflection of problems related to tumor metabolism or to chemotherapy. Levels of calcium, potassium, magnesium, iron, and other electrolytes can be modified by disease or by its treatment.

FISH (fluorescence in situ hybridization)

This test of the DNA contained in blood cells or other tissue uses fluorescent chemicals to mark damaged genes. The chemical consists of molecules constructed to match exactly the gene being sought, so FISH is not practical for broad screening for DNA damage. The probe untwists (denatures) the two strands of DNA and, when a match exists between the chemical probe and a gene, attaches itself to the one piece of DNA being sought, thus the term hybridization. Using a special microscope, the pathologist or geneticist can visualize the gene, its breakpoint, any crossing over with other genes on the same or on other chromosomes, and so on, by viewing the fluorescence it produces. This is an exquisitely sensitive technique for differentiating certain colorectal cancers.

Flow cytometry

This method of examining tissue exploits two principles. First, cancer cells can be tagged with chemicals and so be made to look different from normal cells. Second, these cells can be forced to flow single-file through a narrow tube so that they can be counted one at a time, much like schoolchildren returning from recess. The tagged cancer cells are counted as they pass through a light beam or other tool for detecting whatever tagging agent was used. In this manner, cells can be examined for very specific features indicating cancer, such as abnormal surface antigens.

5-HIAA

5-hydroxyindoleacetic acid is elevated in those with carcinoid syndrome.

Liver enzymes (SGOT, SGPT, ALT, AST)

Unusual amounts of liver enzymes correlate loosely with the presence and extent of liver disease.

Polymerase chain reaction (PCR)

PCR can use many different source tissues as long as they contain genes and chromosomes (DNA). PCR is a method, not a test or substance. It involves taking a very small amount of genetic material and replicating it over and over so that enough exists to run tests that will require large amounts of genetic material.

Prostate-specific antigen (PSA)

This blood test can detect spread of disease to the prostate as manifest by malfunction of the gland, although it is not a specific test for colorectal cancer or prostate cancer.

Tissue polypeptide antigen (TPA)

Like CEA, this product of tumor metabolism rises in the presence of certain types of colorectal cancer. It is not accurate enough to use alone to track the progression or regression of cancer, but it is meaningful in concert with other findings and in the presence of certain symptoms. It is most reliable for signaling the presence of local and peritoneal metastases.

Uric acid

As with creatinine, this substance reflects kidney function and possible effects of the tumor on the kidney, such as tumor lysis syndrome.

Bone marrow aspiration/biopsy

By examining the liquid marrow or the solid core of marrow/bone structure under a microscope, a pathologist can determine if colorectal cancer has spread into the marrow. Bone marrow aspiration involves drawing a small amount of liquid bone marrow into a narrow needle; bone marrow biopsy involves drawing a piece of bone and its attached marrow into a larger needle called a trephine. Although in most people all bones are capable of producing marrow, for these tests the large bone of the hip is usually used. Bone marrow aspiration and biopsy is usually, but not always, an outpatient procedure.

Preparation: A sedative and/or an amnesiac may be given to you in advance—see Pain, later in this section. Bring a heating pad with you, and ask the staff if you can place it over the hip area for ten minutes or so beforehand, as some patients report this reduces pain afterward. If you have had biopsies in the past and prefer the technique of a particular staff member, try to obtain an appointment that matches his or her schedule. Be sure your sedative or local anesthetic has become fully effective before allowing the staff to proceed.

Method: A local anesthetic is injected over the back of the hipbone and a very small incision is made. Into this incision the needle or trephine, or each in turn if both aspiration and biopsy are being done, is inserted to penetrate the bone. For a marrow aspiration, the liquid marrow is drawn into the needle and the needle is removed. For a biopsy, the trephine is pushed through the bone to collect a core of bone and its attached marrow, and is removed. If not enough marrow can be obtained, a second insertion through the same incision but into a different area of bone will be tried. Pressure is applied over the insertion point for a few minutes to stop bleeding. A small bandage is applied.

Pain: Many patients report moderate to severe pain during this procedure. Be sure to ask for a sedative or an amnesiac such as Versed if you know from past experience that you prefer being very much unaware of pain. You may feel unpleasant pressure as the needle is pushed through the bone, especially if your bones are very dense. You may feel a unique, unpleasant sensation as the marrow is drawn into the needle. You may feel pain if the needle slips across the bone surface as it is being inserted.

Recovery: Afterward, your hip may feel sore for a few days. This can usually be relieved with Tylenol-type medications.

Risks: There is a slight risk of infection at the incision site.

Bone scan (scintigraphy)

This outpatient test exploits the fact that some bone irregularities will absorb more of a substance than will healthy bone.

Preparation: A mildly radioactive agent, usually Technetium-99, will be injected and you will be asked to return later, perhaps in three hours, for scanning. You will be encouraged to drink copious amounts of water to spread the agent from soft tissue into bone. Get comfortable after lying down on the table for the scan, because you must hold this position for up to an hour.

Method: Scanning is done by having the fully clothed patient lie on a table that has, above and below it, a camera that is sensitive to the energy emitted by the agent injected. It is important to hold still for the duration of the film exposure. The table is fully open, not enclosed like an MRI machine, and you'll see the arm of the camera passing over your body starting with your head and going toward your feet. The arm is about six inches wide and about as long as the table is wide. It moves slowly: a whole-body scan can take thirty or forty minutes.

Pain: A slight sting may be felt when the scintigraphic agent is injected.

Recovery: There are no recovery issues associated with this test.

Risks: As with other imaging techniques, there are risks of false-positive and false-negative readings.

Bronchoscopy
See Endoscopy.

Catheter insertion (central catheter, central line)

This procedure can be inpatient or outpatient. A central catheter or line is a flexible tube that is threaded into a very large vein near your heart. Its presence in a large vein dilutes chemotherapy drugs amidst a large volume of blood and thus makes chemotherapy safer; moreover, depositing chemotherapy drugs near your heart will distribute them more quickly and more evenly to all parts of your body than is possible when chemotherapy is infused directly into an arm vein. Using a central catheter can eliminate damage to arm veins during chemotherapy, and can eliminate somewhat painful penetration of arm veins for blood testing and for administering other drugs.

Preparation: You need to decide whether a catheter is the right choice for you. You will also need to decide whether to get an external catheter (with tubing emerging from the skin), or a subcutaneous or internal catheter (under the skin). Your oncologist may have very strong opinions on this topic.

Some advantages of catheter use are:

* Chemotherapy is safer when diluted by lots of blood.

* Chemotherapy is spread throughout the body more quickly and evenly with a central catheter.

* Vein damage is minimal or nonexistent.

* Some models can be used for blood transfusions.

* Some models can be used for hemapheresis, the collecting of stem cells for stem cell rescue.

* With an external catheter, there are no needle sticks that hurt.

* With an internal catheter, cleaning is not necessary.

Some drawbacks of catheter use are:

* Surgery is required to install a central catheter.

* External catheters must be cleaned and flushed daily or tri-weekly, and kept dry.

* Infections can lodge in a catheter. Their treatment may entail use of very strong antibiotics with risky side effects such as permanent vertigo, or may require surgical removal with a third surgery for reinsertion at a later date.

* The external types that emerge from the skin of the neck or chest can make the patient feel unsightly.

- The types that do not emerge from the skin still require somewhat painful skin penetration to access the port.

- Central catheters can break and travel through the vein to your heart.

- Central catheters can kink and make drug infusion difficult.

You may be given the choice of a local or a general anesthetic. If you choose a general anesthetic, preparation for and recovery from this procedure may be more complex. On the other hand, some who choose a local anesthetic report that they can feel pain during the procedure. See Chapter 7 for a description of preparation for general anesthesia.

You will be asked to dress in a hospital gown and will be taken to a surgical suite. After the anesthetic has taken effect, two areas, both on the chest, or one on the chest and one on the neck, will be cleansed and two incisions will be made. The surgeon will access the large vein near the heart through one of these incisions. The central line will be threaded through the large vein until it rests near your heart. The other end will be threaded beneath your skin and, for an internal port, secured there. For an external port, it will be threaded through the surface of the skin with an anchor just below the surface.

Pain: Some who have had a central line implanted report pain when moving their arms or when lying in a certain position for several weeks following implantation. Some who elect local anesthesia report feeling pain deep in the body during the procedure.

Recovery: See Chapter 7 for recovery issues after general anesthesia.

You will be taught how to clean and flush your port if you have chosen an external catheter. Redness, swelling, or bleeding that persists at the incision site should be reported to your doctor.

Risks: See "Some drawbacks of catheter use," listed earlier. In addition, surgery entails risks such as accidental penetration of a major vein, uncontrolled bleeding, and slight risks associated with anesthesia.

Two colorectal cancer survivors describe their very different experiences with catheter implantation:

> *I had an awful time getting my port put in. It was done under general anesthesia which was fine with me, but they had trouble getting it in because of the shape of my blood vessels. I had a lot of pain in my chest*

for a few days and was very bruised. They put the port on the inside of my left breast, so I also had a lot of discomfort when they tried to access it. From then on, I made them use painkilling Xylocream to numb the skin and inject a local of xylocaine before they put the needle in.

I think it is always good to know all the facts. I was told that it was a simple procedure, and I was very angry afterwards and had a big fight with the surgeon.

· · · · ·

My port was installed as an outpatient procedure. I sat in a chair like a barber chair, with my shirt off. The procedure took about half an hour. The port was placed in my left chest about two inches below the collarbone. A small incision of two inches allowed access, which was taped (no stitches). I understand there were a couple of stitches under the skin, to hold it in place.

I did have an IV in my arm, and I remember most of the procedure, however, I did go under for some of the time, but really was unaware of it since they can bring you in and out without your being aware. I would compare my awareness to that of having a colonoscopy, meaning you are awake during most of the procedure but can't remember it all. I had no pain at all and healed just fine within a couple of weeks.

Chest x-ray

See X-rays.

Colonoscopy

This test, usually an outpatient procedure, uses a microscope, camera, and light source on a narrow flexible tube to examine and sample the colon, a part of the body that would otherwise require open surgery to access.

Preparation: You may be asked to restrict your diet to clear liquids for two or three days before the test. You will be instructed to use a laxative and/or an enema (about which more later), and to forego certain medications such as aspirin or iron supplements for several days or weeks. These steps of preparation are extremely important, as an incompletely cleansed colon can result in serious or fatal side effects following this procedure, and can block the physician's view of cancerous tissue.

The laxatives required and the resulting diarrheal bowel purge cause distinct distress among those who must follow this procedure. Some patients are told to purchase and drink a very large volume of a commercially prepared liquid containing electrolytes (GoLytely, NuLytely); others are told to use a sodium phosphate laxative or enema. Many patients prefer the less voluminous sodium phosphate product, as consuming a very large quantity of fluid makes them nauseous.

If you are an ileostomate, verify instructions about laxatives with your doctor before using any of these products.

Regardless of the kind of laxative used, most patients are unhappy with the copious and persistent diarrhea that results after using laxatives and enemas. Nonetheless, adequate bowel preparation is very important.

Randall describes his preparation for his first colonoscopy:

> From where I sat (and believe me, on GoLytely I sat a lot) the colonoscopy preparation was the worst part of the colonoscopy. Ginger ale-flavored, strawberry-flavored, hell, even scotch-flavored, it still wouldn't have made the experience any more pleasurable. GoLytely my ass ... so to speak!
>
> Aaack! Rinsing my mouth out with mint Listerine after each gulp helped make some difference. I only managed to choke down three of the four liters. It seemed like a fifty-gallon barrel.
>
> The bathroom was well-stocked with lots of fluffy toilet paper, all obstacles to a clear path were removed, and I wore break-away clothing which could be pulled off my body in a split second.
>
> It was needed.

Discuss sedation with your doctor, as some but not all patients report pain during a colonoscopy.

You may be given large doses of antibiotics to take several days before the procedure.

You will be asked to bring someone with you to drive afterward, if your colonoscopy is done as an outpatient procedure.

Method: A sedative will be injected into a vein of your forearm to relax you. It may be administered with a syringe, or by an IV that will remain in place until you are ready to go home. A self-inflating blood pressure cuff will be used on your upper arm, and a rubber thimble for monitoring oxygen levels will be placed on your finger. You may be asked to lie either on your side or on your back.

Once the sedative has taken effect, the doctor will insert her finger into the rectum to ascertain that there is no immediate obstruction for the colonoscope, to relax the muscle called the anal sphincter, and to lubricate the tissue—steps not performed, of course, if the colonoscope is inserted into a stoma. The instrument is then inserted. During the rectal exam and the insertion of the colonoscope, you may feel the urge to move your bowels. A feeling of pressure may become apparent as the scope is moved inward and air is pumped into the colon. Releasing this air as you feel the need to do so is expected. The examination lasts from 15 to 60 minutes, with best visibility occurring as the colonoscope is being withdrawn. Very small pieces of tissue may be collected painlessly and sent to the pathology lab for testing. While the scope is being used, you may be asleep, or you may be somewhat aware that the procedure is underway. You may feel gassy and crampy, but the sedative may make you feel as if it is happening to someone else.

Pain: Patients report cramping pain that ranges from minor to severe. Those with known obstructions or strictures might expect more pain.

If you have hemorrhoids, you may experience pain during and after this test. Your doctor can give you medicine to relieve this pain.

Recovery: It may take from half an hour to several hours to awaken. For several hours after having a sedative it is unwise to drive, even if you feel able to do so. You will pass a significant amount of gas in the days following this procedure, as the air that was used to expand the bowel for better visibility is expelled.

Risks: There are some risks associated with endoscopy, such as the risk of puncture of the intestine or spleen, or twisting of the intestine. There is a very small risk of the sedative injection site becoming infected. Sites that are biopsied using a colonoscope might, in rare cases, continue to bleed afterward. Transient changes in heartbeat or vascular function may occur. Nausea, vomiting, bloating, or dehydration may follow the use of purgatives to clean the bowel.

The most serious risks, though, relate to having incompletely cleaned the colon beforehand:

- Infection following accidental puncture
- Explosion of methane gases within the intestine upon exposure to the colonoscope, an electric device
- Occlusion of the camera lens with feces, resulting in a cancerous site not being seen

Randall continues:

> *The colonoscopy went well. There was another jokester in the GI lab getting prepped for a flexible sigmoidoscopy at the same time I was in there. We had everybody cracking up (no pun intended). One nurse said, "We don't often get laughter up here."*

> *I was coherent enough to watch the video monitor of my colonoscopy as the doc snipped one small polyp. He sent it to pathology for confirmation but wasn't concerned about it. Everything else looked good. Well ... as good as the inside of a colon can look.*

CT scan (computed tomography, "cat" scan)

An outpatient procedure, computed tomography is a series of many very narrow x-rays taken at many varying depths of tissue and from different angles around your body. These x-ray images are then analyzed and reassembled by a computer into an image of your internal organs. CT scans differ from traditional x-ray imaging in that x-ray imaging can't readily distinguish organs that are lying behind other organs. Imagine looking at several veils hanging one behind the other, each painted with a different design. You can imagine how difficult it might be to discern the design on the farthest veil. CT scans, on the other hand, are able to delineate even those organs that are obscured by other tissue.

Preparation: You may be asked to fast overnight, to use a laxative, or to purchase and drink a contrast agent if a CT scan of your abdomen and/or pelvis is planned.

Your studies may require an iodine-based contrast agent. Be sure to tell your doctor and the staff doing the test if you have thyroid disease or are allergic to iodine in seafood or other sources. A non-ionizing version of the contrast agent can be substituted. Because the iodine contrast agent used may cause a sensation of heat, skin flushing, or rapid heartbeat, be sure to tell the technician if you have heart disease, high blood pressure, or any other health concerns in addition to being a colorectal cancer survivor.

If you have internal staples from a previous surgery or pieces of metal embedded in your body from a previous injury, tell the technician. They represent no danger to you during the scan, but may appear on the film as unexplained phenomena.

CT scanners are open, doughnut-shaped machines that generally do not cause patients to feel claustrophobic.

Method: CT scans are performed while you are lying in a carefully chosen position that has been aligned with the machine. It is important to maintain the position that was chosen until the technician says you can relax. Most CT scan sessions include a fast, initial pass with no contrast agent, followed by a second, slower scan with a contrast agent. The first scan images the entire body to use as a frame of reference for the rest of the scanning. During the first scan, you'll feel the table you're lying on move smoothly through the doughnut-hole of the machine, without stopping and starting.

While the second, slower scan is underway, you may be asked to hold your breath briefly over and over. Some scanning machines take ten to twenty minutes to scan, depending on how much of the body is being scanned. During this time, the contrast agent is slowly dripped into your vein. The part of you being scanned is positioned inside the doughnut-hole, which is about 12 inches thick. You'll feel the table you're lying on move slowly through the machine a few centimeters at a time, stopping and starting.

Newer scanners can do the entire scan very quickly, in about twenty seconds. For these machines, you may have to hold your breath for the entire twenty seconds, and if a contrast agent is injected, it will be pushed rapidly into your vein instead of slowly dripped. This quick administration of the contrast agent may cause stronger feelings of heat and faster heartbeat, sensations that are not considered an allergic reaction. You will feel the table you're lying on move smoothly through the doughnut-hole of the machine without stopping and starting.

For some studies of the stomach or bowels, you may be required to drink a contrast agent just before the scan is taken.

Pain: CT scans are painless; however, when a contrast agent is used, it is injected into a vein, perhaps causing minor discomfort—see Blood tests. As mentioned earlier, the iodine contrast agent used may cause a sensation of heat, skin flushing, or rapid heartbeat.

Recovery: If you have had a study that required drinking a contrast agent, you may experience gas, diarrhea, or constipation for one to three days afterward. Drinking large amounts of water will hasten the removal of the contrast agent from the digestive tract. If you have had a contrast agent injected, you may have a harmless and temporary discoloration of the urine or skin for several days afterward. If you are sensitive to iodine or have a thyroid condition, you may feel fatigue for several days after receiving an iodine-based contrast agent.

Risks: A CT scan, if repeated over and over for many years, may deliver enough radiation to body tissue to cause health problems later in life, such as lung, thyroid, or breast cancers. However, as CT scanning technology has improved, the amount of radiation delivered has lowered.

Endoscopy (bronchoscopy, gastroscopy, sigmoidoscopy)

Colonoscopy is described separately, earlier in this chapter.

These outpatient tests use a microscope and light source on a narrow flexible tube to examine and sample parts of the body that would otherwise require open surgery to access.

Preparation: Depending on the part of the body being examined, you may be asked to restrict your diet, to use a laxative or an enema, or to forego certain medications such as aspirin for a day or more. You may be asked to bring someone with you to drive afterward.

If you're having a sigmoidoscopy and you have hemorrhoids, tell the doctor. She can use medications and lubrication to avoid causing you pain.

Method: For certain of these tests, a sedative may be injected first into a vein of your forearm to relax you. It may be administered with a syringe, or by an IV that will remain in place until you are ready to go home. A self-inflating blood pressure cuff may be used on your upper arm, and a rubber thimble for monitoring oxygen levels may be placed on your finger.

Once the sedative has taken effect, the endoscope will be inserted. If you're having a sigmoidoscopy, air might be inserted to improve visibility. The target organ will be examined, and in some cases very small pieces of tissue may be collected painlessly and sent to the pathology lab for testing. While the scope is being used, you may be asleep or you may be vaguely aware that the procedure is underway. You may retch if the scope's tube is inserted in your throat, but the sedative will make you feel as if it is happening to someone else.

Pain: Some people report a panicked feeling of being unable to breathe during bronchoscopy. If you have hemorrhoids, you may experience pain during and after sigmoidoscopy. You may experience gas after sigmoidoscopy if air was inserted to improve visibility. Your doctor can give you medicine to relieve this pain.

Recovery: If a sedative was used, it may take about half an hour for you to awaken. For several hours after having a sedative it is unwise to drive, even if you feel able to do so.

Risks: There are a few low risks associated with endoscopy, such as the risk of puncture of the esophagus or intestine. There is a very small risk of the sedative injection site becoming infected.

Fecal occult blood test

This test can be performed at home using a kit purchased from a pharmacy, but often it is done in the doctor's office as part of post-treatment surveillance.

Preparation: You may be asked to avoid certain foods and medications for several days prior to the test. Once in the examining room, the doctor will ask you to undress from the waist down, lay on your side, and pull your knees up toward your chest. If you have hemorrhoids, tell the doctor for several reasons: to avoid unnecessary pain, to account for fresh red blood that the doctor may notice, and to help the doctor assess correctly any positive reading the test may give.

Method: The doctor will insert a lubricated finger into the rectum and rotate it to collect fecal samples from all areas that can be reached. The material collected is deposited on a slide that has been treated to react visibly when in contact with blood.

Pain: If you have hemorrhoids you may experience pain during and after this test. Your doctor can give you medicine to relieve this pain.

Recovery: No recovery period is necessary after this test.

Risks: The risk of a false negative is present with this one-time test, as blood passing from the bowels may be intermittent. A risk of false positives is also possible; follow-up with colonoscopy is usually recommended to rule out recurrent cancer.

FISH (fluorescence in situ hybridization)

See Blood tests.

Flow cytometry

See Blood tests.

GI series

See X-rays.

Intravenous pyelogram

See X-rays.

Laparotomy

Laparotomy is discussed in great detail in Chapters 6 and 7.

Mammogram (mammography, breast x-ray)

Women who have had colorectal cancer should have regular mammograms, as this group of women face a risk of breast cancer that's significantly higher than that faced by the general population.

Preparation: If you are still having menstrual periods, schedule your mammogram for the ten days following the first day of your period. This will lessen the chance that your breasts will be tender and will give a more accurate x-ray result. Avoid caffeine, chocolate, and other foods that may contribute to breast tenderness for several days prior to your mammogram.

Request an appointment that includes a patient/doctor consultation directly following the x-ray session, so that you can discuss immediately with the doctor any unusual results, and have repeat x-rays or ultrasounds if warranted. Otherwise, if the results are questionable, you may have to wait several highly stressful days, or even longer, for the staff to find an opening in their schedule for repeat testing or for the doctor's availability.

Tell the technicians and the radiologist that you are a colorectal cancer survivor.

Directly before the mammogram, remove all aluminum-based antiperspirants and all metal jewelry. Be sure the technician is aware of moles, scars, or other skin characteristics that may appear questionable on the films.

You will be asked to remove all clothing from the waist up and to replace them with a gown. While the mammograms are being performed, however, the gown must be partially removed to facilitate placing the breast above the photographic plate.

Method: Mammography is usually done while the woman is standing with the breast resting against a warmed, flat surface that contains a photographic plate. The technician will measure the density of the breast tissue and slowly lower a matching plate from above until the breast is somewhat compressed. While you are holding that position carefully, she will step behind a radiation shield and activate the x-ray machine for about three seconds.

Usually, two x-rays of each breast are taken, each from a different angle, to maximize the amount and location of tissue imaged. It is particularly important to capture the tissue high against the chest wall, approaching the collarbone, because breast tissue extends beyond what we traditionally refer to as the breast. Using equipment commonly available today, tissue compression remains necessary to ensure good visualization of all breast tissue.

You will be asked to wait, wearing the gown, until the films are developed to ensure that films of high clarity were obtained. If unclear, the studies must be repeated. If unusual features are present on one of the films, the x-ray may be redone using a small compression paddle to highlight a particular area of breast tissue. Alternately, an ultrasound may be used to re-image the breast in an attempt to distinguish benign fluid-filled cysts from other lesions.

Pain: Many women report discomfort, minor pain or moderate pain during breast compression. Some women report a great deal of pain. If you have had previous breast surgery or breast implants, you may experience pain that is qualitatively or quantitatively different from that experienced by other women.

Recovery: Many women report a bruise-like pain or a discharge from the nipple for a day or two. Report these aftereffects to your oncologist and your primary care doctor.

Risks: Some researchers believe that the accumulated dose of radiation delivered to breast tissue over a lifetime may increase a woman's risk of getting breast cancer. This, of course, must be weighed against the risk of failing to detect a breast cancer. The risk associated with bruising or discharge from the nipple is thought to be minor or absent.

MRI (magnetic resonance imaging)

This outpatient test uses large magnets and radio waves to cause the different atoms that make up our cells to vibrate at different speeds. The different speeds are then mapped by a computer into an image of the body part being examined. MRI is better than a CT scan for imaging soft tissue, such as cartilage or the brain.

Preparation: You will be asked to lie on a table that moves in and out of the tunnel-shaped MRI machine. The body part being scanned may be positioned within a basket-like brace to help keep the position chosen by the technician.

MRI machines make hammering noises because the magnets are being repositioned constantly while the images are being generated. The technician will supply you with disposable earplugs.

A contrast agent may be injected for imaging certain organs. Imaging the brain, for example, is sometimes facilitated by injecting a very safe agent called gadolinium. Ask the technician about the risk associated with the agent being used, and tell her if you have any allergies or problems with blood clotting.

Some people find the enclosed models of MRI machines claustrophobic. Certain MRI machines have an open gazebo-like design to reduce claustrophobia, with the magnets overhead supported on pillars. Yet others are made of clear plastic. While images from open models may be distinct enough for diagnosing knee problems, for example, they might not be detailed enough for mapping the brain.

If you're claustrophobic, there are several things that will help, such as knowing that there is a speaker inside the machine so that the technician can hear you if you ask for help, and that you, in turn, can hear her. There is also a hand-held beeping summons that you can press if you feel tense. Most facilities have a sound system and will let you choose the music. You may also notice that relaxing photographs have been taped to the inside of the machine. Fans circulate fresh air into the tunnel at all times. It's also possible that, unless your head is being imaged, only part of your body will be within the machine and your head may not. Most relaxing of all may be the thought that this is $17 million of technology, and for one hour, it's all yours.

Some people, on the other hand, report that the MRI experience is comforting, like a return to the womb. In fact, a friend reports that he likes to have an MRI because it's the only place where nobody can interrupt him.

If you still feel that claustrophobia will be a serious problem, ask your doctor whether a sedative would interfere with the imaging process.

Method: An initial scan to set benchmarks is done rapidly using no contrast agent. A second scan for finer detail is then repeated at slower speed. If a contrast agent is to be used, it is injected into a vein in the arm before the second scan. Although sound is muted by earplugs, you will hear hammering noises that vary in speed and pitch. While being scanned, one must remain as still as possible, but breathing is not restricted as it sometimes is during a CT scan.

A scan of the knee or brain, for example, takes about forty minutes. After scanning is complete, there is a five- to ten-minute wait while the computer analyzes and maps the signals generated by the magnets. The technician will check the resulting images to be sure they are readable.

Pain: The imaging process is painless, although you may feel a slight sting or warmth during injection if a contrast agent is used.

Recovery: If a contrast agent is used, temporary changes in the color of skin, urine, or feces is possible.

Risks: There may be risks of an allergic reaction associated with specific contrast agents: ask your doctor or the technician. As always, there is a very slight risk of infection at the injection site, and a risk of minor, painless bruising at the injection site.

OncoScint

See Radioimmunoscintigraphy.

PCR (polymerase chain reaction)

See Blood tests.

Percutaneous guided needle biopsy (fine-needle aspiration, CT-guided needle biopsy, percutaneous biopsy)

This outpatient test might be used as a means of diagnosing colorectal cancers that have spread to other organs such as the liver or uterine cervix. Organs commonly examined using needle biopsy are the thyroid, kidney, liver, lung, breast, uterine cervix, pancreas, salivary gland, spinal fluid, and bone marrow. (Bone marrow biopsies were discussed earlier in the Bone marrow aspiration/biopsy section.)

Preparation: You may be asked to fast for 12 hours before the procedure if a sedative or general anesthetic will be used, or if the tissue being biopsied is part of the digestive system. Prior to biopsy of the uterine cervix, you should not have sexual intercourse for 24 hours. Blood or urine samples may be collected prior to the biopsy. For children, ask the doctor if the procedure can be done under sedation or general anesthesia, or if EMLA cream can be applied at the site of the puncture two hours before surgery. Bring comfortable clothing to wear afterward, and plan on not being able to walk or drive alone after a sedative or general anesthetic are used.

Method: You will be lying flat on a table for most such biopsies, although lung biopsies may be done while you're either lying flat or seated. The skin will be cleaned. A local anesthetic will be injected, or a sedative or general anesthetic may be given by injection or by inhalation, or, if a fine-needle biopsy is planned, no anesthetic may be used. Directly before the biopsy, the area of interest may be imaged by CT scan or x-ray, and the skin above may be targeted with ink or dye. Depending on the organ being examined, you may be asked to regulate your breathing or to hold quite still during the biopsy. A tiny incision is made and the biopsy needle is inserted through the incision. For kidney biopsies, a guide needle may be used first. A small amount of tissue is drawn (aspirated) into the syringe. The needle is withdrawn, pressure is applied to halt bleeding, a bandage is applied—no stitches are required—and the tissue is sent to the pathology lab for analysis.

Pain: A slight sting from injected anesthetic or fine-needle biopsy is common. Depending on which organ is being biopsied, you may feel pressure, a brief, sharp pain, a dull, deep ache, or cramping. For liver or other digestive tract biopsies, you may feel pain in the shoulder. Tenderness or bruising may exist at the site of the biopsy and within any intervening muscle tissue for three to seven days. Some physicians prescribe Tylenol or Tylenol/codeine combinations for the aftereffects.

Recovery: After biopsy of the cervix you may be asked to forego sexual intercourse for seven days. Following kidney biopsies you may be asked to lie on your back for 12 to 24 hours, and you may note red blood in your urine for 24 hours.

Risks: Risks of organ failure while under general anesthesia; of infection; of bleeding, internal or external, at the site of the puncture; or of injury to adjacent organs exist. For lung biopsies, risk of a collapsed lung exists and any difficulty breathing should be reported immediately to your doctor. For kidney biopsies, blood in the urine may persist beyond 24 hours and should be reported to your doctor.

Radioimmunoscintigraphy

This outpatient test exploits the fact that some tumors will attract and retain more of a substance than will healthy tissue. This homing agent is first coupled to a radioactive substance that gives off energy that can be detected by specialized equipment.

Your doctor will choose a radioimmunoscintigraphic agent that works best for the type of tumor you have. Agents often used today for detecting microscopic colorectal cancers are radioactive isotopes coupled with monoclonal antibodies—proteins secreted by white blood cells and made en masse in the laboratory. These antibodies react with CEA, TAG-72, or other cancer antigens found on the surface of colorectal cancer cells.

Preparation: An enema or laxative may be necessary the day before the test. After lying down on the camera table, get comfortable because you must hold this position for about one hour.

Method: An injection of the radioactive agent is made into a vein in the forearm and the needle is withdrawn. Depending on the agent used, the patient may be scanned repeatedly in 2, 4, 24, 48, or 72 hours, or a combination of these times. For tests intended to be repeated, the patient must return to the hospital. No second injection is required before the second scan.

If radioimmunoguided surgery (RIGS) is planned, the scintigraphic agent might be injected as long as several weeks prior to surgery, or perhaps only several days.

Scanning is usually done by having the fully clothed patient lie above or below a camera table that is sensitive to the energy emitted by the agent injected. It is important to hold still for the duration of the film exposure. Some patients are embarrassed to note that, although they are fully clothed, the computer-assembled image on the screen is of the naked body.

Depending on the scintigraphic agent used, this procedure may be performed using a camera that is sensitive to the emission of a single positron (a positron is a piece of an atom). This is called a SPECT (single photon emission computed tomography) scan, and works on a similar principle, that is, the radioactive agent makes your tissue more visible to the camera. If the substance emits gamma rays, a gamma camera might be used, similar to a shield that moves back and forth in half circles starting at the top of the body and working down. It moves close to the body, but does not touch it.

Pain: A slight sting may be felt when the scintigraphic agent is injected.

Recovery: There are no recovery issues associated with this test.

Risks: As with other imaging techniques, there are risks of false-positive and false-negative readings with scintigraphic agents. Anti-CEA antibodies coupled to Indium-111, for example, may concentrate in healthy lymph nodes, liver, or spleen, giving false positive results.

You won't have to stay away from others later to avoid exposing them to radioactivity, as is necessary after receiving injections of some other isotopes.

Because many of these agents are manufactured using white blood cell antibodies from mice, they may cause an allergic reaction in humans, although allergic reactions are rare.

SPECT scan

See Radioimmunoscintigraphy.

Sigmoidoscopy

See Endoscopy.

Sonogram (ultrasound, sonography)

An outpatient procedure, sonography creates a map of how your body structures appear when sound waves echo from them. The sonography equipment includes a wand that generates sound waves and a microphone for sensing the echoes the sound waves generate. The wave signal is passed to a computer that reformats the signals into a picture of body organs on a screen.

Bone interferes with sonography, so scanning the brain with this equipment is not successful using the equipment readily available today.

Color Doppler ultrasound is specialized sonography that can detect the speed and direction of blood flow within the body, called the Doppler shift. The differences are mapped by the computer as different colors. This is useful because some tumors commandeer a large blood supply, and this excessive blood supply may be visible and meaningful using color Doppler ultrasound. A common use today is visualization of the ovaries to distinguish the fluid-filled cysts of ovulation from spread of colon or rectal cancer to an ovary.

Preparation: For a pelvic sonogram, you may be asked to drink large quantities of water, because the urinary bladder acts as a window for sound waves when the bladder is very full.

For transrectal sonography, an enema about four hours beforehand is necessary. If prostate tissue will be biopsied during a transrectal sonogram, an antibiotic may be required for several days prior to the procedure.

Method: You will be lying on a table while the technician gently presses a wand called a transducer over your body. Depending on what body part is being imaged, you may be asked to remove certain items of clothing and to wear a sheet in their place. The technician will first apply warmed gel to your skin to make the wand move smoothly. She may ask you to tilt your body and to maintain the tilt with your muscles, or she may place pillows under you. For transrectal ultrasound, you may be asked to lay on your side with your knees pulled up to your chest.

For transvaginal or transrectal ultrasound, the technician will apply warm gel to a specially shaped wand and ask you to insert it comfortably into your vagina or rectum. Once in place, she will guide it from side to side to visualize the uterus, ovaries, prostate, or rectum. This specialized wand is quite long, which means that the technician's hands are not very close to your private body parts, and, being covered by a sheet, you probably won't feel that your body is overly exposed to a stranger.

If prostate tissue is to be sampled via transrectal sonography, a needle rapidly enters and exits the prostate gland through the wall of the rectum to collect tissue for analysis.

If you are having pelvic sonography along with a second sonographic scan, ask the technician to do the pelvic scan first so that you can empty your bladder.

Many sonography facilities have an overhead screen so that you can see the same image the technician is seeing.

Pain: Most sonography procedures are not painful, but having to maintain a very full bladder for a pelvic sonogram is uncomfortable.

If prostate tissue is sampled during a transrectal sonogram, slight pain or pressure may be felt as the needle rapidly enters and exits the prostate gland through the wall of the rectum.

Recovery: There are no recovery issues following sonography if biopsy was not performed. If prostate tissue was sampled, blood in the stool or semen may persist for a few days after the procedure.

Risks: There are no known risks associated with most sonography procedures, except for biopsy of prostate tissue during ultrasound, which entails a slight risk of continued bleeding.

Ultrasound (ultrasonography, sonogram)

See Sonography.

X-rays (radiographic studies)

X-ray imaging may be used early in the diagnostic process to detect unusual masses and determine the extent of disease, although x-ray studies in the absence of a biopsy cannot positively diagnose colorectal cancer.

During treatment, x-rays can be used to locate intestinal blockages caused by certain chemotherapies or by disease, and to detect other secondary conditions such as blockage of the ureters, the tubes descending from the kidney to the bladder, by tumor growth.

After treatment, radiographic studies of the chest may be done to monitor the lungs for possible spread of disease.

X-ray imaging is diagnostic, and is different from X-radiation therapy in that it delivers much lower doses of radiation to tissue. X-ray studies are an outpatient procedure.

Preparation: You may be asked to fast overnight, to use a laxative, to purchase and drink a contrast agent, or to drink copious amounts of water if x-ray imaging studies of your colon or kidneys are planned.

If your studies will require an iodine-based contrast agent, as is used for certain x-ray studies of the kidneys, be sure to tell your doctor and the staff doing the test if you have thyroid disease or are allergic to iodine in seafood or other sources. A non-ionizing version of the contrast agent can be substituted.

If you have internal staples from a previous surgery or pieces of metal embedded in your body from a previous injury, tell the technician. They represent no danger to you during the x-ray session, but may appear on the film as unexplained phenomena.

Method: X-rays are taken while you are sitting, standing, or lying in a carefully chosen position that has been aligned with the x-ray machine. It is important to maintain the position that was chosen, and to remain very still, until the technician says you can relax.

For some studies of the stomach or bowels, you may be required to drink an additional amount of contrast agent while the x-rays are being taken.

For some bowel studies, an enema may be administered to fill the lower bowel with a contrast agent such as barium or barium and air. Hospitals with the latest equipment will help you retain the fluid with an inflatable bulb that is part of the enema package and is inserted just inside the rectum and painlessly inflated when correctly positioned. If this newer equipment is not available, you will be expected to retain the contrast agent using rectal muscles alone for up to ten or fifteen minutes. While not painful, this may be uncomfortable, because in these circumstances the urge to empty the bowel is quite strong.

Pain: X-ray studies are painless; however, if a contrast agent such as dye is needed, it may be injected into a vein causing minor discomfort—see Blood tests. Some studies require positioning of the body that may be temporarily uncomfortable, if, for example, you suffer from back pain. If you are having a barium enema, ask the technician to let you remove the nozzle of the enema yourself when the test is complete to reduce the chance of rectal discomfort.

Recovery: If you have had a study that required barium in the stomach, small intestine, or large intestine, you may experience gas, diarrhea, or constipation for one to three days afterward. Drinking large amounts of water will hasten the removal of the contrast agent from the digestive tract and will reduce the chance of barium forming an obstruction.

If you have had a contrast agent injected, you may have a harmless and temporary discoloration of the urine or skin for several days afterward.

If you are sensitive to iodine or have a thyroid condition, you may feel fatigue for several days after receiving an iodine-based contrast agent.

Risks: X-ray studies, if repeated over and over, may deliver enough radiation to body tissue to cause health problems later in life, such as lung, thyroid, or breast cancers.

Barium used as a contrast agent in the gastrointestinal tract can cause an impaction if not cleared by drinking copious amounts of water after the test.

Summary

Various tests are used throughout the process of detecting, treating, and monitoring colon and rectal cancers. This chapter outlines only the most common of these; see the bibliography for other sources of information about tests not described here.

Key points to remember:

- Some tests are uncomfortable. You have the right to insist on pain medication if you feel it's needed. Arrive prepared to be comfortable.

- Always inform the staff performing the test that you're a colorectal cancer survivor, and of any other health problems or allergies you may have. Never assume that they have your medical history at their fingertips.

- Discuss in advance how test results will be communicated, to whom, and when.

- If you'll need sedation for an outpatient test, bring someone with you to collect information about aftercare and to drive you home.

- Ask about the risks associated with the test. Ask about safer alternatives.

CHAPTER 6

Modes of Treatment

There are no such things as incurable,
there are only things for which
man has not found a cure.

—Bernard Baruch

HOW COLORECTAL CANCER IS TREATED DEPENDS ON what type of colorectal cancer is found, the location of the tumor or tumors, the pathologic stage of the tumors, the general health of the patient, and on his or her willingness to undergo certain therapies, including promising experimental therapies in clinical trials.

In this chapter, we will discuss treatment for both colon and rectal cancer, and the theories behind surgery, adjuvant chemotherapy, adjuvant radiotherapy, and biological treatments. Typical treatments used today against the various presentations of colorectal cancers will be outlined; however, full details of all treatments cannot be covered in a chapter of this length.

This chapter will not outline which treatment is best for you, as such information changes continually with treatment, research, and time. Nor will this chapter discuss rare treatments used outside the US and Canada, nor treatments classified as alternative. Rather, we list generally accepted standards of care for colorectal cancer at the time this book was written. These descriptions are provided to give you an overview of treatments and a starting point to find out more about the treatments your doctors recommend for you.

The information in this chapter is drawn from the National Cancer Institute's colon and rectal cancer state-of-the-art treatment statements for physicians, and is supplemented from various sources such as Wanebo's *Surgery for Gastrointestinal Cancer* and Cohen's *Cancer of the Colon, Rectum, and Anus*, as well as information from current research papers, pharmacological databases, and our medical reviewers.

A word of caution

Most medical writers approach a chapter such as this one with great caution, and so should the reader. The reason is this: no single publication of this type can possibly reflect current progress in cancer research.

Few formal vehicles of communication, printed or otherwise, can reflect the continually evolving judgment of the finest researchers in the field. None is permitted to publish very early results from promising clinical trials until the results are vetted by peer review. The best any medium can hope to capture is a snapshot of theories and findings as understood at the moment.

For your needs in battling colorectal cancer, that's not good enough.

As you read this chapter, you must keep in mind that, no matter how recent the copyright date in the opening pages of this or any other medical book, you will always get the latest information on the best way to treat your disease from the medical doctors and researchers in the trenches. Your surgeon and oncologist, who know how to tailor your treatment and schedule to suit your circumstances, may recommend treatment options that are different from those you'll read here or elsewhere. You should always verify treatment information that you find with your treatment team, and you should attempt to find the very latest information on treatment using only reliable sources such as peer-reviewed medical journals. How to find this information is discussed in Chapter 24, *Researching Your Illness*.

Theories of treatment

There are several ways to treat colorectal cancer depending on its location and spread:

- Surgical removal of all cancerous tissue is the principal and most effective means by which cure of colorectal cancer is achieved. Although surgical cure is possible in most stages, the chances of cure are highest in earliest stages (0, I, and some stage II). It is possible to cure approximately 40 percent of stage III colon cancer patients with surgery. A small percentage of stage IV patients can be cured with surgery.

- Adjuvant treatment with chemotherapy and/or radiotherapy improves the chances for cure in a significant number of stage III colon and stage II and stage III rectal cancer survivors for whom surgery alone may not eradicate all traces of disease. Some high-risk stage II colon cancer survivors may benefit as well from adjuvant chemotherapy or radiotherapy.

- Biological therapies work in a variety of ways, usually by mimicking or augmenting a natural body process such as immunity.

- Metastatic tumors that have traveled to the liver occasionally can be treated by several means: surgical removal, freezing, several types of heat treatments, or blockage of tumor blood vessels. Generally, however, most metastatic disease is treated with systemic chemotherapy.

Randall explains his decision, informed by his treatment team, not to have chemotherapy:

> *Before resection of my colon cancer, my CEA level was 6.6. After a CT scan and the surgery, I was placed at stage II. No metastasis to major organs was found, no spread to lymph tissue, although the cancer had permeated all layers of my colon. Post-surgery, my CEA level is 1.1. Given two years of symptoms before diagnosis (implying a non-aggressive cancer), my staging, and my pre- and post-surgery CEA levels, my oncologist has decided against chemotherapy: it will not improve my apparently already good odds.*

Surgical removal (resection)

Surgical removal or resection is the chief means by which colorectal cancer is cured if found in stages 0, I, or II. Surgical removal of all visible tumors contributes significantly to cure of stage III disease when combined with adjuvant chemotherapy or radiotherapy. Surgery can cure some survivors who have tumors spread to the liver or lung if these tumors meet certain criteria.

In addition, surgery frequently is the most accurate means to stage disease, although some of our medical reviewers stated that a patient with clear pre-surgical evidence of stage IV disease might not benefit from the additional staging information obtained from surgery, and instead might suffer unnecessary pain and discomfort from surgery that would damage the quality of the patient's life in the time he had remaining.

A survivor of long-standing, uncomfortable ulcerative colitis who developed a stage I colorectal tumor describes his satisfaction with treatment:

> I'm very happy that I had this surgery. I didn't realize just how bad I was feeling until surgery got rid of the diseased organ that was inside of me. Even my nasal allergies have cleared up. If I'd known how much better I'd feel, I would have done this years ago.

Clear margins

The goal of surgery for colorectal cancer is complete removal of all diseased tissue. One of the best determinants of complete removal are clear margins determined with pathologic examination. A clear margin is the presence of a rim of healthy tissue, uninvaded by cancerous cells, on all perimeters of all tissue removed. Clear margins indicate that the entire tumor was removed, totally and intact, without being accidentally divided during removal.

Removing adjoining tissue

Note that proper colorectal cancer surgical procedures include removal of lymph nodes (lymphadenectomy) and blood vessels nearest the tumor. At times, lymph nodes somewhat distant from the tumor also are removed. There is no evidence that removing these nodes causes harm to the patient.

Examination of lymph nodes and other adjacent tissues is an essential step in determining the spread of disease. Removal of adjacent tissue such as blood vessels and lymph nodes might reduce further the chance of recurrence by interrupting the outward path of any cancer cells remaining within the lymphatic or circulatory systems.

Surgery for colon cancer

A considerable number of surgical options exist for treating colon cancer, so you must ask your surgeon for the details of the surgery he's planning. The phrase "wide surgical resection and anastomosis," often used in the National Cancer Institute's State-of-the-Art Treatment Statements, actually encompasses a multitude of surgical techniques and approaches. Generally, when an anastomosis is performed, a permanent colostomy is avoided. Your surgeon will select the surgical technique most suitable for your circumstances:

- **Hemicolectomy.** Removal of part of the large intestine (colon) and rejoining of the two remaining ends (anastomosis). These surgeries can involve the right, transverse, or left bowel, or the sigmoid colon. Correspondingly, they are called:
  - Right hemicolectomy
  - Transverse colectomy
  - Left hemicolectomy
  - Sigmoid resection
  - Rectosigmoid resection
- **Partial colectomy with colostomy.** Removal of part of the colon and creation of an opening in the abdominal wall, a stoma, for passage of feces, using the remaining end of the colon.
- **Total colectomy and ileostomy.** Removal of the entire colon and anus, and creation of an opening in the abdominal wall, a stoma, for passage of waste, using the small intestine. This procedure is most likely to be used on patients with:
  - Familial polyposis
  - Ulcerative colitis
  - Multiple lesions
- **Colectomy with ileorectal anastomosis.** Removal of the entire colon and reattachment of the small bowel to residual rectal tissue or to the anus.
- **En bloc resection.** Partial or entire removal of other pelvic or abdominal organs inflamed by, attached to, or invaded by the tumor.
- **Pelvic exenteration.** Partial or entire removal of all pelvic organs, regional lymph nodes or abdominal organs involved with, attached to, or invaded by the primary or metastatic tumor.
- **Temporary ostomy.** Creation of a temporary single- or double-opening stoma while one or more pieces of the large bowel are healing.
- **Continent ileostomy.** Addition of a manually operated valve to the stoma to allow control of the passage of waste. Generally used only on those with ulcerative colitis or familial polyposis.

- **Ileorectal or J-pouch.** Adaptation of a piece of the small intestine into a pouch that can be attached to the anus to retain feces. Generally used only on those with ulcerative colitis or familial polyposis.

- **Anastomosis.** For temporary colostomies, rejoining of the remaining colon at a later date.

Surgery for rectal cancer

From the standpoint of technical ease, surgeries for rectal cancer can be more challenging for the surgeon than surgeries for colon cancer, owing to the narrow, bony structure of the pelvis, particularly in males. Continuing advances in the development of surgical instrumentation, however, are narrowing this technological gap.

Special surgical techniques might be used for rectal cancer that are not possible with disease located higher (more proximal) in the colon. Means to remove tumors without opening the abdomen, and methods to preserve the anal sphincter and to avoid having a lifelong ostomy are two examples.

The rectum, considered to be ten to twelve inches long, is divided logically into three sections by surgeons specializing in colorectal surgery:

- Upper-third tumors usually can be removed completely, and fecal continence usually can be surgically restored via low anterior resection, described later.

- Lower-third tumors, those closest to the anus, usually require abdominoperineal resection, described later.

- Middle-third tumors may have characteristics of either or both upper- or lower-third tumors, and require a skilled and experienced surgeon to choose appropriately between abdominoperineal resection and reconnection of remaining bowel (reanastomosis).

For rectal cancer, the following surgeries are most typical:

- **Low anterior resection (LAR).** If the tumor is located high enough in the rectum, removal of the tumor and rejoining of the two remaining pieces of bowel, or bowel and anus (bowel anastomosis). A stapler might be used to rejoin tissue, especially if little anal or rectal tissue remains to reattach.

- **Abdominoperineal resection.** If the tumor is located too low to rejoin remaining tissues, or if anal tissue appears to be invaded by the tumor, removal of the tumor and all anal tissue, accompanied by creation of a stoma through which feces will pass. External anal tissue is replaced and closed by suturing pelvic tissue over the opening (called the perineal wound), or, less often, allowed to heal by granulation, a gradual filling of the wound with scar tissue.

- **Pelvic exenteration.** Partial or entire (en bloc) removal of all other organs inflamed by, attached to, or invaded by the tumor. If disease is extensive, removal of all pelvic organs adjacent to the rectum is performed. In men, the bladder and prostate are removed; in women, the bladder and uterus are removed. Pelvic exenteration involves two permanent ostomies: colostomy and urostomy, and involves two stomae— one for the passage of feces and one for the passage of urine.

- **Transanal or transsphincteric resection.** A removal of superficial tumors without opening the abdomen, using instead surgical instruments inserted through the rectum.

- **Coloanal anastomosis.** For selected middle and low rectal tumors, the sigmoid colon that remains after tumor removal can be sewn to the anal muscles to maintain fecal continence.

Other surgical considerations

The following surgical issues and techniques might affect your outcome. Some of these issues have not yet been fully studied:

- The skill and experience of your surgeon.

- Laparoscopic-assisted surgery versus open surgery. Use of the laparoscope, a camera-guided surgical tool containing a microscope, for this surgery is still uncommon, but is sometimes offered to patients as part of a research protocol (clinical trial) at certain major cancer centers. These surgical procedures are not performed totally with a laparoscope, and so are called laparoscopic-assisted surgeries. When a laparoscope is used, the procedure is called laparoscopy instead of laparotomy, the incision is smaller, and healing time is shorter. Some controversy exists regarding the safety of laparoscopic surgery in removing colonic cancers; clinical trials comparing this surgery to traditional open surgery will answer these questions.

- The National Cancer Institute states that colon cancer patients whose tumor extends through the bowel wall and to adjacent structures, once considered a bad prognostic sign, have survival odds equaling those whose tumors are not as invasive if en bloc surgery yielding clear margins—removal of all tumor along with a good portion of healthy tissue on all edges—can be performed.

- Radioimmunoguided surgery (RIGS), still in clinical trials and not yet approved by the FDA, involves the injection of a mildly radioactive isotope some time before surgery, varying from hours to weeks depending on what contrast agent is used and how your cancer center plans these surgeries. In the time that follows, tumors, including microscopic, invisible cancer cells, absorb these isotopes more readily than healthy cells do. During surgery, the surgeon, using a hand-held gamma counter, is in theory able to detect and remove these micrometastases. Long-term survival following this technique has not yet been compared via randomized prospective trials.

- Nerve-sparing techniques can be employed to preserve sexual function. Abdominopelvic surgery frequently affects nerves and blood vessels that connect to the sexual organs and the bladder. A surgeon who has performed many colorectal surgeries is more likely to succeed in sparing nerve function than a surgeon who seldom performs abdominoperineal resection or low anterior resection.

- During surgery for rectal cancer, construction of an intestinal sling might be performed to support and thus spare the small bowel from effects of later radiation therapy. Often the sling is made from material that will dissolve in a number of months or from muscle transferred from the abdominal wall.

- Endorectal ultrasound (ERUS). This preoperative staging modality has become the most accurate staging technique for rectal cancer. It can accurately predict the depth of invasion as well as the extent of lymph nodal involvement.

Adjuvant chemotherapy

Adjuvant chemotherapy consists of preoperative or postoperative treatment with anticancer drugs to eliminate circulating cancer cells before surgery, or to kill any tumors or microscopic cancer cells that remain after surgery.

Several clinical trials involving about 4,000 patients have shown that adjuvant chemotherapy consisting of 5-fluorouracil and leucovorin combined with surgery reduces mortality in stage III patients by 22 to 33 percent compared to treatment with surgery alone. The gains are less clear in stage II patients, but studies are in progress to identify high-risk stage II patients who also may benefit from adjuvant therapy. A recent study comparing several chemotherapy regimens in stage II (Dukes stage B) patients, for example, found a clear survival advantage when adjuvant chemotherapy was used regardless of differing prognostic indicators for stage II patients.[1]

Some studies show better long-term patient survival for continuous infusion of 5-FU during radiotherapy for rectal cancer; however, prolongation of survival is less clear for those receiving continuous infusion of 5-FU for colon cancer in spite of improved tumor shrinkage or disappearance on this regimen.

Chemotherapeutic treatments of liver metastases are discussed separately later in this chapter.

How anticancer drugs are given

Adjuvant chemotherapy can be administered in several ways, and on different schedules:

- Into a vein or a semi-permanent catheter by a doctor or nurse, repeated several times a month for several months. This is called bolus infusion.

- Through a semi-permanent catheter that empties into a vein, throughout the day for several days, using a portable continuous infusion pump that is either implanted inside, or carried on the outside of your body.

- Directly into the abdominal cavity, called intraperitoneal therapy, for microscopic disease that has affected, or may affect, the lining of the abdominal cavity in stage IV disease.

- Directly into an artery supplying the liver, for those with stage IV disease that has spread to the liver (hepatic metastases).

- Before or after surgery, perhaps along with radiotherapy, to reduce tumor bulk.

- Orally, as pills.

See Chapter 8, *Experiencing Chemotherapy*, for the practical aspects of this treatment.

Drugs effective against colorectal cancer

At the time of this writing, the anticancer drugs approved by the US Food and Drug Administration and used against colorectal cancer are:

- 5-fluorouracil or 5-FU (Adrucil, Efudex, Fluoroplex). Prolonged infusion of 5-FU or floxuridine (FUDR) via portable pump worn continuously may have an advantage over briefer infusions administered in the medical center. This advantage is clearer, though, for those receiving continuous infusion 5-FU and radiotherapy for rectal cancer than for those receiving continuous infusion for colon cancer.

- Capecitabine (Xeloda) is an orally administered prodrug of 5-FU which metabolizes to 5-FU preferentially in tumor cells and remains in the body longer than 5-FU administered by IV. These characteristics may spare healthy cells from toxicity, reduce some side effects, and may provide better anticancer coverage. Like 5-FU, Capecitabine appears more effective when combined with leucovorin. In breast cancer patients, it has been moderately effective even when patients ceased to respond to certain other chemotherapy regimens. Small studies of colorectal patients reveal similar results, but larger studies are required to confirm this.

- Irinotecan (Camptosar, CPT-11) has been approved for use in colorectal cancer patients who fail to respond to 5-FU. Studies are now underway to assess the value of combining irinotecan with 5-FU as first-line therapy.

- Leucovorin (Leucovorin, Wellcovorin), the calcium salt of folinic acid, is a faster acting and more potent form of the vitamin folic acid. Leucovorin is used to enhance the activity of 5-FU by enhancing its binding to thymidylate synthase. Leucovorin is not effective against colorectal cancer on its own.

- Levamisole is an immune stimulant used to enhance the activity of 5-FU. Some clinicians believe that leucovorin is more effective with 5-FU than levamisole with 5-FU.

- Mitomycin (Mutamycin) is an alkylating agent that is sometimes used if first-line therapy with 5-FU fails.

- Colony stimulating factors, a form of biological therapy, are used to offset the toxic effects of chemotherapy drugs in bone marrow.

Other drugs already approved for other cancers might also be recommended by your oncologist, as the FDA permits a doctor to use a drug for any illness once it has been approved for one illness, an approach known as off-label use.

Several other promising drugs for colorectal cancer such as oxaliplatin and tegafur-uracil (UFT, Orzel) are currently in clinical trials for advanced-stage or recurrent colorectal cancer. You can get access to these drugs prior to FDA approval by joining a clinical trial, or by petitioning the FDA for "compassionate use" under its Investigational New Drug program. For more information on these approaches, see Chapter 20, *Clinical Trials*.

> *I just finished my third two-week cycle of taking Xeloda. After the first two sessions, my CEA dropped by about 10 percent; I won't know about the current status until the end of next week when I have a blood sample and visit my oncologist.*

> *I think it is helping and the oncologist agrees.*

> *I have metastases to my lungs and liver. For about nine months I was on 5-FU, which was effective initially, but then lost its effectiveness. Then I tried CPT-11 for three times, but it seemed to have no effect.*

> *The Xeloda originally did not give me any side effects. This third time I do have a "foot syndrome" problem (feet feel a bit numb), but it is not serious.*

How anticancer drugs kill tumors

Drugs approved by the FDA for use against colorectal cancer fall into several categories: antimetabolites, topoisomerase inhibitors, DNA adduct formation, alkylating agents, chemosensitization drugs, and rescue drugs.

- **Antimetabolites.** As the word antimetabolite implies, these substances in some way impede the cell's metabolism—its building up and breaking down of cell parts.
  - 5-fluorouracil when administered by bolus infusion is incorporated into RNA in place of uracil, causing malfunction of RNA and protein synthesis.
  - 5-fluorouracil when administered as a continuous infusion is thought to act as an inhibitor of the enzyme thymidylate synthase,

which affects DNA synthesis, but other studies implicate a factor potentially involved in pre-RNA processing, called provisionally ribosomal RNA binding protein.[2]

– Floxuridine (FUDR), an antimetabolite closely related to 5-FU, is sometimes used against disease in the liver (hepatic metastases) because it is removed more quickly from the liver than 5-FU, thus limiting damage to healthy liver tissue.

– Capecitabine (Xeloda) is an orally administered prodrug of 5-FU that shares its mechanisms of action.

- **Topoisomerase inhibitors.** Topoisomerases are enzymes that our cells use to untwist DNA before copying, and to repair breaks in DNA after copying. Topoisomerase inhibitors interfere with DNA replication, causing the cancer cell to die, because damaged DNA cannot be translated into proteins, such as transport and digestive proteins, that each cell needs to breathe or eat. Camptosar (irinotecan, CPT-11) is a topoisomerase-I inhibitor.

- **DNA adduct formation.** Oxaliplatin, a drug used in Europe against colorectal cancer but not yet approved by the US FDA, interferes with the cancer cell's ability to copy its DNA for cell division by forming adducts with DNA. Adducts confuse and derail the enzymes responsible for cell division and replication.

- **Alkylating agents.** Alkylating agents form new bonds within double-twisted DNA strands that resemble ladder rungs. This disrupts many normal functions of DNA, including its ability to divide. Alkylating agents are able to affect a cancer cell's DNA even when the DNA is not uncoiled and separated—in other words, they are not cell-cycle specific—which may explain their relatively high activity against many cancers. Mitomycin, derived from the fungus Streptomyces caespitosus, is an atypical alkylating agent used against colorectal cancer. Mitomycin is also capable of creating oxygen free radicals, which damage DNA.

- **Chemosensitization drugs.** Research has shown that some drugs, while having no direct ability to kill cancer cells, appear to heighten the cancer cell's vulnerability to other drugs. Leucovorin interacts with 5-FU and its metabolites to stabilize their binding to body products called enzymes so that increased cancer-killing activity occurs. In a similar fashion, 5-FU makes tumor cells more sensitive to radiation therapy.

- **Rescue drugs**. Some drugs are effective in offsetting certain dangerous effects of chemotherapy. Colony stimulating factors, described later under "Biological therapies," help bone marrow produce more red and white blood cells and platelets after they have been suppressed during chemotherapy.

Adjuvant radiotherapy

For rectal cancer, and in some instances of colon cancer, adjuvant radiotherapy before, during, or after surgery is recommended to combat the spread of disease.

How radiotherapy is given

Radiation therapy can be administered in several forms:

- Traditional external-beam radiotherapy, administered from outside the patient's body, either before surgery to reduce tumor bulk, increasing the chance of clear resection, or after surgery to kill microscopic remains of disease. External radiotherapy is the most common form of radiotherapy in use for colorectal cancer.

- Radiotherapy given simultaneously with 5-FU appears to work better than either does alone.

- Brachytherapy, the positioning of a source of radiation contiguous to or within the tumor to enhance the radiobiologic effect of the radioisotope. Rectal cancer, for example, might be treated by placing the radiation source within the rectal vault through the anus. This technique is not often used for colon or rectal cancer.

- Interstitial radiotherapy, involving implants of radioactive material within an organ bearing the tumor, stored in capsules, wires, or similar sealed delivery vehicles, often permanent. This technique is never used for colon cancer and only occasionally used for rectal cancer.

- Intra-operative electron beam irradiation (IOERT), which is directed against specific sites of disease while the patient's abdomen is open during surgery. This technique is occasionally used for colon or rectal cancer, and is still considered experimental by some researchers.

- Radioimmunotherapy, an injection of radioisotopes attached to a carrier that binds more selectively to antigens on the surface of tumors instead of to those on healthy tissue. This technique is in clinical trials, not yet approved by the FDA. The most common of these carrier substances are antibodies, proteins produced by our white blood cells in response to perceived invasions such as infections or cancer. The monoclonal antibodies in use today are specifically designed hybrids created to bind preferentially to certain types of cancer cells.

For rectal cancer, especially for tumors that are inoperable or borderline operable, reducing tumor bulk prior to surgery permits safer, more complete surgeries that increase the chance for cure, and permits surgery that better preserves sphincter function thereby avoiding permanent colostomy.

While radiotherapy for some rectal cancers is now considered standard treatment, its use for colon cancers is less common and more controversial. The risk of significant and lasting side effects to the small intestine and other adjacent organs (ureter, liver, kidney, spleen, and so on), the possible formation of abnormal tubes called fistulae between organs, and the development of chronic diarrhea and cramping must be considered. In general, for colon cancer, narrowly targeted irradiation of small areas of the abdomen or spine in stage IV patients is the most common use of radiation therapy.

See Chapter 9, *Experiencing Radiotherapy*, for the practical aspects of this treatment.

How radiotherapy kills tumors

Radiation therapy interferes with the growth and replication of cancer cells by changing the structure of molecules that make up the cell's DNA, after which the DNA strand can no longer be correctly copied, lengthened, paired, and twined.

Similar damage is possible in healthy cells that happen to be in the path of the radiation beam, especially if they are in the process of dividing.

Biological therapies

There are a number of biological therapies, and each works differently, but in general, they are manmade copies of natural body substances, and enhance the action of these substances.

Monoclonal antibodies

Monoclonal antibodies are manmade copies of proteins—antibodies—that our white blood cells secrete. Because a particular cell surface protein, or antigen, attracts a particular antibody, natural antibodies are responsible for attaching to foreign substances in the body, and for initiating an attack against invaders such as viruses and bacteria.

When mass-produced in the laboratory, antibodies can be made all of one type (monoclonal) to target preferentially a certain kind of invader. Because cancer cells are different in some ways from healthy cells, such as in the number or combination of proteins that extend from their surface, manmade monoclonal antibodies (abbreviated moabs or mabs) can be made to aim preferentially for cancer cells by targeting these surface proteins. They are capable of attaching to healthy cells as well, but the aforementioned differences in expression of surface proteins between healthy and cancerous cells result in a higher likelihood of attachment to cancerous cells.

A monoclonal antibody may be naked, or it may be coupled, or conjugated, with another substance called a payload: a toxic substance such as ricin, or a radioactive substance (radioisotope) such as iodine-131 or yttrium-90. When the conjugated monoclonal antibody attaches to a cell's surface protein, the proximity of the toxic substance damages or kills the cell.

Moab 17-1A is a monoclonal antibody being tested in phase III trials for use against colorectal cancer.

Even though the concept of the use of monoclonal antibodies is very promising, there is no well proven data to show their benefit for the treatment of colorectal cancer.

Cytokines

Cytokines are substances the body uses to trigger other immunologic events. Interferon-alfa-2B, for instance, is a cytokine that can halt growth of some tumors, force cells to mature, and interrupt cell motility.

Colony stimulating factors

Colony stimulating factors are substances that cause growth of new blood cells in marrow.

- G-CSF. Granulocyte colony stimulating factor (Filgrastim, Neupogen) is a manmade copy of a protein that causes bone marrow to grow new white blood cells called neutrophils.

- GM-CSF. Granulocyte-macrophage colony stimulating factor (Sargramostim, Leukine), like G-CSF, is a manmade copy of a protein that causes bone marrow to grow both new white blood cells called neutrophils and new monocytes. Macrophages, which develop from monocytes, are cells that surround and digest foreign material and microorganisms in the body.

- EPO. Erythropoietin (Epoetin alfa, Epogen, Procrit), like the colony stimulating factors, is a manmade copy of a substance made by the kidney (and in lesser quantities by other organs, such as the liver and adrenal glands) that causes bone marrow to produce new red blood cells.

- TPO. Thrombopoietin, like G-CSF and EPO, is a manmade copy of a body product that causes bone marrow to grow new platelets. TPO is not yet approved by the FDA as of July 1999.

Tumor vaccines

Tumor vaccines, now in clinical trials for colorectal cancer, are an attempt to re-educate the body to attack tumor cells. For reasons still unknown, at some point the body stops attacking cancer cells, even though evidence suggests that it does mount an immune attack against cancer cells when they are still small and few in number.

Stem cell support

Use of stem cell support in conjunction with chemotherapy for colorectal cancer is in clinical trials. Stem cells are very young blood cells that can repopulate depleted bone marrow. Reintroducing stem cells to the body after high-dose treatment permits very high doses of chemotherapy or radiotherapy to be used—that is, doses high enough to kill all cancer, but also to destroy bone marrow.

For more information on many other treatments still in the experimental stage, see Chapter 23, *The Future of Therapy.*

Treatment of colon cancer by stage

In general, the treatment guidelines listed below were adapted from the National Cancer Institute's State-of-the-Art Treatment Statement for physicians as of July 1999. Not all surgical oncologists, colon and rectal surgeons, medical oncologists, and radiation oncologists agree on all of these points for all patients, however. When differences of opinion were presented by our medical reviewers, their viewpoints were included below.

You should discuss your specific treatment options with your own oncology treatment team. You should consider calling the NCI periodically at (800) 4-CANCER or visiting their web site at *http://cancernet.nci.nih.gov/clinpdq/soa.html* to obtain updated standards of care.

Stage 0 colon cancer

Stage 0 is the most superficial of tumors, and is readily and successfully treated with surgery that aims to be minimally invasive.

Treatment options:

- Local excision or simple removal of polyps using a flexible colonoscope, always with the goal of achieving clear outer margins showing only normal cells on the removed tissue, indicating that all of the tumor has been removed.

- Removal of the section of diseased colon and rejoining (anastomosis) of the remaining colon using open abdominal surgery, again striving for clear outer margins showing only normal cells on the removed tissue, indicating that all of the tumor has been removed. This more extensive, invasive surgical procedure is for larger tumors or other tumors that cannot be treated with local excision: tumors that have invaded the box or stalk of the polyp, or polyps that lie flat (sessile).

Stage I colon cancer

This stage describes a tumor that has invaded the wall of the colon, but has not penetrated through the entire wall. This stage is roughly equivalent to Dukes A or Modified Astler-Coller A and B1. There is no one-to-one correspondence among these staging systems.

Stage I colon cancer is treated with open abdominal surgery that permits removal of the section of diseased colon and lymph nodes, and the rejoining of the remaining sections of colon. Alternately, it may involve the creation of one of a variety of means to capture and pass feces, if necessitated by removal of the rectum and anus. The goal is the achievement of clear outer margins showing only normal cells on the removed tissue, indicating that the entire tumor has been removed.

Surgery for stage I cancer is intended to be curative, but also is a means of obtaining tissue for biopsy to confirm whether disease is truly confined to the bowel, and to what degree the tumor may have penetrated the bowel wall. Lymph nodes also are removed and analyzed in the pathology laboratory to assess whether microscopic disease has spread beyond the colon.

Stage II colon cancer

This stage describes a tumor that has invaded through the entire wall of the colon, but has not spread to lymph nodes. This stage may be equivalent to Dukes B or Modified Astler-Coller B2 and B3. There is no one-to-one correspondence among these staging systems.

Stage II colon cancer is treated in the following ways:

- Open abdominal surgery that permits removal of the section of diseased colon, removal of certain key lymph nodes, examination of other abdominal organs, and either the rejoining of the remaining sections of colon, or the creation of one of a variety of means to capture and pass feces, if necessitated by removal of the rectum and anus. The goal is the achievement of clear outer margins on all removed tissue, showing only normal cells, indicating that the entire tumor visible under a microscope has been removed.

- The National Cancer Institute recommends that, following surgery, patients at stage II should consider clinical trials of systemic or regional chemotherapy, radiotherapy, or biological therapy.

- Medical reviewers as well as several published articles note that only certain stage II patients will benefit from systemic chemotherapy. Please discuss your own prognostic features with your oncology team in order to understand fully what benefits and risks are involved.

Stage III colon cancer

Stage III colon cancer is characterized by tumor invasion of one or more lymph nodes. This stage may be equivalent to Dukes C or Modified Astler-Coller C1–C3. There is no one-to-one correspondence among these staging systems.

- Open abdominal surgery that permits removal of the section of diseased colon with wide margins, along with certain key lymph nodes, and the rejoining of the remaining sections of colon, or the creation of one of a variety of means to capture and pass feces, if necessitated by removal of the rectum and anus.

- Surgery is followed by chemotherapy. As of July 1999, usually fluorouracil (5-FU) and leucovorin are used.

- The National Cancer Institute recommends that, following surgery, patients at stage III should consider clinical trials of newer systemic or regional chemotherapy, radiotherapy, or biological therapy. The NCI treatment statement says, for example, "Improved local control with postoperative radiation therapy has been suggested in patients with adherence or fixation to adjacent structures."

Stage IV colon cancer

Stage IV disease is disease that has spread to distant organs, such as the liver or lungs. This stage generally is equivalent to Dukes D or Modified Astler-Coller D, although there is no strict one-to-one correspondence among these staging systems.

Patients diagnosed at this stage are encouraged by the National Cancer Institute to join a clinical trial. Treatment within a clinical trial may give you access to better treatment prior to FDA approval, before it becomes available to the general public.

Treatment options recommended by the National Cancer Institute and by our medical reviewers follow. Clinicians expressed differing beliefs regarding the order in which these treatment options should be recommended. The National Cancer Institute lists surgical options at the top of the list; others listed chemotherapy and radiation therapy as first choices:

- Chemotherapy to control painful or uncomfortable symptoms (palliative chemotherapy), or to prolong the patient's life span. Although chemotherapeutic agents in use at this time for stage IV disease are not curative, chemotherapy might prolong the life span of certain patients with stage IV disease.

- Narrowly targeted radiotherapy to control painful or uncomfortable symptoms, known as palliative radiotherapy.

- Select patients with stage IV disease benefit from surgery:

    - Patients with symptoms of pain or blockage from a tumor in the bowel may benefit from its resection.

    - Some patients with solitary tumors in other organs can in some cases be cured by their surgical removal.

Recurrent colon cancer

Recurrent colon cancer may be found in a single site, such as a single liver tumor or several small liver tumors in one lobe, or it may recur as widespread disease affecting several organs.

Patients diagnosed at this stage are encouraged by the National Cancer Institute to join a clinical trial. Treatment within a clinical trial may give you access to better treatment prior to FDA approval, before it becomes available to the general public.

Treatment options recommended by the National Cancer Institute and by our medical reviewers follow. Clinicians expressed differing beliefs regarding the order in which these treatment options should be recommended. The National Cancer Institute lists surgical options at the top of the list; others listed chemotherapy and radiation therapy as first choices:

- Chemotherapy to control painful or uncomfortable symptoms (palliative chemotherapy), or to prolong the patient's life span. Although chemotherapeutic agents in use at this time for recurrent disease are not curative, chemotherapy might prolong the life span of certain patients with recurrent disease.

- Radiotherapy to control painful or uncomfortable symptoms, such as pain from a tumor that has spread to the bone. This is known as palliative radiotherapy.

- Select patients with recurrent disease benefit from surgery:

- Patients with symptoms of pain or blockage from a tumor in the bowel may benefit from its resection.
- Some patients with solitary tumors in other organs can be cured by their surgical removal. The five-year cure rate for complete removal of certain liver tumors, for example, is 20 to 30 percent in carefully selected patients.
- Surgical removal, if feasible, of single lung or ovarian metastases can lead to long-term cure in a small percentage of patients, especially if the recurrence comes more than two years after the original surgical treatment.
- Surgical removal of recurrent cancer very near the site of the original tumor (locally recurrent tumor), such as a recurrence at the site where remaining bowel was rejoined (anastomosis).

Treatment of rectal cancer by stage

The National Cancer Institute specifies the following treatments as standard care for rectal cancer as of July 1999. You should consider calling the NCI periodically at (800) 4-CANCER or visiting their web site at *http://cancernet. nci.nih.gov/clinpdq/soa.html* to obtain updated standards of care.

Stage 0 rectal cancer

Stage 0 is the most superficial of rectal tumors, limited to the mucosa without invasion of a deeper layer of the bowel wall. It is readily and successfully treated with surgery that may be minimally invasive.

Treatment options:

- Local excision or simple removal of polyps, always with the goal of achieving clear outer margins on the removed tissue—showing only normal cells on all edges—indicating that all of the tumor has been removed.
- Surgical removal of the rectum for large lesions not amenable to local excision, generally without colostomy.
- Removal of tumors by electrofulguration, a means of burning away tissue.

- Internal (endocavitary) irradiation using one of the various specialized devices available.

- External radiotherapy is uncommonly used for this stage.

Stage I rectal cancer

This stage describes a tumor that has invaded the wall of the rectum, but has not penetrated through the entire wall. This stage may be equivalent to Dukes A or Modified Astler-Coller A and B1. There is no exact one-to-one correspondence among these staging systems.

Treatment options recommended by the National Cancer Institute:

- Surgery to remove the tumor and rejoin the two remaining pieces of bowel, when tumor location ensures that enough rectal tissue will remain to perform such rejoining after tumor removal.

- For tumors that are too low to allow rejoining remaining pieces of bowel, or bowel and anus, surgery to remove the tumor and all anal and rectal tissue, and creation of an ostomy, called abdominoperineal resection.

- One of the two surgical procedures described above to remove the tumor, or local surgery through the anus, with or without external-beam irradiation plus fluorouracil (5-FU) before or after surgery.

- A mesorectal excision, that is, en bloc resection of the rectal tumor and its local lymph nodes with an enveloping fascia.

- Internal (endocavitary) irradiation without surgery, with or without external beam irradiation. Note that special equipment and experience are required to achieve results that are as good as surgery in selected patients. The National Cancer Institute lists eligible patients to be those with:

  - Tumors less than 3 centimeters in size

  - Well-differentiated tumors

  - Disease without deep ulceration, tumor fixation, or palpable lymph nodes

- In very select patients, electrofulguration, a means of burning away tissue, may be as effective as surgery.

Stage II rectal cancer

This stage describes a tumor that has invaded through the entire wall of the bowel wall, but has not spread to lymph nodes, although the National Cancer Institute states that, "the uterus, vagina, parametria, ovaries, or prostate are sometimes involved." This stage may be equivalent to Dukes B or Modified Astler-Coller B2 and B3, although there is no exact one-to-one correspondence among these staging systems.

Patients diagnosed at this stage are encouraged by the National Cancer Institute to join a clinical trial. Treatment within a clinical trial may give you access to better treatment prior to FDA approval, before it becomes available to the general public.

Treatment options recommended by the National Cancer Institute:

- Surgery to remove the tumor entirely, rejoining the remaining pieces of bowel, or bowel and anus, if possible (sphincter preservation). This surgery might include creation of an internal pouch to retain feces. Adjuvant chemotherapy and/or radiotherapy, preferably through participation in a clinical trial, are recommended.

- Surgery to remove all of the rectum and anus (abdominoperineal resection) and construction of a stoma to pass feces. Adjuvant chemotherapy and/or radiotherapy, preferably through participation in a clinical trial, are recommended.

- Partial or total removal of certain pelvic tissue when, rarely, bladder, uterus, vagina, or prostate are involved. Adjuvant chemotherapy and/or radiotherapy, preferably through participation in a clinical trial, are recommended.

- Preoperative radiotherapy with or without chemotherapy, followed by surgery that attempts to preserve sphincter function. Adjuvant chemotherapy, preferably through participation in a clinical trial, should be used in conjunction with surgery.

- Intra-operative electron beam radiotherapy (IORT) targeted to the sites of remaining disease following surgical removal might be used if the tumor could not be entirely removed. This technique is still considered experimental by some researchers.

- Radiobiologically effective pelvic radiotherapy of approximately 50 Greys (Gy) is recommended when radiotherapy is used.

Stage III rectal cancer

Stage III rectal cancer is characterized by tumor invasion of one or more lymph nodes. This stage may be equivalent to Dukes C or Modified Astler-Coller C1–C3. There is no absolute one-to-one correspondence among these staging systems.

Patients diagnosed at this stage are encouraged by the National Cancer Institute to join a clinical trial. Treatment within a clinical trial may give you access to better treatment prior to FDA approval, before it becomes available to the general public.

Treatment options:

- Surgery to remove entirely the diseased rectum, rejoining the remaining pieces of bowel, or bowel and anus, if possible. This surgery might include creation of an internal reservoir to retain feces. Adjuvant chemotherapy and/or radiotherapy, preferably through participation in a clinical trial, should be used following surgery.

- Surgery to remove all of the rectum and anus (abdominoperineal resection) and construction of a stoma to pass feces. Adjuvant chemotherapy and/or radiotherapy, preferably through participation in a clinical trial, are recommended.

- Partial or total removal of certain pelvic tissue when, rarely, bladder, uterus, vagina, or prostate are involved. Adjuvant chemotherapy and/or radiotherapy, preferably through participation in a clinical trial, are recommended.

- Preoperative radiotherapy with or without chemotherapy, followed by surgery that attempts to preserve sphincter function. Adjuvant chemotherapy following surgery, preferably through participation in a clinical trial, is recommended.

- Intra-operative electron beam radiotherapy (IORT) targeted to the sites of remaining disease might be used.

- Radiobiologically effective pelvic radiotherapy of approximately 50 Gy is recommended when radiotherapy is used.

- Radiotherapy and/or chemotherapy to control painful or uncomfortable symptoms. This option is recommended by the National Cancer Institute and some of our medical reviewers as of July 1999, but was not recommended by all of our medical reviewers.

Stage IV rectal cancer

Patients diagnosed at this stage are encouraged by the National Cancer Institute to join a clinical trial. Treatment within a clinical trial may give you access to better treatment prior to FDA approval, before it becomes available to the general public.

Treatment options:

- Surgical removal or bypassing of tumors that are obstructing the bowel or other organs. This approach is used for patients who have been selected as suitable candidates for having their painful or uncomfortable symptoms reduced by surgery. Sometimes it is not surgery intended for cure, but instead for temporarily reducing painful symptoms, bleeding from the tumor, or impending obstruction of the rectum.

- Potentially curative surgery to remove certain tumors that have spread to the liver, lung, or ovaries might be indicated in certain carefully screened patients.

- Radiotherapy intended to control symptoms.

- Chemotherapy intended to control symptoms and possibly to extend survival time.

Recurrent rectal cancer

Recurrent rectal cancer may be found in a single site, such as a single liver tumor or several small liver tumors in one lobe, or it may recur as widespread disease affecting several organs, including bones such as ribs, spine, or pelvis.

Patients with a recurrence of extensive disease should consider joining a clinical trial. Treatment within a clinical trial may give you access to better treatment before it becomes available to the general public.

Treatment options:

- Surgical removal of a recurrent tumor that is very near the site of original disease may be curative in selected patients; in others, it may serve only to reduce symptoms.

- Curative surgery to remove liver tumors for patients in whom liver involvement has been assessed and found to be limited to three or fewer tumors. Five-year cure rate for complete removal of certain liver tumors is 20 to 30 percent in carefully selected patients.

- Curative surgery to remove single lung or ovarian metastases.
- Radiotherapy to control symptoms.
- Chemotherapy to control symptoms.

Treatment of liver metastases

The liver is a common site for the spread of colorectal cancer because part of the blood supply leaving the intestine leads directly to the liver instead of first passing through the lungs.

Surgery

Surgery to completely remove certain liver tumors can result in five-year survival rates in 20 to 30 percent of carefully selected patients who experience liver metastases. At this time, between 11 and 30 percent of patients who experience spread of disease to the liver are found to have tumors that are suitable for surgery. The tumors most successfully treated with traditional surgical removal are:

- Those that affect only a small part of the liver
- No more than three tumors
- A few small tumors that are clustered very near each other
- Tumors with negative margins; that is, with two centimeters of normal liver tissue surrounding the surgical margin
- No other organs concurrently affected by colorectal cancer metastases; that is, no cancer outside the liver
- No liver tumors located very near large blood vessels or other vital organs

Cryosurgery

Cryosurgery, a freezing of the tumor to destroy it, may yield five-year survival rates of 20 percent among carefully selected patients. These patients are:

- Those with localized liver metastases that cannot be surgically removed owing to their location near major blood vessels or other organs

- Those with two lobes of the liver involved, but not more than three to four tumor nodules

Regional chemotherapy

Some studies have shown that chemotherapy with floxuridine (FUDR) directed only into the liver, and combined with surgery, may provide better results than surgery alone. This combination results in a higher rate of tumor regression and greater likelihood that the tumor can be removed surgically. The value of regional chemotherapy still is being assessed; not all researchers agree that it will result in longer survival.

Hepatic arterial infusion (HAI)

Liver metastases might also be treated with infusion of chemotherapy into the hepatic artery. This technique is a form of regional chemotherapy. A drug combination recently shown to be promising is floxuridine (FUDR) and dexamethasone infused into the hepatic artery, plus fluorouracil and leucovorin given systemically.

Tumor embolization

Clinical trials are underway to evaluate methods that cause blood clots within liver tumors. Deliberate formation of blood clots inside the blood vessels that feed liver tumors is also being attempted. Some research centers are combining this technique with infusion of chemotherapy into the hepatic artery.

Radiotherapy

Radiotherapy is used to control symptoms for inoperable liver metastases. The liver is quite sensitive to radiation; the dose that would be required to kill all cancer cells throughout the liver is higher than this organ can tolerate, resulting in significant radiotoxicity.

Radiofrequency ablation (RFA)

Another apparently promising method is the destruction of liver tumors using heat generated by high-frequency radio waves. Results with this technique have been inconsistent, however, and the method requires further study.

I had radiofrequency ablation (RFA) last month for a single 2.5 x 3.0 liver tumor. Excepting for the general anesthesia (I've always had spinals before), its impact seems less than having a wisdom tooth removed—actually a lot less.

I went to the hospital in the morning, and had hardly any prep at all. I just hung out with the surgical staff for 30 minutes or so waiting for the final lab tests to come back. Then into the operating room, awake for 30 seconds, then waking up in post-op 5 hours later.

As I understand it, most of the time was spent removing scar tissue and adhesions from my prior liver resection. I was back in my room in less than an hour, and was able to use oral medications immediately. Amazingly, no tubes. I could probably have escaped for dinner.

At about 5:00 PM my other surgical team who had performed bilateral wedge resection to my lungs a month before stopped by to say hi, asking when I was to have surgery. Even they seemed amazed that surgery had already happened, as I was walking around the floor by this time.

The night went quite well. I even slept for a while, although most of the time, sleeping in the hospital is not possible for me. They served me something that they called food for breakfast. I've built buildings out of more appetizing stuff. By 9:30 AM I was released.

I took a cab home. A great friend picked me up for lunch. I had a wonderful lobster salad at Fabrizio's in Larkspur. Within a day of the surgery!

Okay, I would have rather spent a day at Club Med, but as far as hospital procedures go, this truly was a walk in the park.

Summary

This chapter reflects an effort to digest and summarize the latest information regarding treatment for the various colorectal cancers. New treatments evolve continuously, however, and it's in your best interest to keep abreast of these changes. Your colon and rectal surgeon, medical oncologist, radiation oncologist, the National Cancer Institute, and cancer research journals are your best sources of information for current treatment choices.

If you have questions about the appropriateness of the information you have found here, and in particular if you have a rare type of colorectal cancer that we do not address in the foregoing discussion, please rely on your doctor for clarification and updates.

All treatment information is subject to change as research yields better weapons against colorectal cancer. Currently, here are some key points to remember:

- Surgery is usually the most effective means to cure colorectal cancer. Discuss with your surgeon *before* surgery what procedures will be used to preserve bowel function and sexual performance. Your surgeon should be one trained to perform all of the sphincter-saving procedures available to limit the need for a permanent colostomy or ileostomy. Your surgeon needs to be experienced in treating colorectal cancer and must know when to consult with oncologists, both pre-operatively and post-operatively.

- 5-fluorouracil and leucovorin are the mainstay drugs of adjuvant chemotherapy, and improve survival in patients diagnosed with stage III colon cancer, or stages II or III rectal cancer. Some stage II colon cancer patients might benefit from adjuvant chemotherapy. Irinotecan (CPT-11) sometimes is used when 5-FU fails.

- Adjuvant radiotherapy is most commonly used against stage II and III rectal cancer, either pre-operatively or postoperatively. It is also used to convert inoperable rectal tumors into operable tumors, and to treat residual tumors after an incomplete surgical removal. It is used rarely for colon cancer.

- Liver metastases in those diagnosed as stage IV or with a recurrence of disease can be addressed with a variety of treatments, including second surgeries. Of patients who meet carefully outlined criteria to determine their eligibility for surgery, 20 to 30 percent will survive five years or longer.

- Radiation and chemotherapy often are used to relieve symptoms in patients whose tumors are not considered curable.

- Consider using the steps outlined in Chapter 24 to keep informed about changes in treatment strategies.

CHAPTER 7

Experiencing
Hospitalization

*There shall be no card playing or dicing and
such patients as are able shall assist in
nursing others, washing and ironing linen
and cleaning the rooms and such other
services as the matron may require.*

—Regulations of the Philadelphia
General Hospital, 1790

TREATMENT OF COLORECTAL CANCER ALMOST ALWAYS INVOLVES a hospitalization for abdominal, pelvic, rectal, or perineal surgery. Additional hospital stays might be necessary to administer chemotherapy, radiation therapy, or to address side effects of treatment, such as infections that develop when white blood cell counts drop during chemotherapy. Hospitalization and perhaps surgery might be needed to correct intestinal blockages that may occur following some treatments, to reopen the ureters with stents so that urine can flow from kidney to bladder, or to remove other organs, such as the uterus, if disease recurs. Occasionally, complex exploratory or diagnostic procedures, such as biopsy of a suspected lung tumor, may require hospitalization.

Some people are frightened by the idea of being admitted to the hospital, even while realizing that the best care for a particular problem can be delivered only with the around-the-clock medical scrutiny available in a good hospital. This chapter will attempt to help you view the experience in a positive light, and will highlight the precautions you can follow to make your stay brief yet fruitful. We will examine the experience chronologically, beginning with preparation and admitting procedures, and finishing with discharge and home care. Separate sections on radiotherapy, chemotherapy, ostomy, infection, and abdominoperineal surgery are included.

General concerns

In the US, generally you are limited to using hospitals at which your doctors have admitting privileges. It's best to consider this in advance, as discussed in Chapter 2, *Finding the Right Treatment Team*. Ideally, the hospital should be an NCI-designated comprehensive cancer center as discussed in Chapter 2, or affiliated with a medical school. At the very least, it should be accredited by the Joint Commission on Accreditation of Healthcare Organizations (JCAHO). Call JCAHO at (708) 916-5800, and ask the hospital's administrators about the outcome of their latest evaluation by JCAHO. For more detailed information on selecting a hospital, see *A Cancer Survivor's Almanac*, published by the National Coalition for Cancer Survivorship.

If you have a child who is facing hospitalization, you're probably aware that children face unique fears and misunderstandings about hospital care. You can address your child's concerns using the collective advice of more than 40 parents presented in the book *Your Child in the Hospital: A Practical Guide for Parents,* by Nancy Keene and Rachel Prentice.

You should request in writing that the hospital keep your surgically removed tissue samples essentially forever. Some cancer survivors have discovered that hospital policy specifies that tissue samples be kept for only a number of years. This may become a problem if your oncologist needs to compare a newer tissue sample to the original or if there should arise some question regarding the original diagnosis years afterward. Some of the newer biological treatments now emerging require analysis of tumor cells. This means that if you had a tumor removed years ago and now want to take advantage of a new biological treatment, you'll need your tumor sample re-examined.

Preparation

If you know in advance that you'll be admitted to the hospital, you can plan to make your stay brief and successful. If your admission is for surgery, for example, copious helpful information, including what to bring, will be given to you in advance by the staff. Pre-operative tests such as a chest x-ray, electrocardiogram and blood testing, for example, may be necessary.

On the other hand, you may be admitted via the emergency room if symptoms are unusual, have a rapid onset, or are associated with immediate danger, such as difficulty moving your bowels or pronounced abdominal pain.

You may be taken directly into surgery from the emergency room if an intestinal blockage or perforation is suspected. If you have symptoms of an infection following chemotherapy, your doctor may insist that you proceed directly to an isolation room in the oncology wing while your loved ones deal with the admitting paperwork in the germ-filled front lobby.

You might have little control over some of these happenings, but it's best to avoid the emergency room during treatment, if possible, by careful tracking of symptoms and timely communication with your doctor. Emergency-room care may be greatly delayed, or may vary in quality, based on several factors beyond your control, such as the seriousness of the illnesses of others waiting, or the experience of the medical staff on duty. If you must use an emergency room, be sure to call your treatment team and let them know what's happened.

Sue Browne describes her husband's concerns about hospitalization and surgery:

> Surgery was scheduled for late Monday afternoon, but the entire day was weird for us, not knowing what to do or say, so we just remained mostly quiet. I always fixed things, but this I could not fix. Steve felt out of control as well and definitely out of his comfort zone! He had never been admitted into a hospital for anything his whole life, so he joked about losing his hospital virginity. He also asked the surgery prep nurse if she could find a nurse uglier and older than herself to do the prep work! We were all in tears from laughing! We kissed good-bye as he was being wheeled into surgery. It would be about two and a half hours until I could find out anything. I was thankful for the Hispanic family that was also in the waiting room. We could not understand each other, but that was all right with me because I really didn't feel like talking, but I didn't want to be alone either.

Arrangements

Here are a few general tips for preparing in advance for a hospital stay:

- You can smooth the path of abrupt admissions by having an overnight bag ready that contains much of what you'll need. See "What to bring," later in this chapter.

- If you're being admitted for surgery or any other procedure, call your insurance company to see if the procedure must be precertified. Keep a written log of whom you spoke with, and when.

- If you're being admitted for surgery, verify that the surgeon is board-certified in colon and rectal surgery, or in general surgery with a second specialty in oncology. The Official ABMS Directory of Board Certified Medical Specialists is a publication that can be found in a local library, and the American Medical Association also can verify board certification; see Appendix A, *Resources*. Your state licensing board or state medical society can verify how many years of experience your surgeon has had. If you're having a tumor-affected ovary or uterus removed and time permits, consider consulting a gynecologic oncologist for a second opinion. A gynecologic oncologist is a very highly trained surgeon who specializes in removing cancers of the female reproductive organs. This kind of training can contribute significantly to her skills in removing all disease, consequently improving your chances of long-term survival.

- If you're being admitted for surgery, obtain and review all consent documents. Strike any clauses that connote that staff other than your surgeon may be participating in your procedure, unless you and your surgeon already have discussed who else might be participating and you're comfortable with these additional personnel. There are varying risks associated with surgery done under general anesthesia, including excessive bleeding from the incision site and a very small risk from the anesthesia itself. Your doctor and the hospital staff will explain fully the risks that apply most closely to your surgery.

- Hospitals that receive federal funding or are governed by certain local laws must adhere to federal or local laws regarding informed consent prior to use of human subjects for research. Government-funded hospitals include most university, state, and nonprofit hospitals. Verify whether your hospital receives any federal funding, and phone your state health department to determine if your state has its own laws regarding consent issues. If your hospital is a private for-profit hospital that receives no federal funding and is not governed by similar local laws, question closely any treatment suggested for you. Ask your doctor if your proposed treatment represents state-of-the-art treatment as defined by NCI, or if you'll be treated in an investigational study.

- Ask if you can donate your own blood (autologous donation) in advance of surgery.

- Read as much as you can about the procedure you'll be having.

- Make notes about all health problems you have, related to colorectal cancer and otherwise. Make several photocopies of these notes, because each group of medical caretakers you meet will ask the same questions again.

- Arrange for child care, if appropriate. Most likely this care will be provided by a well informed relative, but if not, prepare abundant information well in advance, in writing, including phone numbers of relatives and pediatricians.

- Contact a pet sitter, if needed. Provide clear written instructions regarding feeding and any health problems. Provide your veterinarian's address and phone number, and those of an emergency all-night veterinary service. Leave all supplies, including carrier and medications, in a prominent place.

- Have the mail and newspapers held if nobody will remain at home. Make arrangements for a plant waterer, if needed.

- Pay any upcoming bills in advance.

- Plan transportation to and from the hospital, allowing plenty of time in everyone's schedules for check-in and check-out procedures. Hospitals are not very good at checking patients out quickly, especially if you need special instructions about home aftercare.

- Call the hospital and ask about parking arrangements, such as less expensive long-term passes for those who will be visiting you during an extended stay, special parking for outpatient units, or discounted or waived fees for those accompanying you during a surgery.

- If you'd like to bring a laptop computer, verify first if the hospital has digital phone lines. If so, borrow or buy an adapter so your modem won't be ruined. Tell email friends if you'd love to receive email during your stay, but point out that you might not be able to respond. Ask them not to be offended, but instead to keep on writing.

- Contact your employer, not only to arrange for use of sick time or disability pay, but to ensure their emotional and professional support when you return to work. Ask for a copy of company leave policies and the federal Family and Medical Leave Act in order to become acquainted with all employment-related options.

- Check your calendar and cancel any commitments that conflict with your hospital schedule.

- Arrange for a visiting or live-in home nurse if you think you or your caretaker will need extra help after your hospital stay. Many insurance companies will pay toward this service if your doctor says you meet certain conditions, such as being temporarily unable to bathe.

- If you're having radiation therapy for rectal cancer that involves placing radioactive material onto or into your body, let your family and friends know that children and pregnant women should not visit you at all, and that others should plan for brief visits only. During the time the radioactive substance is acting upon you, you will constitute a radiation exposure risk to others.

- Discuss with your family and other loved ones what aftercare or special considerations you might need when you arrive home. Abdominal surgery will require that you avoid driving for some number of weeks, for instance, or internal radiation therapy might require that you dispose carefully of body wastes for a few days.

Bowel preparation

If you're being admitted for abdominal surgery or for any procedure that will touch the bowel, such as repair of a fistula, it is extremely important to cleanse the bowel thoroughly beforehand. Many of the serious or potentially fatal side effects of intestinal surgery are directly caused by surgical intrusion into a bowel that contains remnants of feces.

The surgeon's staff will give you detailed instructions about having a clear liquid diet for several days, drinking an electrolytic laxative fluid the day before surgery, using one or more enemas, avoiding iron supplements for a week or more, and avoiding drugs that can interfere with blood clotting, such as aspirin. Follow these to the letter. If an intestinal blockage is suspected, however, no laxatives or enemas should be used.

What to bring

Some people bring too many things or inappropriate things to the hospital; others pack too little, assuming that the hospital will provide everything. Here are a few suggestions:

- Ask the hospital staff for a list of things that will be useful. Remind them of your treatment plan so they can give you detailed suggestions.

- Prepare several copies of lists of your medications, both prescription and over-the-counter: never assume the hospital has spoken with all of your doctors.

- Bring your health insurance card and your certificate showing you donated your own blood for use during surgery, if applicable.

- Bring your own over-the-counter medications if you suffer from athlete's foot, tooth sensitivity, or other conditions not related to colorectal cancer. You must remember to inform the staff first, though, if you need to use these supplies: they are medications, and they may interact unfavorably with medications your doctor has ordered.

- You might feel better in your own clothing if you have someone who can launder it for you. Leave behind any clothing with metal zippers or snaps, because you may need diagnostic tests such as barium x-rays or MRI. Choose clothing that won't press on your abdominal incision or stoma, or cause you undue strain as you dress. Choose shirts with easy sleeves that can accommodate IV lines. Add something dashing or seductive to the overnight bag if you think an ego boost will help.

- If you pack a razor, avoid the plug-in electric variety, as the local fire code or the proximity of hospital oxygen supplies may regulate against these. Battery-operated razors generally are most acceptable; however, a disposable razor may do, provided you're able to manipulate it while feeling less than your usual self.

- Bring eye and ear coverings for sleep. Hospitals can be noisy places at odd hours.

- If music will help you relax and sleep, bring a personal player with a headset to avoid disturbing your roommate.

- If you anticipate a long stay, bring pictures of home, family, pets, and loving experiences.

- Remember warm socks (the nursing staff love wild socks).

- If this is a return trip, bring the phone the hospital may have sold you during your prior stay.

- An old sock full of quarters will help you and your family make post-surgical phone calls, pay for parking, buy newspapers, or buy those dreadful but sometimes unavoidable vending-machine meals. Unlike a purse or a wallet, a ratty old sock doesn't look worth stealing.

- Bring a laptop computer if you enjoy Internet email support from other friends with colorectal cancer. Bring a bike lock to anchor your PC to the bed if the hospital has experienced theft.

- Pack a list of phone numbers of friends and family.

- Most hospitals provide some toiletries such as soap, washcloths, and a toothbrush, but you may prefer your own. Avoid scented products, though, as these may make you or your roommate ill.

- Prepare several copies of your advance directives (living will, durable power of attorney) to inform the staff of your wishes for or against extreme life-support measures.

- Bring books that are lightweight, both tangibly and intellectually. You may be groggy and achy for a spell. Don't plan to read and analyze the Hardy-Weinberg equilibrium or to hold open a seven-pound tax code manual during your hospital stay.

- For females, pack a long, loose shirt or tunic top for the times when you're told to "take everything off, and put on this gown with the opening in the front." Sooner or later you will have to open these in the front, but you'll feel less the victim of someone else's poor sartorial taste.

- For both males and females, pack a pair of baggy boxer shorts for the times when you're told to "take everything off, and put on this gown with the opening in the back." A wild, glow-in-the-dark pair might give your sense of individuality a boost, for instance, and might give others a smile.

What not to bring

Bringing certain items to the hospital can turn into a hindrance:

- Leave all jewelry at home. If you want to wear your wedding band, ask the staff about this first. They may secure it with tape during surgery, for example.

- Scented toiletries. You may feel nausea after certain procedures, and scents may tip you (or your poor, captive roommate) over the edge of gastric comfort. Moreover, you may come to associate your once-favorite scent with a hospital stay.

- Leave your purse, wallet, credit cards, and money, beyond incidental change for newspapers and the like, at home or in a safe-deposit box.

- Leave your worries and your work behind. Let your family and the hospital staff coddle you with back-rubs. Channel-surf and watch sleazy TV shows for the utter decadence of it. When you're allowed to eat, order everything on the hospital menu and share it with your pals.

Admission

Admission will start with paperwork, phone calls, questions about next of kin, phone and TV service preferences, attachment of a plastic ID bracelet, and directions to the correct room and floor. Have copies of all insurance paperwork and medical records ready.

After admission, a volunteer may be assigned to stay with you briefly until you've arrived in your room and become oriented, especially if you're having surgery.

Once you have arrived in your room, the nursing staff will take control and prepare you for whatever care you will need. They'll check vital signs such as pulse and temperature, and may start an intravenous line (IV) for administering drugs, and may help you with one final enema if your surgery is later that day or early the next day. You'll probably find that nurses will return a hundredfold any small effort you make to be friendly and kind.

Ask now about the meal menus, as there is usually a delay in getting meal preferences to newly admitted patients.

If you're being admitted for most procedures, you may be sharing a room with someone else. If you have rectal cancer and you're scheduled to be treated with a radioactive substance, you'll most likely be given a private room immediately or very soon.

The staff

The nursing staff is the first group you're likely to encounter in your hospital stay, but they're just one group of a confusing array of medical personnel you'll meet.

Note that you may refuse care administered by any staff member with whom you don't feel comfortable, and may ask for a more experienced person to attend to you.

Nurses

Hospital nurses will provide most of your care:

- Nurses' aides and licensed practical nurses (LPNs) will help wash you, help you in and out of bed, make your bed, and perform simple nursing tasks such as checking your pulse and temperature. LPNs, but not nurses' aides, have completed vocational training and may provide medication.

- Registered nurses (RNs) have earned a college degree in nursing and passed a licensing examination. RNs are able to provide more complex and critical medical care than LPNs, such as changing wound dressings, communicating with doctors, starting IVs, and administering IV medications.

- Nurse practitioners or clinical nurse specialists are RNs who have undertaken extensive additional training and are licensed to provide many of the same services that doctors provide. In some states they are able to prescribe drugs under the auspices of a physician. In some hospitals or clinical settings they may perform simple surgeries and procedures, such as lancing abscesses.

- Head nurses and nurse managers are in charge of other nurses, entire floors, or patient centers. Although all nurses now face the additional burden of administrative work that deprives them of time they prefer to spend with their patients, head nurses and nurse managers usually handle administrative issues exclusively, and seldom provide patient care unless staffing is inadequate.

- Enterostomal therapists are nurses specially trained to help those who will be having a stoma surgically created. A stoma is a temporary or permanent opening in the abdominal wall to allow waste to exit the body. Your surgeon will discuss with you whether your surgical procedure will include temporary or permanent ostomy.

Doctors

In teaching hospitals, you'll encounter the full spectrum of doctors in various stages of training. In some community hospitals, you'll encounter just residents and attending physicians. In other community hospitals that have agreements with nearby medical schools, you may find an amalgam of the two systems. Doctors in various stages of training include:

- Medical students who have completed four years of college and are undertaking four additional years of medical school. Medical students do not treat patients, although they may accompany an attending physician on rounds, and the physician may elicit their opinions.

- Interns, also called first-year residents, or postgraduate year-one students, have completed four years of medical school and are in the first year of three to six years of primary specialty training. They will not give you care unless supervised by much more experienced personnel, such as the attending physician or a more experienced resident, but that supervision may be distant. If you prefer not to be treated by an intern, say so.

- House officers (once called residents) may be postgraduate year-two students, postgraduate year-three students, and so on. These physicians are still receiving primary training that can last from three to six years, depending on the field.

- Fellows, or teaching fellows, have completed their six years' primary training, and have undertaken three years of additional training in a subspecialty.

- The attending physician is in charge of all fellows, residents and interns. In university hospitals, she is likely to be a faculty member. In community hospitals, she is hired to oversee patient care in her area of specialty based upon her reputation in the medical community.

I was in the hospital for chemotherapy and a very nervous looking medical type—student? intern?—tried to access my port and couldn't. After several tries the sweat ran down his face and he gave up.

Later that evening another guy in a white coat showed up. With my newfound bravery, I asked him, "Do you know how to access one of these things? Have you ever done it before?"

"Not only have I accessed them," he said, "I've installed hundreds."

He then proceeded to put the needle in with one quick jab—no pain, no anxiety. So much for my insisting on knowing who knows what they are doing!

Surgery

The most common surgery for colorectal cancer is laparotomy, an incision into the abdomen and pelvis to remove some or all of the colon or rectum, perhaps nearby organs that might be entangled with cancerous tissue, one or more lymph nodes in the abdomen or pelvis, and a portion of the liver if it has been invaded. Some procedures to remove part or all of the colon or rectum require creation of a temporary or permanent opening in the abdomen, called a stoma, through which feces can exit. The different surgeries used for colorectal cancer are discussed in Chapter 6, *Modes of Treatment*.

Other surgeries for colorectal cancer include:

- Rejoining of the intestine and removal of a temporary stoma.

- Removal of abnormal tubes called fistulas that form between two organs as a result of disease or of the healing that follows some surgeries.

- Removal or bypassing of intestinal blockage.

- For rectal cancer, placement of tubes for later containment of radioactive substances.

- Biopsies of lung, liver, or kidney, although these biopsies frequently are done as outpatient procedures.

You'll receive extensive instructions, meet with the anesthesiologist, and be monitored to ensure that no food is taken before surgery. Certain tests such as CT scans, ultrasound, or MRI may be repeated to precisely target tumors that need to be removed.

You'll meet with your surgeon to discuss what will be done during surgery. If the surgeon is planning to create a stoma, your abdomen will be examined to choose the best place for the stoma, taking into account the natural folding of your skin, the kinds of physical activity you enjoy, the part of the intestine that must be removed, and so on.

If you do not have a central catheter, an IV will be placed in your arm or hand—perhaps upon admission, one day before surgery, or directly before.

Just before surgery

The risks associated with this surgery will be explained to you, and you will be asked to sign a consent form.

If your surgery could affect the intestines in any way, you will be asked to fast for 12 to 18 hours before surgery. You may be instructed to use enemas or laxatives beforehand.

The site of the incision will be cleaned, shaved, and possibly marked for proposed incision lines and stoma placement, if ostomy is anticipated. If you're especially hairy, ask that a large area be shaved, including the IV site on your arm. Sticky bandaging can hurt terribly when it's removed if it pulls against hairs that have not been shaved.

If you're feeling nervous, ask for a sedative. The hour or two directly before surgery are likely to be the most tense.

If you have had nausea associated with anesthesia in the past, tell the anesthesiologist.

You may be asked to walk into the surgical suite, or you may be taken in on a rolling bed and shifted to the table. A rubber oxygen mask may be placed over your face to check for fit. Your arms may be positioned on armrests that facilitate giving medications by IV. A breathing tube will be inserted from your mouth to your upper lungs, but this intubation will be done after you're asleep, as may the insertion of a urinary catheter and a nasogastric tube to keep your bladder and stomach empty. Coating your eyelids with a lubricant while you're asleep to keep them from drying may also be done, as presurgical medication may include drugs to dry body fluids and reduce bleeding.

And now, the good part: you'll fall asleep, and you won't care what they do.

Surgical recovery

When you reawaken slowly, you'll be in the recovery room. You may notice that you've acquired rubber support stockings or a series of tubes attached to various body parts—but you won't care too much, because you'll be groggy for several more hours. You may also notice that your hearing returns first, well before sight does, and that you can remember odd or humorous things the staff said as the surgery was ending.

You may feel some pain too, upon waking. Be sure to make clear your need for pain medication as soon as you are awake and are experiencing pain, as excessive pain can interfere with healing. The nursing staff will not administer painkillers, though, until you're clearly awake, in order to avoid overdosing a patient possibly still affected by anesthesia. This means that, if you're feeling pain, you must tell them distinctly as soon as you are able. Groaning, for example, is not considered a clear indicator that you're awake. The nurses will attempt to get you to speak to be sure you're awakening normally.

Eventually you'll be returned to your room, but the first 24 hours may be a hazy memory if you've received general anesthesia. If you received a sedative instead of general anesthesia, you'll be groggy, too, but it will resolve more quickly than the aftereffects of general anesthesia.

Additional pain medication from day one will be given freely if you ask. Most patients find they need a minimum of three days of strong pain medication after abdominal, pelvic, or rectal surgery. Many hospitals now use patient-controlled infusion (PCI) pumps, as they yield a more even dose— about twenty microdoses per hour—than pain medication given by tablet or IV. PCI pumps also will yield a limited amount of additional medication if the patient pushes a button on the pump for this purpose. Don't worry about overdose. The pump won't allow it. The minicomputer within the pump counts the number of patient pushes so that the staff will have a good idea of your need for pain medication.

If you feel any nausea at all, even transient nausea, tell the nursing staff immediately. Vomiting, especially with a fresh incision, is a very unpleasant experience.

esia and painkillers slow the activity of various organs, includ-
ys, urinary bladder, and intestinal tract. Your liquid and solid
monitored after surgery until the staff note that your body sys-
again functioning as they should.

147

For the first few days after intestinal surgery, the contents of your stomach will be emptied by a nasogastric pump to ensure that no food or waste travels through the intestine. This is necessary because the intestine is a sulky organ that stops working after even a small injury. When the doctors and nurses begin to hear gas rumbling in the intestine, they know that its natural contractions, called peristalsis, are resuming, and that the nasogastric tube can be removed and a liquid diet attempted. If liquids stay down and do not cause pain, fever, or abdominal swelling (all signs of intestinal leakage, a serious complication of intestinal surgery), soft foods such as Jell-O can be added. If this succeeds, solid food can be introduced gradually.

Do the physical therapy, walking, coughing, or breathing exercises you're given as soon and as often as possible. Exercise will help you heal more quickly, and will reduce the chance of developing complications such as the form of pneumonia that's associated with lying flat for long periods. If you have an abdominal incision, hold a pillow against it for comfort while you cough.

Max describes how successfully he has recovered from surgery:

> I had a colon resection during which they took seven lymph nodes. A trace of cancer was found in four. I had very little pain after surgery. In fact, I played two rounds of golf five weeks after surgery. My doctor stressed the fact that I should not be in pain. He encouraged me to walk immediately after surgery and I was up to about one mile by the third week. I only needed pain medication for about two to three days after I left the hospital. Believe me, I am a weenie and would have been yelping if there had been pain.

If, after surgery, you have trouble getting in and out of bed, ask the nursing staff to tie something rope-like to the footboard so you can experiment with using arm muscles instead of abdominal muscles to pull yourself up and, especially, to lay yourself back down.

> I sailed through the surgery and was home four days later. I had the morphine pump, which worked wonderfully. Had an uneventful, rapid recovery. The surgeon was pleased that the presurgical radiation therapy had completely shrunk the tumor. Three weeks later I began six months of chemotherapy.

Abdominoperineal resection

Your surgeon will do his best to preserve tissue in the anus and rectum that control bowel movements, but at times the location, aggressiveness, or spread of the tumor makes sparing this tissue unsafe. Removal of all anal and rectal tissue, and the supporting structures near the rectum and anus, is called abdominoperineal resection. For rectal cancer, it might be the only surgery needed; for certain colon cancers, it's generally considered one half of the procedure, the other half being removal of part or all of the colon through an opening in the abdomen.

Two techniques exist for repairing the damage caused by removing this much tissue: a patching together of the tissue that remains, or packing the open wound as if it were an abscess, and waiting for new tissue to regenerate and fill the open area over several weeks. Today, most experts believe that the open wound should be patched with surrounding tissue as best as possible, instead of being left open to heal.

Because so much tissue is removed from such a sensitive surface area, significant and lengthy discomfort may accompany recovery from this surgery. If you're having difficulty sitting, be sure to tell the doctor and the nursing staff so that adequate levels of pain medication are supplied, and other aids are made available to you, such as sitz baths.

This pain may persist for some time after you've left the hospital. Some colon or rectal cancer survivors consider this part of post-surgery recovery more painful than an abdominal incision.

One survivor of ulcerative colitis that resulted in a stage I tumor describes his surgical experience:

> Before surgery I tried to stay in shape and exercise. I had an advantage that I wasn't on any medication prior to the surgery. I think it made recovery an easier experience for me. It probably made the surgery a more successful one, too.
>
> The days before surgery we came up with our own top 10+ list of why I didn't need my colon. I had printed it to take with me to the hospital. I realized I had forgotten it before we got out of the neighborhood. I went back and got it. I gave it to the nurses as I was going into surgery. That got a good laugh. I was pretty nervous. I was told that they posted it

down by the operating rooms. We managed to come up with quite a few good and funny reasons why I wouldn't need the equipment I was born with.

A funny thing happened while preparing for my stay in the hospital: I'd decided to get a room in the deluxe wing of the hospital to make this painful experience better. The fancy room had several advantages: private nursing, fax machine, early American decor, but its best offering was the gourmet menu—and I couldn't eat any of it! By the time I was able to eat, it was time to discharge me.

The surgery went very well. No nerves were damaged, so my sex life is as good now as it was before surgery. I didn't know that I had cancer until they had biopsied the removed colon and all points in between. A tumor was found contained in the interior colon wall. All the biopsies and colonoscopies hadn't seen this particular location. The lymph nodes were free of cancer. It's a good thing I had surgery when I did.

Sitting was a problem for a while, until the area where my rectum used to be healed. I had painkillers for the first few days. The area that hurt the most was my abdomen. My surgeon said I would feel like I had been hit by a truck, and I did. I was sore and stiff in all the places they operated. It took a couple of months before I was really moving normally. I was up and ready to walk in the malls as soon as I got home. The problem was I got tired pretty quick.

Ostomy

You might be told before surgery that an artificial opening called a stoma will be created in your abdomen. You might be told that it definitely will not be—or you might be told that the surgeon just won't know until the abdomen is open, and the full extent of disease can be evaluated.

Just after surgery and for a day or so afterward, you may be too groggy and sore to remember or to care whether you have a newly created stoma. While you're recovering, the nursing staff will do the initial care for you, until you're willing and able to do it on your own. Eventually you'll be visited by a nurse—an enterostomal therapist, it is hoped—who will help you learn how to clean the skin around the stoma, change the bag or patch, and irrigate, if necessary. The stoma itself is self-cleaning, as it is internal epith tissue that continually produces mucus.

If your hospital does not have an enterostomal therapist, contact the United Ostomy Association at (800) 826-0826 for help. Colorectal cancer survivors report both very good and very bad experiences regarding training in ostomy care from nurses who are not specialists in enterostomy.

> *The United Ostomy Association has trained visitors who will talk to you and help you feel better about what you've been through. Usually you don't have anyone to talk to while you're in the hospital who's actually gotten an ostomy. The biggest thing is that you need a live person to stand in front of you, going, "Hey! There's life after surgery. You, too, can look and act like nothing's different: at the spa, snorkeling, laying on the beach—no more issues than I have sitting in the office all day."*

Your first sight of your stoma may be profound, insignificant, or an anticlimax. You may feel extremely relieved that cancerous tissue is removed, and consequently you may feel grateful that ostomy saved your life. You may be afraid to look at the stoma—and then relieved after you have. You may be horrified. You may be sad or angry, or have feelings of great loss. You may feel dirty, or you may be afraid that others will think you are. You may feel much more interested in your abdominal incision, which may be painful, than in the stoma. If all anal and rectal tissue was removed—abdominoperineal resection—you may be fully occupied with doing basic things, like sitting without pain, and inspecting the stoma will wait for later.

Expect the stoma to look bright red and a bit swollen at first. As time passes, it will shrink a bit, but distinct red coloration and continual production of cleansing mucus are characteristic of a healthy stoma.

> *My ostomy is on the side of my navel, two inches to the right, and two inches down. Mine's an ileostomy. It's in that general location because there's a muscle wall there that stays pretty flat almost all the time. It's a functionality point of view: the appliance glues on. You need a flat surface for this, because what is called the wafer is a little bit flexible but it usually doesn't bend in half. It'll bend a little, but the bottom line is that the flatter, the more constant the surface that doesn't flex too much, the better luck you'll have with the appliance staying on.*

Expect the surgeon to inspect your stoma and preen over the good job that was done. Surgeons have been perfecting ostomy since the days of ancient

Egypt, and are happy when it's perfectly round, protruding just a quarter or a half-inch beyond the skin of the abdomen. Chapter 10, *Ostomy*, covers this topic in detail.

Hospitalization for infection

If you're being treated with chemotherapy for colorectal cancer, you might also need to be hospitalized to treat infection.

About seven to ten days after certain chemotherapies are given, it's common for your white blood cell counts to drop to dangerously low levels. Without adequate numbers of white blood cells, the body cannot fight infection.

If you're hospitalized for infection, most likely you'll be placed alone in a hospital room, a procedure called isolation. The air may be scrubbed with a high-energy particulate air (HEPA) filter or controlled via laminar airflow.

Although some studies have shown that infection during neutropenia most often arises from pathogens already within the patient's body, restriction of visitors, gifts, and certain foods will be enforced. For example:

- All who enter will be expected to adhere to safety measures such as vigorous handwashing and covering the mouth with a mask.

- Gift plants with pollen-bearing stamens, potting soil, or silk plants with mossy, fungus-bearing camouflage at their base may be returned or held outside your room.

- Certain foods, such as fresh fruit or yeast breads, may be denied to you.

Isolation procedures may seem odd—after all, you're already infected—but the goal is to prevent your coming in contact with additional and potentially very serious infectious agents.

You'll be given oral or IV antibiotics, antivirals, or antifungals, depending on your symptoms and the results of various cultures. You may also be given drugs to help you grow new white or red blood cells.

You'll stay in isolation until your white blood cell counts rise and the infection is bested, either by the antibiotics you're given, or by the infection-fighting ability of your own increasing white blood cells.

Chemotherapy

Some chemotherapies are given in the hospital in order to simultaneously administer additional agents that offset the damage to healthy organs, or to monitor the state of affected organs. Examples are the use of Mesna to prevent damage to the bladder when the anticancer agent cyclophosphamide is used, and the administration of intraperitoneal chemotherapy.

The procedures used will vary, of course, depending on the agents being given, but most likely you can expect an IV line to be inserted if you don't have a permanent venous catheter, and you'll receive frequent and perhaps somewhat embarrassing attention from nurses regarding normally routine and personal phenomena such as blood pressure, how much urine or feces you've passed, whether bowel movements are painful, and so on.

If copious oral or IV hydration accompanies your treatment, unless a urinary catheter is in place, you'll be compelled to rise frequently to urinate, and you may become quite tired owing to lack of a full night's sleep.

For certain subtypes of colorectal cancer that might have escaped from the primary tumor site and spread along the lining of the abdomen, injections of chemotherapy directly into the abdominal cavity, called the peritoneal cavity, might be used. This treatment is called intraperitoneal chemotherapy.

Access to the peritoneal cavity is achieved either by implanting several tubes and drains during the surgery to remove the tumor, or during a subsequent surgery, or by insertion of a catheter each time the treatment is given.

Once tubing is in place, the administration of anticancer drugs may begin as early as during surgery and continuing the day after for five days while you are still hospitalized. The drugs are infused through the tubes, left in place for many hours, then drained.

The medical staff administering the chemotherapy also may do imaging studies such as CT scans during or after infusion to be sure that all areas of the peritoneum are exposed to adequate amounts of anticancer medication.

Radiotherapy

For those with rectal cancer, several types of radiation therapy usually require a hospital stay. In addition to the more common treatment of rectal cancer with external beam radiotherapy, radioactive substances also can be used by:

- Implanting a radioactive material embedded in wires, seeds, capsules, or needles permanently into rectal and surrounding tissue during the surgery that removed the primary tumor or, less frequently, in a second surgery (interstitial radiotherapy).

- Placing a small container housing a radioactive substance temporarily inside the rectal cavity (brachytherapy).

This means that you might be hospitalized for a surgery to implant tubes or small containers that will contain the radioactive substance.

If your implants are not permanent, a stay in a lead-shielded isolation room might be necessary while radioactive materials are inserted, left in place for a few minutes or a few days (depending on the dose required), then removed. Containment measures will be engaged while the radioactive substance is being handled, and while in place. Visitors will be limited, kept at a distance of six feet, or forbidden altogether. Although hospital staff will provide you with all the care you need, for their safety during this time they must minimize their contact with you.

In order to avoid having implants shift, you might be asked to stay in bed while the implants are in place.

Once the radioactive substance is removed, you are no longer a risk to others.

When treatment has ended, implants might be either left in place or removed. Often, implants, tubes, or canisters that are temporary can be removed with little or no pain at the end of treatment, but you should tell the hospital staff if you are experiencing pain or discomfort during or after removal.

The rectum, perineum, and parts of the internal pelvis might be sore for days or weeks following radiation therapy.

Thriving versus surviving

Very few people look forward to being hospitalized. The goal is to make the stay short and successful by remembering that ultimately it's your life, and, in spite of perhaps temporarily diminished capacities, you're still very much in charge.

Here are several key points:

- Read your medical chart. Ask questions if anything is unclear. Ask for definitions of terms the staff may use, such as NPO (*noli para os*, or nothing by mouth). If you're not well enough to do this, have a friend or relative do so.

- Verify all drugs and treatments given to you. Ask about oral medications before swallowing, and read the contents of the IV bags on your pole. If you're not well enough to do this, have a friend or relative do so.

- Tell the nursing staff right away if something seems wrong. Don't let seemingly simple things, like feeling constipated, become major problems.

- If you are permitted to get out of bed, move about your room and the corridors as much as possible, especially if you've had surgery. You'll heal faster and diminish the likelihood of serious complications if you move about. If you feel too bad to get out of bed, flex your arms and legs a good deal. If you're neutropenic, ask if you and your IV pole can cruise the corridors wearing a mask and surgical slippers. (If you feel conspicuous wearing a mask, you might try making a prank of it by adding a toothy grin with waterproof ink.)

Additional ideas for dealing with your hospitalization follow:

- If you're not on a restricted diet, coerce friends and loved ones into bringing you your favorite foods. This will make you feel better, and will help those friends who would otherwise not know what to do feel useful and loving. Most hospitals now permit outside food to be brought into the patient's room, a change more in keeping with the European model of families caring for patients. Bringing food will help family members feel a part of your care if they are not permitted to do much else; for instance, if their time with you is restricted during certain radiation therapy treatments.

- At first, take pain medication on schedule if it is prescribed, even if you think you won't need it, because you'll heal better, and will be more mobile, if pain is adequately controlled. As time passes, you'll be a better judge of how much painkiller you really need.

- Befriend the staff. They'll repay you tenfold for your kindness. It's surprising how much can be asked of others if it's done in a nice way.

- If you're a caretaker, pitch in and do what you can to help the nurses help your loved one. Stay overnight if at all possible; if the staff decline, insist.

> *When my husband was hospitalized after his abdominal surgery, he was on morphine which slowed his ability to urinate. Often during the night he needed to use the john, and he and his IV pole would stand there in front of the toilet doing not much of anything for ten or fifteen minutes. Because I stayed with him overnight, I was able to help him in and out of bed repeatedly without his calling a nurse.*

Discharge and departure

Discharge may be an anticlimax after your hospital stay, but you should use this time to have the staff answer all of your questions about aftercare. Make sure you understand:

- First, whether you're really going to be able to handle being at home. Hospitalization times vary based on the patient's condition and the type of insurance in effect. If you feel you need to stay longer in the hospital but your insurance policy limits your stay unless the doctor requests otherwise, be sure to make your needs known to your doctor and the nursing staff.

- If your spleen was removed, you should discuss with your doctor the need to be revaccinated every few years with pneumococcal, Haemophilus influenzae type B, and meningococcal vaccines. The risk of being overwhelmed by agents capable of producing encapsulated infections is higher in those lacking a spleen.

- The medications you may be taking. When you are discharged you probably will be given a prescription for oral pain medicine, for example.

- Whether the hospital pharmacy can fill your prescriptions before you leave. If not, get the doctor to phone your pharmacy, or get a family member to fill them beforehand.

- How to care for your incision if you've had surgery.

- How to care for your stoma if you've had one created.

- What side effects or aftereffects you should watch for that might signal a problem.

- What follow-up appointments should be scheduled, and any diet restrictions.
- Your bill. Always ask for an itemized bill.

> *After surgery it would be best to set up a bed downstairs if you can. We have a half bath downstairs, so the second day home I opted for a sponge bath downstairs. After that, as long as I went slowly, stairs were fine.*

> *Any way that you can make it easier for yourself, go for. I slept on the sofa downstairs because it's cooler, and because I was worried if my hubby tossed and turned too much my catheter, inserted at the same time as resection surgery, would get jabbed by an elbow! After three or four days I did move back upstairs and it was no problem—really.*

> *But if you can set up downstairs very comfortably, that is probably best in the beginning when you first get home.*

The person helping you with your trip home should bring the car to the exit in advance, and should make as many preliminary trips as necessary to remove your personal effects and gifts from your room, perhaps warming or cooling the car in advance as well. Most important, though, is that by leaving you for last, your escort can devote attention to you alone as you're exiting. This is a useful arrangement because you may need help getting into the car, for example, but the hospital's assistance and liability end at the door.

Use the restroom before you leave, even if you think you don't need to. Even a small amount of stress on the trip home or cold temperatures, for example, can cause the brain to signal the bladder or bowel to empty.

Most hospitals have a regulation stating that you must be escorted to the door in a wheelchair. This reduces the chance that patients, possibly weakened by extended bed rest, will pass out or suffer a mis-step while exiting. While many people leaving the hospital find using a wheelchair embarrassing, it safeguards both you and the hospital. Fortunately or unfortunately, you'll have plenty of chances to prove you're mobile again once you're out the door.

After many surgeries, one is restricted from driving for several weeks. Certain activities such as climbing stairs may also be restricted. Full recovery may take as long as six weeks and may include pronounced fatigue.

After radiation therapy, you may be surprised to feel more tired over time instead of less tired. This is normal and will reverse eventually. The areas irradiated may feel sore or burnt for days or weeks after therapy.

Summary

Current treatment for colorectal cancer almost always includes hospitalization and abdominal, pelvic, or rectal surgery. The colorectal cancer survivor also might face hospitalization for infection, or for receipt of radiotherapy or chemotherapy. This chapter offers insights and several checklists to help make your stay brief and successful.

For several good books that deal exclusively and in depth with being hospitalized, see the bibliography. For many excellent ideas on dealing with surgery and recovering afterward, read *Surgery and Recovery* by Kaye Olson, RN.

If you want detailed knowledge about the surgery that will be performed, see Cohen's 1995 text, *Cancer of the Colon, Rectum, and Anus*, or Wanebo's 1997 text, *Surgery for Gastrointestinal Cancer.*

CHAPTER 8

Experiencing Chemotherapy

Surely every medicine is an innovation,
 and he that will not apply new
remedies, must expect new evils.

—Francis Bacon

THIS MAY BE THE FIRST CHAPTER YOU CHOOSE TO READ, as the specific chemotherapy treatments one might face to treat colorectal cancer are of consuming interest to many people after having heard negative stories about chemotherapy.

The goal of this chapter is to acquaint you with a typical chemotherapy experience, and with events that may unfold. As most chemotherapy for colorectal cancer is administered in the outpatient setting, and because portable infusion pumps usually require visits to the doctor for refilling, we will walk you through an outpatient treatment, beginning with your preparations and scheduling, entering the treatment office, encountering certain medical personnel and other patients, advancing through the treatment itself, and finishing with what you can expect afterward. Keep in mind, though, that what you experience may differ from what you read here.

Use of certain standard and experimental treatments categorized as biological therapies and biological response modifiers—monoclonal antibodies, interferons, colony stimulating factors, anticancer vaccines, and the like—are also discussed in this chapter. Biological response modifiers often are injected as are other chemotherapies, and pose some of the same risks.

The theories behind colorectal cancer treatment and the side effects of treatment are discussed separately in other chapters.

The information this chapter provides is not a substitute for your doctor's knowledge. Always ask your doctor when an aspect of your treatment is unclear, and report immediately to your doctor any adverse reactions that arise during or after treatment.

Preparation

People can have a wide range of responses to chemotherapy, even if they're receiving the same drug and dose. You don't know for certain how you'll respond, so it would be best to make sure you have certain supplies and assistance if you need them. Some of the drugs given for chemotherapy or to prevent side effects can cause drowsiness or affect concentration, for instance, or you might be sitting for many hours in a room that is overly warm or too cool.

> *My advice is to begin receiving treatment with an open mind and the attitude that you will have no side effects. You may not have any. I've been on 5-FU/leucovorin for nine months so far, and I've not had any mouth sores. Chemotherapy is different for each patient, and sometimes each treatment is different. My experience is that my first few treatments were without any side effects at all. As I continue (I have it every other Thursday) sometimes I have what I call chemo sickness. I just feel bad, no vomiting or trots to the bathroom as some patients have, I just feel tired and don't want to do much. I don't always get those feelings, and oftentimes when I do, I force myself out of the house and mow the lawn or get busy with something to take my mind off how I'm feeling. It really works for me.*

For these and other reasons, during your first treatment visit it would be wise to have a friend or loved one along, not only for emotional support, but to handle issues such as safely tucking away written instructions for diet and aftercare; understanding and remembering verbal instructions; communicating insurance information; handling the co-pay, if any; and assisting with the drive home. As you adapt to treatment, you may need someone to drive if you take medication for nausea before leaving home, as many of these drugs cause drowsiness.

Comfort should be high on the list of priorities for anyone facing chemotherapy. Come prepared for a few hours' testing or treatment by wearing comfortable, layered clothing; bringing relaxing buddies or music cassettes; and asking in advance what to expect. Don't arrive with an empty stomach. Eat light food up to two hours before treatment.

I experienced many of the side effects of chemotherapy: mouth ulcers, nausea, vomiting, fatigue, a metallic taste. But there were medications to counteract these problems. We had to try more than one, but finally hit on a combination of Zofran/Decadron drip with Phenergan pills. By midweek a shot of Ativan IV was added for nausea. That really worked well. My dentist prescribed a mouth rinse of Triamcinolone mixed with water and absolute alcohol that really numbed it.

I completed my chemotherapy a week ago. I have a glorious five weeks off before beginning Camptosar for added protection, as I am at high risk for future pelvic recurrence.

Although the antinausea drugs in use today are excellent, store a bucket in your car against the possibility of nausea during the ride home. Call the doctor a day or two in advance to get nausea medications, and take them beforehand if instructed to do so.

Before your initial treatment, ask about wearing cosmetics, jewelry, or nail polish, because skin and nail bed color are useful ways for the medical staff to assess your well-being and response to drugs. Ask about using lotions or aftershave, as these may cause skin irritation depending on the treatment being given. If you feel strongly about wearing cosmetics and nail polish to treatments to improve your frame of mind, ask them about a compromise, such as leaving one fingernail bare for visibility or for using the thimble-like oxygen sensor that slides over your finger.

Ask if your chemotherapy will be administered into an arm vein. If so, plan to wear a short-sleeved top, and bring a cardigan for the parts that needn't be uncovered and might get chilled.

Tell the staff about dental appliances, contact lenses, surgical staples, pacemakers, and other manmade materials that may interfere with treatment.

Certain drugs used for chemotherapy may react badly with certain foods or food supplements. Ask your doctor if you should avoid certain foods such as grapefruit for a week or two before or after treatment, as grapefruit interferes with metabolism of some drugs by the liver. Vitamins, antioxidants, or supplements should also be approved by your doctor before use. Potassium supplements may trigger a dangerous metabolic imbalance, tumor lysis syndrome that imperils the kidneys if you have a large tumor that is killed rapidly by treatment.

You may also receive instructions about avoiding other possibly dangerous circumstances such as excessive sunlight or crowds. Some of the drugs used for colorectal cancer cause skin to become overly sensitive to sunlight. Protective clothing, sunglasses, and sunscreen lotions may be recommended.

Scheduling

The schedule on which chemotherapy is administered is based on years of research that determine a drug's effectiveness at a certain dose and interval. Some chemotherapies are given daily; some are given weekly for several months; some are given once a month for many months. Those delivered via portable pumps may enter the body throughout the day for many days. Oral medications taken at home may be taken once a day or several times a day.

If you can't afford or don't want to miss time from work, you might prefer scheduling your treatment to occur just before the weekend so you'll have a couple of days to adjust and recover without the additional stress of meeting work responsibilities.

Don't be surprised if the schedule on which your chemotherapy is administered differs from the schedules you hear others discussing, because your schedule is likely to be tailored to your particular circumstances. You may, for instance, be receiving a drug that might be toxic to the heart, but on a less condensed schedule that is intended to lessen toxicity.

Depending on what drugs are being used, the timing of subsequent therapy may be influenced by the quantity of blood cells remaining in your bloodstream after your last treatment. Thus, for certain regimens, your blood will be tested when you arrive (or perhaps a few days in advance, if your doctor recommends or you prefer) using a standard measurement known as a complete blood count, or CBC. If your blood counts are too low, treatment may be delayed a few days or a week.

A delay of one week is not likely to affect the success of treatment, but a great many delays, or a delay of long duration, may. For this reason, oncologists sometimes prescribe either blood transfusions or injections of colony stimulating factors to bring your blood counts up to safe levels. Colony stimulating factors are manmade copies of natural body products that cause bone marrow to produce more new blood cells than it otherwise would.

Shelly describes how important it is to get treatment on schedule:

> *Just the other week I had a cold, but had chemotherapy anyway. I spent one whole day in bed sleeping. In general the 5-FU/leucovorin infusion knocks me down for at least two full days. It's something I've learned to expect after chemo. I guess I will never get really used to it.*
>
> *I've just learned to tolerate it and look forward to tomorrow which can always be better. Keep up the spirits and the attitude, the rest will be easier.*

For therapy administered from an IV bag or syringe rather than by infusion pump, it's not unusual for one chemotherapy session to last for several hours. High-dose therapies that must be administered over several days (with or without stem cell rescue) may require a hospital admission, but the trend is toward outpatient treatment for all but the most rigorous procedures or the sickest patients.

Arrival

Often, your treatment is not started until a doctor, nurse, or medical technician has weighed you, taken your blood pressure and temperature, done a brief physical, asked you about symptoms and side effects, and drawn blood to check blood counts.

If you have a portable pump, however, you might simply be examined, refilled, and discharged.

Your first visit is a good chance to begin to make friends with the nursing staff. Oncology nurses are a unique breed, generally cheerful and unusually kind. Often they'll have great ideas for helping you that might not occur to your doctor to mention, such as where to buy satin pillow covers to reduce hair loss. Interaction with a good nurse may well be one of the finest and most rewarding experiences in life, exemplifying the best that humans can offer each other. Many oncology nurses say that they get much more from their patients than they give.

You may find as well that your fellow patients in the waiting or treatment areas have good insights to share about experiencing chemotherapy. Often, those waiting in an oncologist's office are reluctant to start a conversation with others because the people nearby seem very worried or withdrawn, or because they themselves have so much mental and emotional processing underway. You might find, though, that deep and instructive friendships are formed among cancer survivors in this setting.

After you're settled in the treatment area, waiting or being treated, consider having your companion visit the pharmacy to buy ice bags or a pill organizer, fill any prescriptions, or buy any over-the-counter drugs, including stool softeners and anti-diarrheals, that you'll need later. With this arrangement, if you feel bad or fatigued after treatment, your medications and supplies will be immediately available.

The setting

Chemotherapy may be administered in a doctor's office, in a hospital outpatient setting, or, if given in the form of tablets or a portable pump, actively or passively in your home. If it is administered in a doctor's office or outpatient department, it may be administered by a chemotherapy nurse or by the doctor. It may be administered in a large room with other cancer patients who are seated in reclining chairs in partitions divided by curtains, or it may be administered on a bed or chair in a private room.

Sometimes the setting in which chemotherapy is given is dictated by what insurance companies will pay for. Injections of colony stimulating factors, for example, which may be necessary to stimulate bone marrow, may be administered safely and easily by the patient or another at home. Some insurance companies, however, will pay for these injections only if they are administered by a doctor.

Some chemotherapies and some tumor types are known to be associated with risks that are best handled in a hospital setting. Cyclophosphamide (Cytoxin), for example, is known to damage the bladder, and is best administered simultaneously with heavy bladder irrigation such as that provided by intravenous fluids. Large tumor masses of the chest or abdomen that die quickly when treatment is started may require IV fluids to protect the kidneys only at the start of treatment. For this reason, you may be admitted to the hospital to receive these treatments. See Chapter 7, *Experiencing Hospitalization*, for what to expect.

> To tell you the truth, so far the chemotherapy has not been bad. I've only just had my second week of it, but I look at it this way: At the end of each week, I get to go into a quiet, peaceful room, read a good book, watch Oprah if I desire, suck on ice chips and 7-Up, and even call a

friend on my cell phone if I feel so inclined, while my combination of 5-FU and leucovorin drips into my veins. Okay, okay... I will admit I had a small bout with diarrhea when I got home last evening, but nothing to complain about. For me, I think I made the right decision to have chemotherapy, and a positive attitude makes it all the easier.

How chemotherapy is administered

There are several different forms of chemotherapy for colorectal cancer, and different ways to administer it.

Portable (Ambulatory) Pumps

Some studies have shown that, for certain patients, a continuous infusion of anticancer drugs for colon and rectal cancer is more effective than a single weekly administration. By using a portable infusion pump, it's possible to have certain anticancer drugs administered throughout the day for many days, or to have multiple drugs delivered at the same time. These pumps can be programmed to deliver, or not deliver, a steady or varying dose of drugs for hours, days, or weeks.

If you have a venous access device such as a central (chest or neck) catheter or a peripheral (arm) catheter, most likely it can be used for delivering drugs via portable pump. If you don't have a venous access device, almost certainly one will be put in place before treatment starts. A very small battery-powered pump—about the size of a paperback book—is connected to this line. The pump can be implanted under the skin, or carried in a satchel that you can wear around your waist or over your shoulder.

I am 72, and am in the sixth week of a six-month course of continuous infusion of 5-fluorouracil and leucovorin. I had a hemicolectomy three months ago; I was diagnosed as stage III with two of 35 nodes containing tumorous tissue that had spread, but no other metastases were detected.

My 5-FU is infused continuously 24 hours a day through a Mediport implanted in my chest and powered by a battery-operated pump contained in a fanny pack weighing about 1-3/4 pounds. It's a nuisance I've gotten used to, and I have no trouble sleeping, driving, shopping, working in my shop, showering, and so on. I get new batteries, a 5-FU refill, and a dose of leucovorin every Wednesday at the USCF/Stanford Oncology clinic. So far, the entire process has been completely painless and I've had no nausea or diarrhea. The only side effects have been a painless rash on the backs of my hands and some irritation in my windpipe during week four. Every week of continuous infusion is followed by one week off.

I definitely recommend my Mediport central catheter rather than a PICC (peripherally infused central catheter) line, although the Mediport was more expensive and required a surgical procedure for installation.

Portable pumps also can deliver drugs under the skin or directly into the abdominal cavity, but delivery via a vein or directly to the liver via the hepatic artery is most common.

The advantages of a portable continuous infusion pump are:

- The possibility of a better anticancer response to chemotherapy.
- Fewer and shorter doctor visits, yielding less disruption to your schedule.

Disadvantages are:

- The possibility of greater side effects with continuous infusion, entailing a temporarily reduced quality of life.
- The inconvenience of having to adjust to and carry an attached pump all day long.
- The need to have a venous access device put in place. See Chapter 5, *Tests and Procedures*, for a description of this experience.
- If an implanted pump is used, it might need to be put in place while you are under general anesthesia.

Implanted and portable pumps have advantages and disadvantages as well. Implanted infusion pumps might be more expensive and require a surgery to implant, but are less likely to clot or become infected as a central venous catheter might when it is attached to an external pump.

The reservoir in your pump can be refilled weekly or on some other schedule determined by your oncologist. Implanted pumps might be accessed through the skin; external pumps and balloon reservoirs might just be replaced.

There are several kinds of portable infusion pumps, and many different regimens for delivering drugs at optimal levels. A search of the medical literature reveals some of the techniques attempted by various researchers in the last few years. These examples are given so that you'll be aware of this variety of approaches, and so that you'll have less concern if you hear of someone whose treatment schedule or pump type is different from yours:

- A 60-milliliter reservoir pump with variable flow rates of 2, 6, 8, or 12 milliliters every 24 hours, and refilled weekly.

- An implanted reservoir giving low-dose infusion over six to seven days for several months to two years, using balloon-style continuous infusion. Access to the body was via central venous catheter, aortal infusion, or both.

- Two disposable balloon pumps connected to an implanted pump via a central venous catheter.

- A pump connected to the hepatic artery via a prior surgery delivering first floxuridine continuously for seven days, and followed by a weekly one-dose pump of 5-fluorouracil for three weeks.

- Continuous infusion via portable pump for 21 days, ceasing for 7, and repeated every four weeks.

- Prolonged infusion for six weeks with a one-week rest period.

- Continuous infusion for five days, followed by weekly one-hour intravenous infusions, all for seven weeks.

- Continuous infusion for five days, followed by five-minute intravenous injections on days 12 and 19.

Intravenous therapy

Chemotherapy for colorectal cancer often is administered once a week into a vein using a temporary or semi-permanent IV line in the forearm, or by any one of a number of venous access devices (VADs), such as a central catheter that has been implanted into a large vein in your chest.

If you have difficulty finding a usable vein, see Chapter 5 for suggestions that may make this easier. If you continue to experience trouble with inaccessible veins, or if they worsen during treatment, discuss with your doctor the advantages and disadvantages of venous access devices such as central catheters.

Some of the drugs used will be in plastic bags that are hung from your IV pole. They may be mixed with a saline drip to dilute them as they enter your vein. Others may be injected directly into your IV line from a large syringe. This method is called a bolus push.

Some drugs used for intravenous chemotherapy are damaging if they come in contact with skin. Notify the medical staff immediately if you experience any pain, swelling, redness, or burning near the injection site.

You may feel a warm flush when certain drugs are administered. Verify with the medical staff that this is normal for your drug regimen.

> My husband had severe sweats during the administration, and so took atropine about 30 minutes into treatment, and again an hour later. This helped with the sweats and with immediate onset diarrhea.

Monoclonal antibody therapy

Monoclonal antibodies are a manmade version of a natural body product secreted by our white blood cells. They are injected into a vein via an IV line or catheter.

It's possible to have an allergic reaction to monoclonal antibodies, because often they are formed from combined human and mouse antibodies. This is a very common reaction that is easily controlled, but it must be addressed immediately to keep it from becoming serious. To avoid this allergic reaction, antibodies usually are injected very slowly over several hours.

Intraperitoneal chemotherapy

For a few subtypes of colorectal cancer that escape from the primary tumor site and spread along the lining of the abdomen, injections of chemotherapy directly into the abdominal cavity, called the peritoneal cavity, might be used.

Intraperitoneal chemotherapy requires access to the peritoneum. Access is achieved in one of two ways:

- Implanting of several tubes and drains during the surgery to remove the tumor, or during a subsequent surgery

- Insertion of a catheter each time the treatment is given

Once tubing and drains are in place, the administration of anticancer drugs may begin as early as during surgery and may continue for five days beginning the day after surgery while you remain hospitalized. Typically thereafter, cycles are repeated for five days of each month for several months. The drugs are infused, left in place for almost 24 hours, then drained.

The medical staff administering the chemotherapy also may do imaging studies such as CT scans during or after infusion to be sure that all areas of the peritoneum are exposed to adequate amounts of anticancer medication.

Hepatic artery infusion (HAI)

Hepatic artery infusion is the delivery of large doses of chemotherapy directly to the liver, either as a multi-hour dose during surgery or in the doctor's office, or at home via a portable infusion pump. When it is administered in the doctor's office, your experience will resemble that described previously in the section called "Intravenous therapy," whereas administration by portable infusion pump is described in the section "Portable (ambulatory) pumps," earlier in the chapter.

> *In October of 1997 I had an operation for hepatic arterial infusion. This necessitated wearing a fanny pack whereby chemotherapy was infused directly into the liver for two weeks, then I had a rest of two weeks off. At the same time, I was given once a week treatments of CPT-11, 5-FU, and leucovorin. By January of 1998, I had a 50 percent reduction in size and number of my tumors (eight tumors averaging 5-8 cm). By April, my CT scan showed no evidence of liver involvement.*

Oral therapy

Your chemotherapy regimen may include oral medication along with or in place of intravenous injections, or you may be given oral medication to offset nausea. You might be given tablets to take at home, perhaps several times a day, or perhaps every other day. You may be given prescriptions for antidiarrheal or antinausea medications to take with your chemotherapy.

Although taking pills may seem easy, there are several potential issues of which you should be aware.

The chemotherapy drugs can cause some problems in swallowing pills. After several days or weeks of treatment, you may notice your mouth becoming increasingly dry as the rapidly dividing cells in your mouth die. A good habit to cultivate is wetting your mouth before attempting to swallow a tablet.

It's easy to forget what medications you've taken when you have quite a few, and when some of them are making you drowsy. Each day, keep a new list of what you must take, and check them off as you take them. Consider buying a plastic pill organizer to assure that all doses are taken.

Subcutaneous injections

Colony stimulating factors such as granulocyte colony stimulating factor (G-CSF), thrombopoietin, or erythropoietin (EPO) frequently are injected under the skin or, less often, into muscle.

If your insurance company will pay for the drug, you may be able to give yourself these injections at home. The medical staff will teach you the quick, painless poke-in-the-thigh, using pinching, stretching, or slapping to anesthetize the area first. Small syringes of the type used for insulin usually will do; they'll give you a "red bag" for needle disposal, which should be returned to the doctor's office when full, not put into the trash.

If your insurance company will only pay for these injections if they are administered in a doctor's office, you may have to make twice- or thrice-weekly trips to the doctor.

Departure

Before leaving the doctor's office, be sure you have received written instructions regarding any necessary dietary or behavioral changes, information about possible side effects, prescriptions, and phone numbers for emergencies.

Do not leave feeling unwell. If you are feeling unwell, tell the medical staff.

Use the restroom before leaving if you received your treatments via IV line. Often, IV drugs are accompanied by a saline drip. The volume of fluid that your kidneys have processed from this treatment may surprise you halfway home.

Most chemotherapy treatments do not result in infection or side effects that require hospitalization. However, occasionally such problems do occur. Carefully note all symptoms and communicate immediately with your doctor if problems arise.

Dosages

If you feel inclined to do so, you can verify your chemotherapy dosage. Most chemotherapy drug dosages are calculated based on body surface area, but some are based on other parameters such as renal function. Keep in mind that any variation you note may be planned deliberately by your doctor or may vary based on how the drug is administered—that is, by IV line, pump, or intraperitoneal infusion.

See Appendix C for a chart of common heights and weights, and the corresponding body surface area in square meters.

If you have a personal computer, you can access Glaxo-Wellcome's DoseCalc web site, *http://www.meds.com/DChome.html,* to calculate dosages automatically given your weight, height, and a drug name. DoseCalc also lists the current chemotherapy regimens used against colorectal cancer, and the milligrams per square meter needed for each drug.

If you notice a substantial difference between the calculated and actual dose given, ask your doctor why. Often there are very good reasons for differences.

Summary

Not surprisingly, many people have concerns about what chemotherapy will be like, and how they'll make it through treatment. This chapter, in combination with Chapter 11, *Side Effects of Treatment*, aims to make the experience a less frightening one.

Many of the topics we touch on in these chapters are well described in other books. See the bibliography for several excellent books that can offer you much more information.

Key points to remember:

- Plan in advance for side effects by purchasing prescriptions in advance and taking antinausea medications as prescribed.

- If your insurance plan provides a liberal allowance for prescriptions, ask your doctor to prescribe the most effective antinausea medication (antiemetic), regardless of cost.

- Take along an advocate who can ask questions and take notes.

- Dress for comfort, avoiding clothing that will interfere with access to veins, ports, or pumps.

- Report any unusual feelings or discomfort immediately to the medical staff.

- Talk to the other survivors in the waiting and treatment rooms.

- Consider scheduling your first few treatment appointments near a day off so that you can recover before attempting to return to work or other responsibilities.

- After treatment or during continuous infusion via pump, report to your doctor immediately any illness, fever, or unusual side effects.

- If you note blood in the line leading from a vein to a portable infusion pump or in the catheters that access the peritoneum, notify your oncologist.

- If you will be having hepatic arterial infusion or intraperitoneal chemotherapy, it might also be useful to review the chapter on hospitalization.

CHAPTER 9

Experiencing Radiotherapy

Poisons and medicine are oftentimes the same
substance given with different intents.

—Peter Mere Latham

BY NOW YOU HAVE CONSULTED WITH SEVERAL TYPES OF ONCOLOGISTS and have decided that radiation therapy is a good choice for treating your colon or rectal cancer. Perhaps it will be used before surgery to shrink a rectal tumor; perhaps one of several sites will be irradiated to alleviate unpleasant symptoms; most likely radiation will be used in conjunction with other therapies such as chemotherapy or surgery.

We are justifiably afraid of radiation. We know that sunlight can burn us, that x-ray technicians leave the room and wear lead aprons when they treat us. We know we should be wary of too many diagnostic x-rays, and that large amounts of radiation caused tremendous damage at Hiroshima, Nagasaki, and Chernobyl. In spite of fears about radiation, many colorectal cancer patients are pleasantly surprised to find that radiation therapy is a smooth, quick, silent, painless treatment.

As was done in the prior chapter for chemotherapy, in this chapter we will acquaint you with a typical radiotherapy experience. Most radiotherapy used for colorectal cancer is external radiotherapy and is administered in the outpatient setting, so we will walk you through an outpatient treatment. We will begin with your preparation, including treatment simulation; scheduling; arriving at the treatment office; encountering certain medical personnel and other patients; advancing through the treatment itself; and finishing with what you can expect afterward.

For those with certain rectal tumors, however, radiation implants might also be used. We will discuss these techniques briefly. See Chapter 7, *Experiencing Hospitalization*, for more information regarding experiencing this form of radiation therapy.

The theories behind radiotherapy as treatment for colorectal cancer, and the side effects of treatment, are discussed separately in Chapter 6, *Modes of Treatment* and Chapter 11, *Side Effects of Treatment.*

The information this chapter provides is not a substitute for your doctor's knowledge. Always ask your doctor when an aspect of your treatment is unclear, and report immediately to your doctor any adverse reactions that arise during or after treatment.

If you would like greater detail on radiation therapy, *The Chemotherapy and Radiation Therapy Survival Guide,* by Judith McKay, Nancee Hirano, Myles Lampenfeld, *Making the Radiation Therapy Decision,* by David Brenner and Eric Hall, and *Coping with Radiation Therapy: A Ray of Hope,* by Daniel Cukier and Virginia McCullough, are books that focus on radiation therapy from the patient's perspective.

Types of radiotherapy

Although there are different kinds of radiation, including x-rays and electron, proton, or neutron beams, for the sake of readability we will not distinguish among them. We will use only the term "radiation."

There are several ways to administer radiation therapy:

- External radiotherapy, also called external beam irradiation, involving narrow x-ray beams aimed at your body while you lie on a table. This is the most common form of radiotherapy used for rectal cancer.

- Radioimmunotherapy, an injection of radioisotopes into a vein. The radioisotopes are attached to a carrier that homes preferentially to tumors instead of healthy tissue. The most common homing substances in use today are monoclonal antibodies, proteins produced by white blood cells and capable of traveling preferentially to tumors. Use of this technique against colon and rectal cancers is still in clinical trials.

- Intra-operative radiotherapy, which is aimed directly and only at the tumor bed, the empty spot in your body where the tumor once was. This is done while your body is still open during surgery, but after tumor removal. This technique is not discussed in this chapter, as the patient needn't prepare for or anticipate it in ways that differ from preparation for and anticipation of surgery.

- Brachytherapy, the positioning of a radioactive substance within the body very near or within the tumor. This technique might be used for rectal cancer, but not for colon cancer.

- Interstitial radiotherapy, involving implants of radioactive material, often permanent, stored in capsules, wires, or similar sealed delivery vehicles.

- Endocavitary radiation therapy, which utilizes a wand that emits radiation of very short wavelength that is placed in the rectum or vagina. This is expensive, specialized equipment that is not yet widely accessible, and is not discussed in this chapter as it is not often used for colorectal cancer.

All of these delivery techniques are used for rectal cancer. For some colon cancers at certain stages, external radiotherapy is used, but use of abdominal radiotherapy for colon cancer remains controversial owing to the significant risk of permanent damage to the small bowel and adjacent organs.

External radiation therapy

External radiation therapy might be used before rectal surgery to shrink tumors, or after surgery to kill any remaining microscopic tumor cells.

The following sections will walk you through preparation and treatment simulation, scheduling, receiving therapy, departure, and the days that follow treatment.

Simulation

Your first one or two treatment visits to the radiation oncology treatment offices will be spent determining precise details of how best to treat you: positioning you on the treatment bed, marking your skin with small dots of temporary or permanent ink, taping body parts in place for stability, and creating lead shields for sensitive organs. If you have rectal cancer, the bed you'll be lying upon may have an opening for your abdomen so that the small intestine will drop down out of the path of the radiation beam, or you may be positioned head-down to shift the small intestine upward. All of these preparations are called simulation, and may take several hours spread over one or more visits.

Several medical specialists are involved in this stage of your treatment: your radiation oncologist, the radiation therapy technician who will administer the treatment, a dosimetrist who calculates the correct dose, and the radiation physicist who calibrates the machine. Some of these staff members may work behind the scenes.

For these initial visits, which may be lengthy, make yourself as comfortable as possible by wearing clothing that doesn't bind, that goes on and off easily, and has no metal zippers. Bring a cassette player if you like, and use the restroom before the simulation starts.

None of these preparations are painful, but they may be embarrassing or unpleasant, for instance, if the staff decides that the best access to a rectal tumor is achieved by taping the buttocks into an open position, or if you are asked to drink a barium contrast solution to clarify the position of the small intestine.

Special shields or blocks may be made to shape the radiation beam to match exactly your tumor's shape, or the shape of nearby surgical scars. Beams of invisible radiation generated by the machinery are usually emitted shaped like rectangles, from two to fifteen inches in any dimension. If these beams were trained against your tumor, nearby healthy tissue within the two- to fifteen-inch rectangle would be irradiated, too, suffering damage. To avoid this effect, shields or blocks with cutaways in the silhouette of your tumor are created using your x-ray films as guides.

The shields made for you are used only by you. You may see the same kinds of devices belonging to other patients hanging nearby or in other treatment areas.

The machinery used during simulation looks and moves just as the genuine radiation equipment does, but instead it generates only a plain light beam to verify positioning, ink markings, and the fit of shields.

After all shields and blocks are made and your skin is marked, the entire simulation will be repeated with all pieces in place—exactly like a dress rehearsal.

As your treatment progresses and your tumor shrinks, new blocks may be made to match the new shape of your tumor, and these simulations may be repeated.

Preparation

Radiation therapy often makes many patients increasingly tired as it progresses. For this reason, once treatment starts, it would be wise to have a friend or loved one along, not only for emotional support, but to handle issues such as saving written instructions for diet and aftercare; understanding and remembering verbal instructions; communicating insurance information; handling the co-pay, if any; and assisting with the drive home.

Ask the medical staff about avoiding products such as skin lotion before treatment. They may interfere with treatment, or they may cause your skin to become hypersensitive if they are exposed to radiation. Ask as well about pacemakers, surgical staples, and clothing with metal zippers.

Scheduling

Years of research have shown that a large amount of radiation can be delivered to a tumor safely if the dosage is spread out over several weeks. This is called fractionating the dose, or simply fractionation. It spares healthy tissue from unnecessary damage and gives it time to recover.

Dosage fractionation means that you will have to visit the treatment center several times a week, or perhaps every day, for several weeks, depending on your treatment plan. It also means that each dose of radiation lasts only two to four minutes. If your tumor is irradiated from several different angles (and most are), each angle may take two to four minutes after the machine is repositioned. After the lengthy time spent in simulation, you may feel that ten to thirty minutes of treatment time is an anticlimax.

Don't be surprised if the schedule on which your radiotherapy is administered differs from the schedules you hear others discussing, because your radiation schedule *always* is tailored to your particular circumstances, based on the size, number, and location of tumors; your overall health; your body size; and the type of cancer you have.

Depending on what treatments are being used, the timing of your radiation therapy may be influenced by the quantity of white blood cells remaining in your blood after your last chemotherapy or radiotherapy treatment. Your blood may be tested when you arrive, using a standard measurement known as a complete blood count, or CBC. If your white blood counts are too low, treatment may be delayed a few days or a week.

For each treatment, you might want to call the treatment center before leaving home or work. Radiation therapy machines sustain heavy use, and must be taken offline periodically for recalibration or repair. You can save time by calling first to see whether appointments are running on time.

After a few treatments, you may begin to feel that most of your time is spent traveling or chatting in the waiting room, because treatment itself is so brief.

Arrival

Make a point of discussing nausea and diarrhea medications with your doctor *before* treatment starts. With the excellent anti-emetics (antinausea drugs) available, you shouldn't have to endure nausea. If you become nauseous after treatment, though, request a change in medication. Although the new anti-emetics are excellent, ask for suppositories in case oral medications won't stay in your stomach. If nausea becomes a problem, subsequent treatments may be preceded by an injection of one of the new antinausea drugs, such as Zofran.

Ask your doctor if you should avoid possibly dangerous circumstances such as excessive sunlight or crowds.

Ask about skin care, too. External beam radiation must pass through your skin to reach tumor sites, and irritation may result. Newer, higher voltage equipment used today causes less damage to skin because the damaging rays concentrate in deeper layers, but some skin reaction still is possible, particularly in sensitive areas such as the skin between anus and genitals. See Chapter 11, *Side Effects of Treatment*, for a discussion of radiation therapy's effects on skin and other tissue.

The setting

The source of radiation will be a machine that either safely contains a radioactive substance such as Cobalt 60, or generates its own radiation as needed. Like a CT scanner or a gamma camera, the radiation machine is designed to move around you and your bed as you hold still. Many models are almost silent, but some make a sound like a vacuum cleaner, and of course they may click and whir as they reposition.

The room in which treatment is given has thick walls and is lead-clad to prevent the very small amount of radiation that bounces off your shields, known as scatter, from affecting the medical staff, those in the waiting room, and random passers-by. For the safety of the staff, the treatment room will contain only you when the machine is engaged. (The small dose of radiation they would sustain if they stayed with you would probably not harm them, but if they stayed with all patients, all day, every day, the dose from scatter would indeed accumulate to dangerous levels.)

The staff can see and hear you at all times, because there are microphones and cameras connecting you and them. If you feel at all bad, just let them know. Music and wall art sometimes are available in the treatment room to lower your boredom and stress levels.

Delivery of external radiation therapy

External radiotherapy is administered using the blocks and shields made expressly for you, and perhaps on a special table that will shield the healthy parts of your intestines if needed, perhaps with sandbags to hold your arms and legs still, and blankets to keep you warm. If you have a rectal tumor, your buttocks may be taped into an open position so that the radiation beam targeting the rectum or lower pelvis will avoid healthy skin.

You may have your bladder filled with saline water prior to treatment in order to lift the small intestine away from the treatment area, thus protecting the small intestine.

You should feel no pain, no heat, no sensation at all during treatment, although some survivors say that they feel a sensation of energizing—not quite a tingling—in the area of the tumor during treatment. It may indeed be that some of us can sense a highly active biological entity such as a tumor reacting to the disruption of its DNA.

Some find the absence of sensation eerie, but most people are grateful that the treatment is comfortable and brief.

Dosages

Dosage of external radiation therapy always is tailored to the patient's specific circumstances, depending on where the rectal or colon tumors are located, and how much radiation a given organ can withstand. The liver, for instance, is very sensitive to radiation, and cannot survive doses high enough to kill most tumors. Moreover, doses for control of symptoms differ from those used for cure.

A typical curative dosage for rectal cancer is 180 to 200 centiGreys (cGy) per day, repeated a few times a week for several weeks until a total dosage of 4,500 to 5,000 cGy is achieved. Additional radiation boosts of 540 to 900 cGy to smaller areas occupied or once occupied by tumor, called the tumor bed, are sometimes added. A variation sometimes introduced is delivering 120 to 160 cGy twice a day, 4 to 6 hours apart, for several weeks. In patients at high risk of recurrence of disease, a total of 6,000 to 7,000 cGy might be used in areas local to the tumor if the small bowel and other sensitive organs can be shielded. It's important to remember, though, that your radiation oncologist will adjust dosage to suit your individual needs.

If a higher dosage is required for certain sites, more sessions are added, but the dose per exposure is not raised. Because external beam radiation often must pass through healthy tissue to reach the site of the tumor, a moderate dose per exposure has been determined to be the best means for killing colorectal cancer cells while allowing healthy cells to recover.

Some patients question why lower doses over a longer period of time aren't used in order to reduce the side effects of treatment. Doses lower than those outlined above might allow a surge of cancer growth to go unchecked, as some researchers have noted accelerated growth in head and neck cancers apparently stimulated by radiotherapy. While this finding is not directly applicable to colon and rectal cancers, the risk of cancer regrowth after reducing the single fractionated dose is considered too great in the absence of more solid information.

Departure

After each of your first few treatment sessions, make sure before leaving the doctor's office that you have received written instructions regarding any necessary dietary or behavioral changes, information about possible side effects such as possible inflammation of hemorrhoidal tissue, prescriptions, and phone numbers for emergencies. Often, side effects of radiation therapy do not emerge until you've had two or more weeks of treatment. If you have prepared for these possibilities by asking questions during the treatment visits when you feel well, side effects may be easier to deal with.

You are not likely to feel unwell after your treatments, but if you do, do not leave without telling the medical staff of your problem.

Radioimmunotherapy

Radioimmunotherapy is a new treatment, still in advanced clinical trials, but promising. It combines the principle of radiation therapy with one of the newest treatments available, tumor targeting with monoclonal antibodies, which are discussed fully in Chapter 6.

Radioimmunotherapy involves linking one molecule of a radioactive substance, a radioisotope such as iodine-131 or yttrium-90, to a monoclonal antibody. The proposed benefit of radioimmunotherapy over existing radiation treatments is that less healthy tissue is exposed to radiation because the antibody attaches preferentially to, but not only to, cancerous tissue. Some healthy tissue is affected because the radioactive substance decays as the antibody travels to the tumor and because monoclonal antibodies also will attach to some antigens on healthy cells, but it is thought that this effect is less than that sustained during external beam therapy. Radioimmunotherapy is administered into a vein, like chemotherapy.

The correct dose of radioimmunotherapy must first be determined. To calculate this dose, a small "tracer" amount of the substance will be injected first, and visualized using a CT scan or other imaging device. Based on what is seen, the doctors in charge will determine the total dose you should receive.

You will be kept in a lead-shielded hospital room throughout this treatment, and your body wastes will be disposed of in accordance with rules for handling hazardous waste. Face-to-face family visits will be very limited or denied entirely. The nurses who care for you may wear protective clothing and will limit contact with you.

If the radioisotope iodine-131 is to be used, your thyroid gland will be shielded first. The radioactive isotope, I-131, will destroy the thyroid gland if it is absorbed.

To shield the thyroid, large doses of *nonradioactive* iodine, iodine-123, are given to you first. This substance is taken up by the thyroid in excess compared to other body tissues. After the maximum amount has been absorbed, the thyroid cannot absorb more iodine for several days. This protects the thyroid gland from absorbing subsequent doses of I-131.

This method of treatment is not likely to be used for those who have had previous allergic reactions to iodine in shrimp, other foods, or in other medications.

Interstitial therapy, brachytherapy

Although external beam radiation is the most common form of radiotherapy used for rectal cancer, for some rectal tumors, a radioactive substance placed very close to or within the tumor may offer the best chance for cure. Often this treatment is combined with surgical removal of as much tumor as possible.

Interstitial radiotherapy

Permanent implantation of a low-dose radioactive material often is done during the surgery intended to remove the tumor. If not done at that time, implants can be inserted in a second surgery while you're under a general anesthetic or a sedative. Radioactive agents chosen for this type of treatment are those with an active range of just a few centimeters, which ensures the safety of nearby healthy tissue and of others around you.

Brachytherapy

For brachytherapies that involve implanting vessels that will temporarily hold a radioactive substance, surgical implantation of small canisters or tubes usually is done first in the absence of any radioactive substance.

Once the vessels are in place, the patient is returned to his hospital room. After sufficient healing, the patient is moved to a lead-shielded isolation room if not already so housed. A team specially trained to handle radioactive material arrives dressed in protective clothing to insert the radioactive substance into the vessel. It might be left in place for only a few minutes, or for a few hours, or a few days, depending on the dose required and the isotope used.

Typically, a high dose of radiotherapy for a short period is delivered by brachytherapy. This means that, while your body contains the radioactive substance, the radiation will pass through your tissues and will continue to travel beyond your body. Your bodily wastes might contain radioactive byproducts. Consequently, during this time you will represent a radiation hazard to others. Visits from family and friends will be discouraged or denied, and nursing staff will wear protective gear and limit their contact with you. They will provide you with all the care you need, but they may, for example, speak to you from the doorway instead of the bedside.

After the designated amount of time has passed, the team will return to remove and dispose of the radioactive substance. Once the agent is out of your body, you are no longer a risk to others. You may be discharged from the hospital the same day, or very soon after.

Summary

Radiation therapy confuses and frightens some people. An advance glimpse at what it's like may help to alleviate this stress. This chapter is intended to address your concerns and fears.

As always, you should ask your doctor about any issues that concern you, and report immediately any untoward effects to the medical staff.

CHAPTER 10

Ostomy

> *If God had stopped to think a bit,*
> *He would've put them on the*
> *abdomen to begin with.*

—Anonymous colostomate
The Ostomy Book

NOT EVERYONE WHO HAS SURGERY TO REMOVE COLORECTAL CANCER will need to have an ostomy. When it is possible to do so, your surgeon will remove all of your cancer and reconnect your remaining intestine to the rectum or anus so that you can continue to eliminate solid waste as you always have. Newer surgical techniques permit preservation of the anal sphincter, for instance, in rectal cancer patients who would have had to have an ostomy in the past.

At times, however, surgery for more extensive disease requires removal of rectal and anal tissue as well. This absence is remedied by a manmade opening in the abdomen through which solid waste can exit.

In this chapter, we first describe what an ostomy is, when an ostomy is needed, and what types of ostomies there are. Then we discuss how to care for your body and its new elimination path following ostomy surgery. Technology has made caring for an ostomy much easier and more comfortable, and improvements continue. Here are a few insights from one ostomate:

> *I fly a lot for my job. Traveling is a lot easier now than it was before when I was dealing with ulcerative colitis. I'd get on an airplane and something would happen, and they'd end up sitting on the runway for 45 minutes or an hour. The flight attendants didn't want anyone getting up and walking around, much less locking himself or herself in the bathroom, because they can get a call at any time to take off.*

> *I flew down to a business convention in New Orleans about eight weeks after my surgery, though, with no problems. (Unfortunately, I didn't realize I'd be too tired to do much carousing.)*

As far as how an ostomy under clothes looks to others, it looks—unless you know exactly what you're looking for—maybe just like somebody's shirt is bunched up wrong on one side. If someone is staring at your pants that much to start with, they've got other issues to deal with, so I wouldn't worry about it anyway!

When I went to a vacation spa, I questioned the nurse there about restrictions. She suggested the only thing I shouldn't do was the thing where they use a hose to squirt you from a distance, a water massage. She didn't think it would be a good idea to pound the stoma with water. She also suggested I skip the seaweed wrap, which might dehydrate me—dehydration can be a problem for ileostomates. I did it anyway, but they kept the seaweed away from the stoma. I did the algae whirlpool baths, too. I just left my appliance on, just like I do when I'm swimming.

There are people who are so hung up on body image and looking like supermodels—they can't deal with it. I knew somebody who was a nurse who died of colon cancer basically because she knew her husband—and therefore her life—couldn't deal with it if she had an ostomy.

What is an ostomy?

Ostomy is the surgical creation of an opening through the abdominal wall to allow feces or urine to exit. During colorectal cancer surgery, part or all of the colon or rectum is removed in order to remove the cancer. If there is not enough intestine or rectum left to reconnect the remaining tissue, or if the anus is removed, an ostomy will be created in the abdominal wall so that waste can exit. The surgeon will make an opening and attach the end of the intestine to that opening. See Figure 10-1.

A person who has had an ostomy is called an ostomist or ostomate.

Types of ostomies

Most ostomies involve surgical creation of an open stoma. Waste passes out of the open stoma and is collected in a pouch. However, in some cases a continent ostomy can be performed.

For colorectal cancer, ostomies are further divided into colostomies and ileostomies, depending on how much of the colon must be removed.

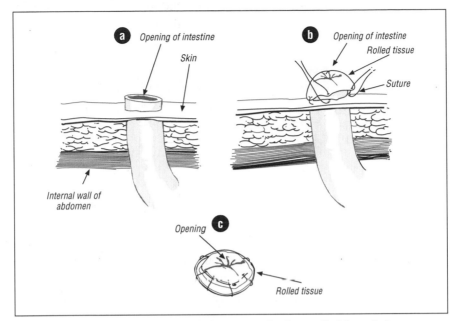

Figure 10-1. Construction of a stoma: a) the intestine has been pulled through the abdominal wall so it protrudes from the body, b) the tissue around the opening of the intestine has been rolled outwardly and stitched down, c) top view of the completed stoma.

During a partial colectomy, only part of the colon is removed and the remaining colon is reattached to the ostomy. Because part of the colon remains to remove moisture from waste after it passes through the small intestine, the waste will be more or less solid.

Removal of the entire colon (total colectomy) necessitates an ileostomy. The ileum, the portion of the small intestine nearest the colon, is what remains to create the ostomy.

Because the colon is not present to remove water from feces, the waste that passes out of an ileostomy will be more liquid.

Temporary ostomy

Sometimes one's colon and rectum need to heal before they can safely process waste. Surgery for colorectal cancer has advanced beyond the point of performing colostomies or ileostomies on all colorectal cancer patients. Today, many alternatives exist, such as creation of internal ileorectal pouches, and stapling surgeries to reconnect the remainder of the intestine to the anus within the narrow bony space of the pelvis that rules out traditional suture surgeries.

For some surgical procedures, a temporary ostomy will be used. This might also be true, for instance, if pre- or postsurgical chemotherapy or radiation therapy is planned, as these treatments can slow healing, or if an obstruction or perforation was caused by the tumor.

If you receive a temporary ostomy, you might have two closely positioned stomas instead of just one:

- One from the top portion of the intestine, which will remain active in the digestion of food, and from which waste will exit.

- A second for the temporarily inactive lower portion of intestine, called the mucus fistula, from which only mucus will emerge. (A fistula is an abnormal tubelike body tissue that erroneously connects two organs, or one organ and skin, usually developing as the result of disease. In this instance, it is manmade.)

> *I still wear a colostomy bag. I tried to have the ostomy reversed back in November after wearing the bag for more than fourteen months. However, because of lack of muscles, the operation did not go as planned and I am still wearing a bag.*
>
> *The surgeons were going to try to reverse it again, but due to CEA levels climbing from being off chemotherapy so long while recovering from surgery, my oncologist said that I have to wait.*

J-pouch (ileoanal anastomosis with reservoir)

In this surgical procedure, the small intestine is folded back onto itself to form a J shape, then stitched together to create a wider reserve. The sphincter muscle and the anus are left intact. The end of the constructed pouch is connected to the anus.

Continent ileostomy

Certain patients who have had most or all colon tissue removed may be candidates for a type of ostomy called a continent ileostomy. This variation on ostomy surgery involves creation of an abdominal stoma implanted with a valve that remains closed until the patient opens it to drain the intestine.

The advantage of this implant is that no pouch is needed for collection—just a stoma cover, a sound awareness of body function, and reasonable manual dexterity. The disadvantage is that continent ileostomy works well only for ileostomy and the liquid waste that results—not for sigmoid colostomy's more solid waste.

Why ostomy is necessary

Most patients realize quickly that a colorectal tumor that's found very low in the colon, or in the rectum itself, might require surgery that entails removal of all rectal and anal tissue along with creation of an ostomy. It's sometimes difficult, though, to comprehend why a tumor that's farther up in the colon requires what seems like drastic surgical treatment, including an artificial opening. The answer depends on several factors:

- Healthy tissue must be removed along with diseased tissue to ensure that no microscopic cancer remains. If several tumors or a very large tumor that has invaded deeply are found, a great deal of healthy tissue, including many lymph nodes and blood vessels, must be removed. The relatively small portion of healthy intestine that remains after radical surgery might not heal or function if it were reconnected to the anus or rectum.

- Tumors that are associated with certain diseases, such as ulcerative colitis, or that occur in family members at risk for inherited colon cancer, often are best treated by removing all colon and rectal tissue to avoid recurrence of disease.

- Severely inflamed colon and rectal tissue, such as that crushed by a nearby tumor or affected by the body's inflammatory response to the tumor, will not heal if surgically cut and repaired. Thus, in some cases, a temporary ostomy is created to allow the intestine to heal, after which the remaining pieces of intestine are rejoined, and the opening in the abdomen is surgically reversed.

Appearance and location

The ostomy's exit through the skin of the abdomen is called the stoma, a Greek word meaning mouth. The most visible portion of the stoma is actually a portion of the inner lining of the intestine. When healthy, the stoma is pliant, painless, red, and moist. It has these characteristics because centuries of surgery and research—colostomies have been performed since ancient Egyptian times—have shown that the most workable, infection-free ostomies are made by pulling intestinal tissue through the abdominal opening and rolling it outward to form a ridge.

Although directly after surgery the stoma may appear large and swollen, in time the healthy stoma will shrink, protruding a bit past the skin of the abdomen and developing a puckered appearance. Ileostomies will protrude farther than colostomies, because ileostomy must accommodate more liquid waste than colostomy, as the removal of the entire colon changes the ability of the body to remove water from the stool. This liquid waste is more likely to "travel" and irritate nearby skin than solid waste; the protruding stoma is intended to be a larger barrier between waste and skin.

Where the ostomy is positioned on the abdomen is determined by several factors:

- The location of the tumor
- The extent of disease
- The kind of surgery performed—that is, how much of the colon is removed
- Certain physical characteristics of the patient, including weight, posture, and skin folding

The typical stoma location for an ileostomy is a little below and to the right of the navel. For a colostomy, there is more variety in location, but often it is on the lower left side of the abdomen.

If time permits before surgery, you should discuss with your surgeon any preferences or concerns you might have regarding the proposed position of the stoma, such as your desire to remain active in a certain sport, and the subsequent possibility that the position of the stoma might interfere with this activity. Most surgeons will do their best to accommodate their patients' concerns, but the overriding consideration must be the positioning of the stoma to facilitate proper functioning of the intestine after removal of all cancer.

Caring for an ostomy

While you are still in the hospital, the nurses, and especially a nurse trained as an enterostomal therapy (ET) nurse, will help you learn to care for your stoma, the skin around it, and the health of your altered digestive tract.

If your hospital does not have an ET nurse, contact your surgeon or medical oncologist for a referral, or contact one of the ostomy associations, such as the United Ostomy Associates, and ask a volunteer to visit you to discuss up-to-date tips and techniques. Often the regular nursing staff haven't time to keep abreast of new advances in ostomy appliances and care. You'll save time, money, and peace of mind by learning the best ideas as soon as possible.

Issues with which these professionals can help you include:

- How to clean and care for the skin around the stoma. The stoma itself is relatively tough tissue compared to the skin nearest it, which must be protected from intestinal enzymes, bacteria, and potentially irritating ostomy products.

- How to choose, empty, and clean appliances that attach to the stoma to collect waste.

- How to select clothing that will not injure the stoma or interfere with its emptying.

- How to eat to avoid constipation and diarrhea, and how to choose foods to cause bowels to move at your convenience.

- How to irrigate your bowel through the stoma, if you have a sigmoid colostomy and choose to irrigate instead of using a collection pouch. Irrigation, which is similar to an enema, is a means to remove waste from the remaining colon on a schedule that's convenient for you.

Before I was discharged, an ET nurse helped me learn to care for my stoma and showed me various ostomy appliances. I spoke with a few people about this and it still was a shock for a while. I haven't had too many problems caring for my new body part. I did do some shopping around and experimenting to find things that would work best for me. Finding the right combination of appliance skin preps is very important.

I heard an older couple, obviously retired, talking about how they take care of things. They irrigate every 48 hours, and spend four hours doing it. The first thing I thought of was, "Man, you are wasting a lot of time." They say "we" do it, so his wife has to be there to take care of him, so every two days ...

A young man in my Ostomy Association group was talking about his colostomy. He irrigates and still puts on a closed-end pouch in case it leaks. He irrigates every night and changes his bag every day, so that's one way to do it. One of the first things I thought of was that my equipment costs about five or six dollars every time I change it. I've gotten so mine lasts seven or eight days without skin irritation or problems. But if people are changing these things daily, even if they're two or three dollars a day, that mounts up pretty quick. To change it every day is expensive.

One of the things the Ostomy Association points out is that just because one guy says irrigation works for him and he's been doing it for five years doesn't mean that you should also start out doing irrigation if your system is working fine and things are moving through. You need to figure out what's best for you. Just because someone else does it doesn't mean you should switch your style to do it.

Ostomy appliances and supplies

An ostomy appliance consists of two parts: a collection pouch and a positioning plate that surrounds but does not touch or enter the stoma.

If you've had an ostomy for years, you may remember how few products used to be available in the past, and you may note happily how many are available now. The era of the leaky rubber pouch that smelled odd even when clean and didn't accommodate gas episodes is over. Today's options include:

- Disposable pouches.
- Reusable pouches that empty from the bottom, or from the top, while still attached. These are the most practical choice for ostomies that produce liquid waste.
- Pouches with filters to control odor.
- Pouches that hang sideways instead of down for use when jogging or playing tennis. This might be a more suitable option for sigmoid colostomates who will manage solid waste rather than other colostomates and ileostomates.

- Small patches similar to Band-Aids to cover and protect the stoma during swimming. These are suitable only for sigmoid colostomies or those with continent ileostomies. An ileostomate with a traditional stoma and many colostomates with liquid waste would have the patch pushed away from the body by the constant flow of diarrhea from the small intestine.

- Ornamental stoma covers for romantic interludes.

- Pouches that glue in place.

- Pouches that are held in place with a belt, for those who are allergic to some adhesives.

- Hypoallergenic gluing and skin-sealing products made from vegetable matter.

- Neoprene pouch belts for use during sports activities.

- Irrigation tubes (catheters) for those who prefer to empty the bowel by irrigation (enema) instead of collecting waste in a pouch. This applies only to sigmoid colostomates; many other colostomies as well as ileostomies produce continuous liquid waste.

- Catheters for opening and draining the continent ileostomy.

- Skin barrier creams to protect the skin nearest the stoma, which must be shielded from bacteria and digestive enzymes (to which the stoma itself is impervious).

- Appliances geared either to the continual liquid waste of ileostomy or the more solid and periodic waste of sigmoid colostomy.

- One-piece appliances, or two-piece appliances with a stoma-surrounding attachment that stays glued in place, but a bag that's detachable.

- Appliances in different sizes to accommodate individual stomas and more copious flow overnight or during travel.

Many of these products are preferred by some people, but disliked by others. Some people say, for instance, that certain pouches with built-in filters that are intended to allow gas to escape without odor don't work as advertised. The best way to find what works for you is to contact a local branch of one of the ostomy associations and talk to a volunteer (many of whom have ostomies), to join a support group for colon cancer survivors or ostomates, and to try various products. Products can be purchased by mail until you feel comfortable talking about your needs with your pharmacist.

It took me a while after both operations to find the correct bag that fit properly. The last operation left me with an open wound near the new stoma and that caused the bag to keep coming loose. I had problems for about a month with that, but eventually it cleared up and everything is fine now.

Cleaning the stoma and skin

The stoma will clean itself by producing and shedding intestinal mucus, but the skin near the stoma, called peristomal skin, must be kept gently and scrupulously clean. There are several reasons for this:

- Its juxtaposition to both feces and digestive enzymes makes it very likely to become infected, as digestive enzymes are capable of breaking down skin, which is then very likely to be infected by fecal bacteria. Fecal bacteria are common, abundant, and necessary for digestion, but not at all healthy for skin.

- The peristomal skin is more likely to be scratched or scraped owing to the amount of activity it sees in its new role: pouch attachment, cleaning, removing adhesives, and so on. These scratches and scrapes make it more likely to become infected or to develop allergic reactions.

Most people find it easiest to clean the stoma and its surrounding skin when the digestive tract is least active. For many, this is in the morning before breakfast.

The stoma can be rinsed with water and patted dry, if you wish, although it is not necessary to clean it: as mucus-shedding intestinal tissue, it will clean itself. Exposing the stoma to the spray from a shower will not hurt it. A stoma should never be scrubbed.

Peristomal skin should be cleaned gently with very mild soap and patted dry—never rubbed. If you use a skin barrier or a skin sealant, cleaning is done every few days to once a week, dictated by your own skin's tolerance for the barrier substance. If a bit of skin sealant or barrier remains after washing and rinsing, leave it until the next cleaning, provided the skin beneath looks healthy. Rubbing away residual barrier or sealant is more likely to harm your skin than leaving the residue in place.

If your stoma was placed amidst body hair, trim it regularly so that removing the pouch or adhesive will not pull hair, causing pain and opening the skin to infection.

Peristomal skin should look just like the skin anywhere else on your abdomen: not red, wrinkled, grey, or chapped. Changes in peristomal skin should be discussed with an ET nurse and reported to your oncologist.

Skin barriers and seals

A skin barrier or seal is a liquid, powder, paste, or membrane that rests between your skin and the stoma attachment in order to protect the skin from bacteria, moisture, and the irritants in adhesives. These are excellent products that truly save the skin; many varieties are available, and should be used no matter what model appliance you prefer. Each comes with its own instructions and precautions for use.

> People normally gain weight after surgery, especially if they've had ulcerative colitis, because they feel better. They warn you not to gain too much weight because then the stoma can pull inside, it doesn't protrude like it's supposed to, and it makes life interesting. But they have appliances that will work around that. The barrier spray goes on to protect the skin from any irritation.

> I had trouble with yeast infections under the wafer. I got little blisters and it was irritated all the time. I had to change the wafer every couple of days because it got itchy, and I had to spray cortisone on it. Basically once I got the rhythm down for the combination of products I use, I haven't had any trouble like that for a year or longer. How much you sweat and what kind of food you eat can also come into how well the appliance stays on.

Even if you've never had a skin allergy before, you should assume that these products might cause an allergic reaction because:

- Humans develop more allergies as they age.
- Skin that is repeatedly injured is more likely to develop sensitivity.
- Chemotherapy and radiation therapy are known to cause skin to become more sensitive to a variety of substances.

When trying a new product, it's wise always to do a patch test first on a part of the abdomen well away from the stoma. The instructions packaged with the barrier or seal will explain how to do a patch test.

Emptying the pouch

The pouch should be changed when it's about one-third full. Accumulating excessive material increases the pouch's weight and may cause it to pull away from the skin. Leakage, odor, and infection of nearby skin may result.

> Many pouches are what is termed "drainable," or open ended. The "open" end hangs down. There is a plastic clip that folds the pouch end back and keeps it closed. The seal created by the clip is water/liquid- and gas-proof. I couldn't change the appliance every time it starts to fill! It would cost a fortune and take a lot of time. Drainable pouches come in one- and two-piece models. Most appliances are designed to be left on for up to two weeks. I change mine about every seven days or earlier if it starts coming loose.

> One man in our ostomy support group was using a two-piece system that had a drain. He was not told to leave it on and just open the bottom to let out the waste. He was very pleased to hear there was a faster, cleaner way to deal with the equipment.

At times, the pouch should be emptied before it's one-third full:

- If you're traveling and won't be able to empty it easily en route, it should be emptied first. Some ostomates report that air travel in particular may cause the pouch to expand as the cabin is unevenly pressurized during takeoff and landing.

- If you're having a spell of diarrhea.

- If you've prepped for a colonoscopy.

- If you're about to engage in sports or any physical activity.

Gently remove all pouch models, but especially the one-piece models, to avoid damaging the skin beneath the attachment plate.

> As far as wearing the bag is concerned, it does get better. However, I find that I empty my bag still about eight times a day some days, and usually at least four or five times. However, after a while you learn to live with it and you are able to go out and do things.

Discarding waste

If you are using disposable pouches, you can empty the pouch into the toilet first, then wrap it and put it in the trash, or you can dispose of it, well wrapped, while it's still full. What you choose to do depends on how well you're feeling, what trash collection facilities are available, and the sensibilities of those you live with.

If you have a reusable pouch, you can empty it while sitting on or standing in front of the toilet. Put some toilet tissue into the toilet bowl first to act as a cushion for the material you're discarding—this helps prevent splashback. For emptying, some reusable pouches open from the top, some from the bottom. All come supplied with directions for emptying.

A reusable pouch must be carefully cleaned and deodorized. Fortunately, this is easy today, as many very good products are available for these purposes. A few points to remember are to avoid hot water, as this will cause the pouch material to expand and hold odors, and to dry the pouch thoroughly. Empty the pouch into the toilet (you might need to squeeze the outside of the pouch to get all material out); give it a good rinse; soak it for a spell; then scrub the inside gently with a bottle brush. Add a few drops of mineral oil to the bottom of the bottom-opening type to make the next emptying easier. It might be useful to purchase three reusable pouches at once: one for wearing, one for washing, and one for emergencies.

If you share a bathroom with others, take an extra minute to clean splashes and stow away supplies and trash.

Attaching or reattaching the pouch

How the pouch is attached or reattached depends on which model you're using. Most people find it easiest to reattach any pouch while seated.

For either the two-piece or one-piece pouch, you may need to adjust the stoma opening in the skin plate to match the size and shape of your stoma— they differ among people, and may change as age and weight change. Some appliances come with a template that you can match to your stoma to choose the correct size opening. The skin plate then can be cut carefully to match your needs.

Two-piece pouch

If you're using a two-piece pouch, you can simply continue to reattach fresh pouches to the skin plate for several days or a week until it's time to change the skin attachment.

Your own body will dictate the schedule for changing the skin plate, based on your skin's sensitivity. In general, the skin should be left undisturbed by plate changes for as long as possible in order to avoid irritation by too-frequent changes.

One-piece pouch or pouch plate

The skin plate of a one-part pouch that's glued in place must be changed whenever the pouch is changed. A skin barrier is a must in this instance; otherwise, skin layers are stripped away whenever the adhesive is removed, leaving exposed newer, more tender skin that's increasingly likely to become irritated or infected.

Most people find that placing the bottom of the skin plate under the stoma and "rolling" the plate upward provides a better fit around the stoma, because visibility is better using this method.

Odor

The improved pouches available today hardly ever emit odors. When odors exist, they are identical to the odor of gas and feces of those who have an intact colon.

There are steps you can take to be very certain that odors will not become a problem:

- Use deodorant tablets or liquids in the bottom of the pouch, as recommended by the manufacturer.
- Clean and dry reusable pouches carefully.
- Pretest pouches that contain charcoal filters to be sure they work as advertised.
- Ask a sensitive, helpful, honest person if he or she notices any odors.
- Eat yogurt, parsley, and other foods known to ameliorate odors in the gastrointestinal tract.

- Avoid foods such as cabbage that increase gas if you'll be with people who object to tummy rumbles and possibly an aroma.

- Ensure that the skin attachment fits well and is firmly attached. Most people don't have the ideal flat tummy that allows no gas to escape; firm attachment can remedy this.

- If your pouch has a "burp" valve, engage it in the bathroom or use a room deodorizer.

> *I've never had a problem with gas in my bag when on an airplane, as some ostomates report. It depends more on what you eat first: you'll only have gas in your bag if you've eaten something that causes gas to form ... and you can take care of releasing it from the bag in the bathroom.*

Noises

Passage of waste material and gas through the stoma can create wheezes, sighs, rumbles, or gas-like noises. Do try to be gentle with yourself when assessing these: are they really any worse than the stomach noises your body made when you had an intact colon?

But suppose one of the "healthy unaware" notices and is rude enough to comment? You might explain that it's just your intestine, that your digestive tract has been noisy all your life, which is a true statement for many of us. As Miss Manners says, those who ask nosy questions deserve to be lied to.

If your stoma regularly makes noise as gas passes, you may be able to anticipate it. If the setting is less than ideal for such noise, you can suppress it temporarily by subtly moving your forearm over the stoma and holding it there.

Other sensations

You will undoubtedly have other observations or will note other sensations:

- You may see the pouch expand as material, especially gas, pass into it. It's unlikely anyone else will notice this unless you point it out to them.

- You may feel warmth against your skin as waste material collects in the pouch. At first, you may think this is a leak.

- Your remaining gastrointestinal tract will continue to behave as before, with sensations of movement or mild gas pains. Any pronounced pain should be reported at once to your oncologist, even if it's transient.

Resuming activities

Everything you enjoyed doing before surgery can continue to be done after ostomy. Sunbathing, swimming, dancing, sexual activity—all of these are still possible; all have appliances and techniques developed to allow the gastrointestinal tract to go about its healthy business while you have fun.

Shelly Weiler describes his way of dealing with his ostomy:

> I carry an emergency kit with me, which includes a towel, a fresh bag, a new wafer, scissors, remover pads, skin prep pads, and a roll of paper towels. I am very open about my "emergency kit" and take it anytime I'm going anywhere that is too distant from my house to get back quickly. No need to worry about odor. The modern appliances are tighter than crazy glue and no odor escapes unless the wafer is broken.

> I'm happy the surgeon didn't put the darn contraption on my forehead.

> Of course I can't wait to have it reversed, it is a pain to have to think about it, clean it, and be prepared for that inevitable emergency.

For activities that require lots of skin to be bared, a sigmoid colostomate might consider a stoma plug and a patch that can be used. For ileostomates who have a continent ileostomy, this might also be an option; for other ileostomates and for colostomates with liquid waste, however, the constant flow of diarrhea from the small intestine would push the patch away from the body. For strenuous physical activities, pouches with special capacity and belts that wick away sweat have been developed.

> I'm an RN who had ulcerative colitis for years and knew my risk for colon cancer increased with each year. I swore I would never have a colostomy. I even had it written into my living will at one point. But when it came to the point of having it done or dying with a bowel obstruction, I chose the baggie.

And it really isn't all that bad. It hasn't stopped me from doing any-thing I really want to do. I swim, hike, go to social functions, whatever. No one outside my immediate family and a few close friends even knows it's there.

For the best tips and news of advances in ostomy care, join a local support group. In addition to learning of new products, you'll likely find it an immense relief being able to share feelings with others who know exactly what you're going through.

After a few months I found out about and started going to monthly United Ostomy Association meetings, and I still do. The meetings range from presentations by doctors, presentations by appliance manufacturers, discussions about problems and solutions. We compare stories and share what we've learned about cleaning the skin, using different moisture bar-riers and glues, special appliances for sports, and the like. My local group also has an additional meeting to discuss quality-of-life issues. I've met a lot of good people, and also some people who aren't as lucky as I am: peo-ple who were much sicker, who had no partner and can't seem to find one now. Two women in the group from vastly different cultural backgrounds have had partners divorce them. In my case, my wife has been great throughout this ordeal. We've taken up ballroom dancing and are basi-cally doing everything we did before, and more.

Summary

The creation of a new and essential body opening in an easy-to-reach place has allowed many people to survive colorectal cancer and resume their lives. Adopting this new body part as part of yourself and learning to care for it properly require a forward-looking attitude and a willingness to shed old thinking about private matters.

Unfortunately, we can only touch upon the many compelling issues concern-ing living with an ostomy, but two excellent books and a magazine for osto-mates exist. *The Ostomy Book,* by Barbara Mullen, an ostomate, and Kerry McGinn, her daughter and an RN, is an up-to-date and practical book with copious useful details. *Coping with an Ostomy,* written by psychologist Robert Phillips, does a splendid and timeless job of addressing emotional issues, and also addresses practical issues. The magazine *Ostomy Quarterly,* published by the United Ostomy Association, is an excellent ongoing source of information about products and advances in ostomy care.

Key points to remember:

- Engage the services of an enterostomal therapy nurse while you are recovering from surgery, or as soon as possible after your return home.

- Join a support group or subscribe to *Ostomy Quarterly* to learn about the best products and techniques.

- Wearing an ostomy appliance will not change your enjoyment of life permanently unless you allow it to do so. Activities that you enjoyed before surgery can be done with an ostomy, using special products that have been developed to allow normal lifestyles to continue.

CHAPTER 11

Side Effects of Treatment

The worst about medicine is that one kind
makes another necessary.

—Elbert Hubbard

TOO OFTEN WE RECALL PEOPLE WHO HAVE HAD TERRIBLE EXPERIENCES while receiving cancer treatment, yet remarkable progress has been made in alleviating this suffering. This chapter will describe side effects of colorectal cancer treatment, and what can be done about them. Side effects of surgery that might occur during hospitalization are not discussed here, as medical personnel are likely to notice these before the patient does.

Please be encouraged that, although we list many side effects here, you may have very little reaction, or no discernible reaction at all, to treatment.

Although this chapter has been reviewed by medical doctors, the author of this book is not a medical doctor, and is not familiar with the individual characteristics that make you and your illness unique. The information this chapter provides should never be substituted for your doctor's knowledge. Report immediately to your doctor any adverse reactions that arise during or after treatment, and direct all questions to your doctor, regardless of other sources of information available to you.

If you don't find the information you need in this chapter, see Chapter 17, *Late Effects, Late Complications*. Some late effects occur earlier in some people, at times even before treatment ends.

Several excellent books are available that focus on treatment from the patient's perspective, including dealing with side effects. If you'd like much more detail about dealing with side effects such as nausea, diarrhea, hair loss, appetite changes, or fatigue, these books, listed in the bibliography, are wonderful resources.

Why do side effects arise?

Side effects of treatment can arise for several reasons.

First, the treatments commonly used today for colorectal cancer affect not only cancerous cells, but many healthy cells as well. Radiotherapy and many chemotherapy regimens target cells that divide rapidly, as many cancer cells do. This targeting of fast-growing cells means that many healthy cells that divide rapidly—cells in the mouth, intestinal tract, hair, fingernails, and others—will be affected, too. During treatment, these cells die all at once, instead of passing through the life cycle just a few at a time. This rapid turnover of cells causes some of the most common side effects of cancer treatment, such as mouth sores and hair loss.

Other side effects come about owing to the body's attempt to heal itself. Tumor lysis syndrome, for instance, is a side effect of the body's attempt to clear itself of dying tumor cells after certain treatments.

Many side effects of treatment are normal and pose no danger to you. Fatigue and changes in fingernail growth are common side effects of treatment that do not necessarily herald problems. Your oncologist should give you fact sheets to provide you with information about side effects that are very serious, and about which you should telephone as soon as you notice them. If your doctor doesn't offer this information, ask.

> *I had CPT11 for a year. I didn't have too many side effects. I took the CPT11 together with 5-FU and leucorovin. I didn't lose my hair and unfortunately, didn't lose any weight either. In fact, I gained 30 pounds. When I am given my chemotherapy, the doctor also puts in a Kytril and Decadron drip. This completely eliminates any nausea, at least for me. I have been off chemo for four months now, so I am hoping when I get back on it, it doesn't affect me differently since the first go-round was relatively easy.*

Side effects by drug

Each drug commonly used against colorectal cancer has, in certain people, one or more side effects, which are listed briefly here. For more detail, see the sections below that describe each side effect.

It's wise to keep in mind that even commonly used drugs are known to have numerous side effects. Aspirin, for instance, is known to cause any of the following in certain people: vomiting; diarrhea; confusion; drowsiness; severe stomach pain; unusual bruising; bloody or black stools; gastrointestinal bleeding; dizziness; hearing loss; ringing in the ears; swelling of hands, face, lips, eyes, throat, or tongue; difficulty swallowing or breathing; or hoarseness. Like most other drugs, chemotherapeutic agents also are known to cause a large number of both common and rare reactions.

It's noteworthy as well to remember that, as my pharmacist says, any drug you swallow can cause nausea, and almost all drugs can cause dizziness in certain people.

Fluorouracil (5-FU) and related fluoropyrimidines

At this time, related fluoropyrimidines used against colorectal cancer are fluorouracil (5-FU), floxuridine (FUDR), and Xeloda. Uracil-tegafur (UFT, Orzel) is in clinical trials.

Fluorouracil (5-FU) administered by continuous infusion pump produces fewer side effects, or similar side effects in different proportions, than 5-FU administered by bolus push in the oncologist's office. Xeloda and Uracil-tegafur produce fewer side effects than 5-FU.

Side effects for the fluoropyrimidines are listed in the following paragraphs.

Serious side effects: Pain, redness, or swelling at the injection site; vomiting; diarrhea; unusual bruising or bleeding; sores on the mouth or lips; rash; yellowing of the skin or eyes (jaundice); joint pain; painful urination; blood in the urine; lower back or abdominal pain; chest pain; fever; chills; or sore throat.

Bothersome side effects: Increased sensitivity to the sun; nausea; loss of appetite; fatigue or weakness; headache; dry skin; eye changes; nail changes; hair loss; balance problems; numbness; redness, pain, peeling, and tingling in the hands and feet.

Irinotecan (CPT-11, Camptosar)

Serious side effects: Allergic reaction; shortness of breath; vomiting; fever; sore throat; fainting; lightheadedness; pain, redness, or swelling at the injection site.

Bothersome side effects: Fatigue; pain; headache; chills; appetite changes; weight loss; water retention; hair loss; cough; dizziness; or trouble sleeping.

Leucovorin

Serious side effects: Allergic reactions.

Mitomycin-c

Serious side effects: Allergic reactions; pain, redness, or swelling at the injection site (extravasation); or fever.

Bothersome side effects: Pancytopenia in the absence of fever.

Oxaliplatin

Oxaliplatin is in advanced·clinical trials, and is available outside of clinical trials through the FDA's Investigational New Drug program.

Serious side effects: Allergic reactions.

Bothersome side effects: Numbness; tingling; and sensitivity of hands to cold.

Panorex (monoclonal antibody 17-1A)

Panorex is a biological therapy in advanced clinical trials.

Serious side effects: Allergic reaction.

Raltitrexed (Tomudex)

Raltitrexed is in advanced clinical trials.

Serious side effects: Pain, redness, or swelling at the injection site; decreased urination or dark urine; dry, unproductive cough, shortness of breath, or other breathing problems; unusual bruising or bleeding; sores on the mouth or lips; skin rash; vomiting; diarrhea; abdominal pain; black tarry stools; yellowing of skin or eyes; swelling of feet or legs; joint pain; fever or chills; sore throat; or cough.

Bothersome side effects: Nausea; loss of appetite; or hair loss.

Side effects by type

Listed alphabetically below are many side effects of treatment. Although great variability exists in patients' reactions to treatment, the most commonly occurring are nausea, diarrhea, abdominal cramping, mouth sores, hair loss, and fatigue. Included within the various sections below are tips from colorectal cancer survivors for dealing with side effects.

Abdominal pain

Abdominal pain or cramping is common following surgery, chemotherapy, or radiotherapy for colorectal cancer.

As abdominal pain also can be a sign of intestinal blockage owing to tumor regrowth, you should notify your doctor of this pain, especially if cramping persists or worsens.

Many good medications are available for abdominal cramps, ranging from mild over-the-counter remedies to narcotic substances, but often what works for one patient does not necessarily work for another. Ask your doctor for an appropriate treatment, and be persistent until a good remedy is found.

Dietary changes sometimes are helpful in controlling abdominal cramps. Some patients have found that dairy, soy, fat, or wheat gluten products are not tolerated well following treatment for colorectal cancer. Modify your diet slowly and judiciously, and only with your doctor's approval.

Various other causes of abdominal pain exist, and are discussed in the subsequent sections of this chapter.

Randall describes abdominal pain that persists several months after surgery:

> My colon resection was many months ago. I still have gastroenterologic weirdness. I'm talking stools, gas, and cramps. No blood in stools, but not "normal." The first couple of weeks after surgery, things were back to normal. First time in two years. But then…
>
> My colon-rectal surgeon says that there is usually a tightening of the colon at the anastomosis, or "that-place-where-the-two-healthy-ends-of-colon-were-stitched-back-together." As it heals, it constricts. As it constricts, size, frequency and other characteristics of stool change. He had

me doing high-dose Metamucil to try and "stretch" the opening back out. So far, no progress. My anastomosis is located about halfway down of what is left of the descending colon.

Occasionally, I will have fold-me-in-half cramps in my lower gut which immobilize me until I can get to some place where I can at least pass gas.

Abscess

Following radiation therapy for rectal cancer, abscesses within the pelvis may develop. This usually occurs as a late effect if at all, but may develop earlier in certain people.

If you have unusual and pronounced pain, fever, nausea, difficulty with bowel movements, or the appearance of pus from the vagina or rectum, notify your doctor immediately.

Acid indigestion

See Nausea.

Allergic reactions

It's possible to have an allergic reaction to almost any drug, depending on a host of poorly understood factors. Allergic reactions are more likely to occur with high doses of a drug that is administered rapidly.

In the past, most allergic reactions were detected in the doctor's office as chemotherapy was being administered through an IV line by drip bag or bolus push (a bolus is the back end of a syringe, the reservoir that holds the medication). With the advent of the continuous infusion pump, however, it's possible to have an allergic reaction at home, hours or days after the pump has been restocked with medication.

Allergic reactions are highly individualized to substance type, but the symptoms are similar and include any of these: hives; itching; difficulty breathing; tightness in chest or throat; sore throat; fever; or chills.

Appetite or taste changes

Chemotherapy and radiotherapy can affect your taste buds to the extent that you can't taste food, or that it tastes metallic or even disgusting.

I find so many of the foods I used to love are now repulsive. Even stopped adding sugar to my decaf. Sweet is too sweet. This scares me more than the cancer. I always liked to eat, now I'm avoiding meals in any way I can.

I just had breakfast that consisted of two slices of whole-wheat toast and butter. Still like the taste of salted butter, thank God.

Adequate nutrition in spite of food aversion is a very important part of your recovery. Eat what you like, but eat as much nutritional food as you can. Ask your doctor about vitamin supplements and liquid supplements such as Nutrical or Ensure.

We went to a wedding today and I thought I wouldn't be able to have the good time I used to have at affairs. Too many things driving me down: fatigue, lack of appetite, and now a little depression over the whole situation. I haven't had diarrhea in a week, so at least that's good. Hey, there is a bright side.

I took Zofran and Imodium tablets before leaving for the wedding, and in an hour or so, the pill kicked in, I regained my appetite and lost most of the nausea just in time to enjoy the wedding. I had the chicken. Maybe for the first time in my life I'm eating "healthy." (That's when I can eat.)

I praised the Zofran god last night. I still have seven sample pills left and will ask my doctor for a prescription this Wednesday.

Some colorectal cancer survivors note that, rather than craving particular foods, they are repelled by them, particularly by meats. Foods that once were favorites now have repugnant or metallic taste and scent.

I am on 5-FU with leucovorin and the taste bud problem has been progressive. I find that some foods totally turn me off now. I used to love meat, but now have no taste for it. I used to love bacon cheddar cheeseburgers! The idea turns my stomach now. Used to love especially sweet drinks, can't stand them now, they almost make me gag.

I like salt now more than ever. I have a desire for a hot dog, but I'm afraid to try it because that too might taste different. Had pizza last night and at least that still appeals to me. I hope I never lose my taste for pizza. One of my joys in life was eating; now it seems a chore.

Blood clots, pulmonary embolism

At the beginning of treatment, a large abdominal tumor may shrink rapidly in response to therapy, and may dislodge a pre-existing blood clot. Blood clots also may form around a central catheter at any time during treatment.

If you have a central catheter, or have a large abdominal tumor and have just started treatment, be especially aware of deep pain or difficulty breathing that may signal a dangerous blood clot dislodging, or capable of dislodging and traveling to the lung.

Bone pain

The colony stimulating factor G-CSF (Neupogen, Filgrastim) can cause aching bones and joints. Ice packs may relieve this pain; if not, ask your doctor if the dose can be lowered. Bone pain associated with G-CSF is temporary.

Severe back pain may be associated with degenerative changes to the spine following radiation therapy. The spine is not able to sustain as high a dose of radiation as some other organs can. Surgery to fuse spinal discs may alleviate this pain.

Bone pain should always be reported promptly to your doctor, as colorectal cancer can travel to and lodge in bone, and can affect abdominal and pelvic nerves that cause pain in the spine.

Bowel obstruction

Following surgery or radiation therapy for colon or rectal cancer, one or more bowel obstructions may develop and persist over time.

Bowel obstruction is a painful, life-threatening event. Contact your doctor immediately if you have difficult or absent bowel movements, pain, fever, or a small amount of diarrhea in the presence of these symptoms.

An ostomate describes how a less-careful diet almost caused him serious problems:

You can eat things that will block your intestine and keep things in there for much too long. Then you need to go out and get the medical equivalent of Drano or a sump pump. I ate raw pecans and my digestive tract wasn't quite up to that yet, and it got about 95 percent through and stopped, and the intestine got distended. They literally go in with a tube and suck out what's clogging things up. I wasn't admitted to the hospital for this. I went to the ostomy nurse and said, "I feel bad," and pointed to my stomach. They said, "Yeah, you screwed up." They go through the stoma with a tube about six inches long and an inch in diameter and flush water in—I think 100 ccs—then they suck it out and loosen up whatever's there.

If you have an ileostomy, only a blockage makes it hurt. The nerves in the small intestine seem to be much different from the large intestine. Things like volume and pressure of gas buildup don't hurt like they do in the large intestine. The small intestine just keeps pushing things on through. It doesn't hold material like the large intestine.

Breathing problems

Call your doctor immediately if you have trouble breathing.

Many treatments for colorectal cancer, such as monoclonal antibodies, radiation, or certain chemotherapy drugs that affect the heart, such as 5-fluorouracil, can cause difficulty breathing.

Rapid breathing (tachypnea) can be the body's effort to lower levels of excessive acid, called acidosis. Acidosis is a very early sign of certain conditions such as serious infection, kidney damage, or diabetic complications that should be treated immediately.

Rarely, circulatory or respiratory distress can be linked to untreated, intractable constipation.

Bruising, bleeding

If your chemotherapy is administered directly to the liver via portable infusion pump, you might experience gastrointestinal bleeding, which should be reported to your doctor immediately.

See also Pancytopenia.

Chest pain

Report this symptom to your doctor immediately.

Those receiving 5-fluorouracil therapy may experience a constricting type of chest pain known as angina.

See Heart damage.

Cognitive changes

Many patients report that treatment makes them feel fuzzy-minded or forgetful. These symptoms should go away over time.

Rarely, more serious cognitive changes may occur. Fluorouracil and certain platinum-containing drugs are capable of causing delirium or dementia.

Call your doctor if these symptoms are very disturbing, or if you or a loved one feel that these side effects represent a danger to the patient or the family.

Constipation

Constipation can be a very serious problem during colorectal cancer treatment, because inactivity, tumor regrowth, other illnesses, and certain drugs such as painkillers, antidepressants, or antihistamines may slow or paralyze the intestine, or mask the urge to move one's bowels.

Constipation in its most serious form, a total blockage of the intestine called fecal impaction, can present as circulatory or respiratory distress. Call your doctor immediately if you feel constipated for more than three days, or if you have difficulty breathing or symptoms of heart failure. Fecal impaction can be fatal even in the absence of a tumor.

If your doctor agrees, experiment with small amounts of different foods until you have a sense for what will maintain a balance between constipation and diarrhea. This balance is especially important directly after surgery, when dietary roughage can cause too much soft stool before adequate healing has occurred.

Increased fluid intake, regular exercise, increased dietary fiber, warm or hot drinks, privacy and quiet time in the bathroom, easy access to toilet or bedside commode, and stool softeners may be tried to ease constipation. Do not make dietary changes or greatly increase your fluid intake without first verifying these choices with your doctor.

Dehydration

If you suspect you are dehydrated, call your doctor immediately.

Dehydration is a very serious side effect of vomiting or diarrhea, for cancer patients must have adequate fluid to remove from the body toxins as well as proteins released by dying cells. Moreover, the quantities of electrolytes and minerals such as phosphorus, calcium, potassium, magnesium, and sodium may be disrupted in the colorectal cancer patient, both by disease and by treatment. Dehydration exacerbates this imbalance.

The most reliable symptom of dehydration is thirst. Other signs include the inability to urinate about once an hour, the production of very little urine, or the production of urine that is both dark and low in volume. Other symptoms, such as faintness, dry lips, thick saliva, or loss of appetite resemble the side effects of some chemotherapies too closely to be reliable indicators of dehydration.

Take in as much fluid as possible, but do not drink products containing electrolytes (as do the products marketed to sports enthusiasts) unless your doctor says that your kidneys are in good condition and that these drinks will do you no harm.

Diarrhea

Removal of most or all of the large intestine frequently results in diarrhea. Radiotherapy targeting the abdomen or chemotherapy also may cause diarrhea, as dying cells are shed from the intestine.

> About halfway through my chemotherapy treatments I suffered terrible diarrhea. I thought my colon would turn itself inside out. The oncology nurses kept telling me the usual things like low fiber, small frequent meals, no dairy, and so on, and had me taking double, then triple strength doses of Imodium. This was useless! Finally my oncologist prescribed Lomotil twice daily. It only took about three or four doses to get it under control. After that I only took it as needed.

Phone your doctor immediately if diarrhea is combined with a fever more than 1.5 degrees higher than your normal temperature, general malaise, severe chills, night sweats, burning or pain while urinating, headache, neck stiffness, coughing, or trouble breathing.

Your doctor can recommend anti-diarrheal drugs, which you will have to balance carefully with drugs such as stool softeners to control constipation. Experiment with small amounts of different foods until you have a sense for what will maintain a balance between constipation and diarrhea.

> The dietician, whom I met with weekly, and the doctor gave me a restricted-residue/low-residue diet that really helped when the multiple bowel movements returned from irritation from radiation. I never really got bad diarrhea once I started on the diet.

> As treatment neared its end, my hemorrhoids flared up terribly and my doctor gave me Anusol HC suppositories. Ah, relief.

Administration of the drug CPT-11 (irinotecan) can cause immediate diarrhea in some people. Addition of atropine offsets these symptoms.

> My husband had diarrhea during the cycle, but managed pretty well. He had a positive response to the drug that made it easier to tolerate. It is very important to have an oncologist who will listen to your concerns and adjust things to meet your needs.

· · · · ·

> One side effect of radiation was diarrhea. I couldn't be too far from a bathroom; my back end got really sore. I used baby wipes, the non-alcohol type, and Balmex cream. You can find both in the baby aisle of your drug store. Both were a godsend, as were the sitz baths. If you don't have one, get one, plus a reading rack for the bathroom with your favorite magazines or books.

Dry mouth, difficulty swallowing

Chemotherapy for colorectal cancer can at times cause dry mouth.

Normal saliva contains an antibiotic. In the absence of saliva, dry mouth can lead to serious dental problems that result in whole-body (systemic) infection and tooth loss. Thus, gentle but scrupulous dental care is a must. Avoid spicy, sour, or acidic foods. Examine your mouth daily for fuzzy white patches that might be a fungal infection. Ask your doctor for drugs to increase saliva flow, or for instructions for a homemade mouth rinse that can be used several times a day.

Marsha Center, RDH, describes her dental care during treatment for colorectal cancer:

> I am a registered dental hygienist who has worked 20 years in private practice. I was diagnosed with colon cancer, had a resection and six months of continuous infusion of 5-FU through a Groshong catheter. While I was undergoing the continuous chemotherapy my oncologist cautioned me about any dental work, especially not to have my teeth cleaned. The problem is the introduction of bacteria into the blood stream via the sulcus area surrounding the teeth. That in turn could travel to the central catheter or weak point in my body. Then infection would develop, requiring removal of the port, massive doses of antibiotics, and so on. So I waited to have my teeth worked on until I was through with chemotherapy. I am not a periodontal patient, but this caution is even more significant for those who are.
>
> As far as discomfort, the dentist or even the oncology staff should have access to products [that can help]. I had mouth sores that made eating uncomfortable. A rinse made by the oncology pharmacist made of benzocaine, tetracycline, and other bacteriostatic ingredients was extremely helpful. Peridex has chlorhexadine in it which kills bacteria in the mouth, but also contains alcohol, and that was a no-no for my mouth, because it's too strong. Some fluoride preparations can also be helpful.

Extravasation

Sometimes, chemotherapy that is administered by IV or catheter can leak out of the vein into surrounding tissue, an adverse event called extravasation. The reaction of the body to a high concentration of chemotherapy in the skin or other tissue can be serious and painful. The artery or vein may be unusable for chemotherapy thereafter; the skin may die, slough off, and fail to regrow.

Symptoms of extravasation include pain, redness, swelling, or burning at the IV or catheter site, during or after the administration of chemotherapy. Notify the medical staff immediately if you have these symptoms during or just after treatment.

Eye changes

Administration of the drug CPT-11 (irinotecan) can cause production of excess bodily fluids in some cases, manifesting as watery eyes. Addition of atropine offsets these symptoms.

Administration of the drug 5-fluorouracil can cause watery or dry eyes.

Eye drops might help with these problems. If they do not, you might consider consulting an ophthalmologist who is a lacrimal (tear) specialist. In extreme cases, a surgery can be performed to reopen scarred tear ducts.

> *About seven months into my treatment I started experiencing constant tearing from my right eye. My ophthalmologist said I had very small tear ducts, she probed it, and everything was fine for about a week, when the left eye began to tear.*

> *After repeated probing failed to correct the problem, she sent me to a lacrimal specialist. (I didn't even know such a specialty existed.) My oncologist said this was totally unrelated to the chemotherapy. However, when I saw the lacrimal doctor, his first comment was to ask if I was taking 5-FU. I have since had duct surgery (ouch! I'd rather have another bowel resection), and I possibly face reconstruction surgery in the next few months.*

Fainting, lightheadedness, dizziness

Although dizziness is a known benign side effect of many drugs, these symptoms can be serious side effects of chemotherapy. Notify your doctor immediately if you experience these symptoms.

Fatigue and sleep disorders

Those being treated for cancer list fatigue as the most debilitating symptom they experience. Ninety-five percent of those being treated for cancer report fatigue.

Shelly Weiler describes his difficulty dealing with fatigue:

> *I used to have only about two or three throwaway days, as we call them. Now I'm having as many as five throwaway days in a seven-day week. The fatigue is so overpowering I can't really describe the feeling. It*

leaves me lifeless at times and all I want to do is sleep. To me it feels like I could suddenly sleep standing up. It comes on rather quickly and is totally overpowering. This is more scary to me than having the cancer.

At first I even believed I would eventually get back to work. As the time goes on this has become more than impossible because of the fatigue. I couldn't possibly work a full day five days a week. If I went back to work even for one day a week I'd lose my disability benefits.

I know there are a lot of caregivers who have loved ones experiencing this fatigue. It can't be described as being "tired." That's different. It's not like being tired from working hard or having a long day.

It's more like a hood has been put over your head and you are experiencing almost an out-of-body experience of complete body exhaustion. It comes on suddenly, and sometimes just a quick nap lifts the cloak from your head and you feel refreshed. At other times it's enough to put me to sleep for nine to twelve hours. My muscles don't ache from overwork or exhaustion, it's just a drained feeling. At these times I'm too tired to eat even if I'm hungry. I'm actually having difficulty describing the feeling, but I'm sure all cancer survivors know what I'm trying to express in words.

I sometimes sit here and cry when I feel the fatigue overtaking me. I literally have tears rolling down my face. My wife will say, "Shelly, are you okay?" I just answer, "The fatigue is killing me. It doesn't let me enjoy the life I have left." I'm in no pain from either the colon surgery nor the liver damage from the disease.

Here it is almost 8:00 AM and I've been up since 5:00 AM; slept last night about nine hours. I feel like I haven't slept at all. Does this feeling ever go away? There is so much I want to do today and my body is just not ready.

While being treated, you may be able to offset some of the effects of fatigue on well-being and performance by getting as much rest as possible, eating well, and exercising moderately. Nonetheless, you may do best to adjust your demands on yourself to these new circumstances: let the less critical things go, and attend only to what matters the most.

Symptoms of fatigue should improve after treatment ends; however, many cancer survivors report fatigue years after treatment.

Sleep disorders also are common, and in some cases persist years after treatment. Insomnia, "night horrors," and corresponding daytime sleepiness plague many colorectal cancer survivors.

Because fatigue can have so many causes—nutritional deficit, drug interactions, tumor activity, tumor death, inability to exercise, depression, changed sleep patterns—it is difficult to treat fatigue with other than trial-and-error methods. Ask your doctor for suggestions for dealing with this problem, and see Chapter 12, *Stress and the Immune System*, for additional ideas.

A web site staffed by oncology nurses for cancer survivors suffering from post-treatment fatigue can be found at *http://www.cancerfatigue.org*.

A discussion group for those suffering from cancer fatigue exists on the Internet. Visit *http://www.acor.org* to enroll in the Cancer-Fatigue discussion group.

Fever, chills, sweats

Fever should always be reported to your doctor, especially if other signs of illness accompany fever.

Fever can be the first symptom of life-threatening infection when white blood cells have been destroyed by therapy. Unattended fever in the absence of sufficient white blood cell numbers can be fatal, and is a medical emergency requiring immediate attention.

> *After my first treatment I experienced neutropenia and was hospitalized for five days in isolation and received antibiotics IV. Yuck! During this time they started me on G-CSF (granulocyte colony stimulating factor) to help the white count. The doctor decided to keep me on these shots after the remainder of my treatments. He said most people don't get neutropenic from these treatments, but he thought I might have between the radiation and starting treatments perhaps a little too soon after surgery. I would give myself the shots for four days, beginning two days after chemotherapy ended. One time per day was not bad after the first time I did it.*

I did become very neutropenic again after the last treatment, but my doctor did not make me stay in the hospital. I just had to go in every day for five days and get IV antibiotics. During this time I also developed a blood clot so I went on blood thinners for six months.

Fistulae

After surgery, chemotherapy, or radiation therapy—or simply as a result of disease in the abdomen or pelvis—an abnormal tubelike connection called a fistula can form between internal organs such as the bladder and the vagina.

If you notice unusual discharges, such as urine leaking from the vagina or fecal material or odor when you urinate, notify your doctor at once.

Hair loss and growth

Radiotherapy and many chemotherapeutic agents cause hair loss—alopecia—although there is a wide range of individual responses to treatment in this regard. Some people lose just a little hair; others lose all hair, including body hair, eyebrows, and eyelashes. Others report losing grey hair earlier than hair that contains pigment. Those receiving radiation therapy may lose hair only on the spots irradiated, such as pubic hair.

New hair should regrow in the weeks or months after treatment. In some instances, it might not regrow, although this is more common after radiotherapy than after chemotherapy.

Methods to spare the scalp from exposure to chemotherapeutic agents, such as ice-packing or tourniquets, are not recommended, because small amounts of cancer may be sequestered in the skin or blood vessels of the scalp. Denying chemotherapy the opportunity to kill all colorectal cancer cells may result in failed treatment or relapse.

Conversely, interferons sometimes used for colorectal cancer may cause excessive growth of hair, called hirsutism. Some women taking interferon-alfa-2B report growing long eyelashes for the first time in their lives.

Sue Browne retells her husband's experience with chemotherapy:

Chemotherapy was to start five weeks after surgery. His chemotherapy was the standard first-round therapy, 5-FU plus leucovorin. After four months, it was determined that this was not doing anything, and that the tumors in his liver had continued to grow. This was too bad, because he was tolerating this chemo pretty well, with only slight fatigue and some diarrhea, which we could control with medications. (It has been determined that side effects and treatment efficacy are not related; in other words, just because one has no side effects does not mean the treatment is not working, and severe side effects do not mean that it is working.) This news was very disheartening, and we had to pick ourselves up and dust ourselves off to move on. Time for Plan B.

We then started CPT-11 plus Mitomycin. This time we were not so lucky on side effects. The very next day was hiccups day; day 4 was the start of severe diarrhea; day 8 was his "nadir" point (lowest white blood cell count and he ended up in the hospital); and day 12 he started losing his hair. By day 19, we had to shave it off completely because there were just wisps left. His moustache and goatee are a part of his "signature," so he is hanging on to them even though they are quite thin. I love to touch and kiss his shaved head, but I can tell he is not comfortable with it, so I try to respect his space until he is more at ease with his new look.

Hand-and-foot syndrome

Hand-and-foot syndrome, known medically as palmar-plantar erythrodysesthesia or PPES, is a collection of symptoms of tingling, pain, soreness, loss of feeling, swelling, and skin peeling on the fingers and on the soles of the hands and feet. This is a common side effect following 5-FU therapy.

This syndrome usually recedes when fluorouracil therapy ends. Occasionally therapy is halted if the symptoms become very severe. Research has shown that PPES occurs more frequently when a continuous infusion pump is used to administer 5-fluorouracil.

One thing to watch out for that the doctors didn't tell me about was "hand-and-foot syndrome" or neurotoxicity. My hands and feet became very sensitive to any type of pressure. It was painful to walk, to open a jar or bottle. When I told the doctors about this, they became very concerned and lowered the dose of 5-fluorouracil that I was receiving in the continuous infusion pump.

Headache

Headache can be associated with administration of certain chemotherapy drugs used for colorectal cancer, such as irinotecan (CPT-11). Although headache usually is not considered serious, you should notify your doctor, particularly if pain is severe.

Heart damage

Call your doctor immediately if you experience any symptoms that resemble a heart attack, such as chest tightness or pain, difficulty in breathing, or numbness in the left arm or shoulder.

Fluorouracil, a drug used for colorectal cancer, can be cardiotoxic in certain vulnerable people when used in high doses.

Hemorrhoids

Radiation therapy can exacerbate the painful symptoms associated with existing hemorrhoids. Common treatments for this condition include steroid foam, steroid suppositories, and sitz baths.

High blood pressure

Phone your doctor immediately if you notice rapid pulse, fluid retention, headache, or other symptoms of high blood pressure. High blood pressure can develop temporarily while one is receiving 5-fluorouracil.

Incontinence

If you have had radiation therapy to tissue in or near the rectum, or certain surgeries that remove either all of the colon or most of the rectum including anal muscles, you may experience temporary or permanent incontinence involving escape of fecal material or gas.

The solution to this problem depends on the cause. Ask your doctor what options are likely to help.

Indigestion

See Nausea.

Infection

If you have a fever of more than 1.5 degrees higher than your normal temperature, general malaise, severe chills, night sweats, burning or pain while urinating, headache, neck stiffness, coughing, or trouble breathing, phone your doctor without delay.

Infection can result when leukopenia, a lowering of white blood cell counts, occurs after treatment. The danger period for most patients is five to ten days after treatment. In general, chemotherapy is more likely to cause leukopenia than radiotherapy.

Preventive measures include hand-washing; avoiding scratches and cuts via gentle handling of the skin, such as using an electric razor and patting skin dry, rather than rubbing; thorough cooking of food; reducing human contact; and avoiding gardening and handling kitty litter.

If an infection develops, your doctor will examine you, and you may be admitted to the hospital, placed in an isolation room, and given a combination of immunoglobulin therapy, antibiotics, antiviral agents, or antifungal agents.

Insomnia

See Fatigue.

Jaundice

See Kidney damage and Liver or gallbladder dysfunction.

Kidney damage

Notify your doctor immediately if you have symptoms of kidney failure such as unusually high or low levels of urination, difficulty urinating, swollen limbs, yellowing skin, decreased sweat, or heart or circulatory symptoms.

Temporary or permanent damage to the kidneys may occur from tumor pressure against the ureters that drain the kidneys into the bladder, or with administration of certain drugs such as methotrexate.

Leg weakness

Following radical surgery for rectal cancer, unsteadiness, reduced strength, and numbness in the legs and feet may develop. It is thought that this is linked to surgeries that touch upon certain pelvic nerves. This side effect should diminish in about three months if physical therapy is diligently used.

Leukopenia

See Infection.

Liver or gallbladder dysfunction

Mild liver or gallbladder problems sometimes develop when you are fed only by IV line (TPN, total parenteral nutrition). These problems usually go away when you resume eating normally.

Scarring of the liver, called biliary sclerosis, can occur when an infusion pump delivers chemotherapy directly to the liver. Transient liver problems might result. Thus, if you are receiving chemotherapy directly to the liver (hepatic artery infusion or HAI) via pump, the side effects listed in the following paragraph are particularly germane. Some researchers believe that concurrent administration of corticosteroids such as prednisone can reduce scarring of the liver.

Because liver problems can be a sign of relapse, you should notify your doctor immediately if you notice any combination of symptoms of liver dysfunction: nausea, jaundice, swollen abdomen, pain in the upper abdomen, or mental confusion.

Mouth or rectal pain (stomatitis, mucositis)

Most people remember stories about vomiting when they think of chemotherapy, but treatments for colorectal cancer and other cancers actually may affect the entire gastrointestinal tract, from mouth to anus.

If you experience severe mouth sores, rectal pain that feels like hemorrhoids, or painful or bloody bowel movements, don't suffer in silence. Painkillers, suppositories, and perhaps IV feeding for about a week will help immensely. Some oncologists may prescribe a rinse called Magic Mouthwash that contains a painkiller, an antibiotic, and an antifungal.

> Sucking on ice cubes or ice pops helps reduce or prevent the development of mouth sores and sore throat. I think that the idea is to cool the mouth down to reduce blood flow to the mouth area and thus reduce the amount of chemotherapy going to that area. In any event, it works. The suggestion is to start ten to fifteen minutes before treatment, continue during chemo and for about ten to fifteen minutes after. The down side is a keen aversion to ice pops! I cannot look at, or think about, that particular brand of ice pop without getting the shivers. Maybe it will pass with time.

Nail changes

Many colorectal cancer survivors report differences in the quality of fingernail and toenail growth during and after treatment. This problem is temporary, and will resolve on its own after treatment ends.

Nausea and vomiting

Phone your doctor immediately if nausea and vomiting are combined with any of the symptoms described previously under Infection.

Nausea and vomiting are the result of some, but not all, of the drugs and radiation treatments used for colorectal cancer treatment. Nausea associated with radiation therapy usually occurs only if the area just above the navel is irradiated. Nausea accompanying 5-fluorouracil administration is common.

It's important that nausea and vomiting are controlled, not just to reduce suffering, but to allow your body to absorb nutrients to heal, to keep you well hydrated and thus able to flush chemotherapy drugs from your body, to support your kidney function, and to allow for uninterrupted sleep during which the immune system is rebuilt. You should not suffer nobly through nausea and vomiting as a mark of strength: you may harm yourself if you do.

Fortunately, excellent drugs are available today to control nausea and vomiting. Zofran (ondansetron) and Kytril (granisetron) are two such anti-emetics, and anti-anxiety drugs such as Xanax, a drug similar to Valium, may work for brief episodes of nausea. Some steroids such as Decadron also work, for reasons that are unclear. Older, less effective drugs, such as Compazine, are also still in use, sometimes in combination with newer drugs.

Take your antinausea medications on time, even if you feel well. They work by priming your body *before* nausea sets in. Moreover, if you wait to take them until you feel bad, you may lose them as you vomit.

Keep your doctor informed about the success of these drugs, because they can be recombined and substituted by others until a good solution is found.

Some oncologists start by prescribing older, less expensive nausea drugs because their use is more acceptable to insurance companies—even though many patients report that drugs such as Zofran are more effective than other drugs. If your pharmaceutical insurance option is liberal, tell your doctor so that he will feel free to prescribe his best choice first.

Sometimes just the aroma of food can bring on nausea. If so, you might try eating foods that have been chilled.

If you are unable to keep food down in spite of nausea medication, feeding by IV line for a period of time will give your stomach a chance to recover.

Anticipatory nausea also is normal for many cancer patients. If you had treatment in the past that made you ill, during subsequent visits your central nervous system may react with nausea to visual cues or odors in the doctor's office before treatment is begun. You're not crazy: many people report this reaction, even years after treatment. Chapter 12 describes this subconscious and unbidden learning process more fully.

> My husband took CPT-11 for seven months. He was on the four-weeks-on, two-weeks-off schedule. To help with side effects, we lengthened the infusion time from ninety minutes to two hours. In addition to the Decadron and Zofran which he took prior to the infusion, he often took Zofran every eight hours for several days after. Some people have their nausea controlled better with Kytril or Ativan rather than Zofran.

Neutropenia

See Infection.

Numbness and tingling

Peripheral neuropathy, which may include numbness, tingling, or pain in hands and feet, is sometimes seen after platinum-based therapy, such as oxaliplatin. Peripheral neuropathy associated with oxaliplatin is temporary; no treatment exists yet for this side effect.

Neuropathies of the pelvis may follow radiation therapy for rectal cancer, including pain, loss of sensation, or loss of bladder or anal control. These side effects are more pronounced when intraoperative radiotherapy (IORT) is used.

See also Hand-and-foot syndrome.

Pain

Pain can be caused by surgery, by drugs used for colorectal cancer, or by radiation therapy.

Postsurgical pain may persist for months or years following treatment. Although advanced surgical techniques are used to reduce pain, chiefly by avoiding nerve groups, the surgeon's primary concern is the curing of cancer by removing all diseased tissue. At times, healthy tissue must be sacrificed in order to achieve this goal. As a result, a variety of persistent painful phenomena might be experienced by colorectal cancer survivors, such as pelvic pain that spreads to other body parts, perineal pain, or phantom anus syndrome, a sensation of pain in nonexistent tissue after anal tissue has been removed.

Severe back pain may be associated with degenerative changes to the spine following radiation therapy targeted near the spine. Surgery to fuse spinal discs may alleviate this pain. Painful radiation fibrosis, a reaction of the immune system after exposure to radiation, can develop in any tissue that has been irradiated. Burning perineum syndrome, a sensation of burning pain in or near the scrotum, vagina, or near the anus, is known to occur in some colorectal cancer survivors treated with radiotherapy.

Pain in the hands and feet or abdominal cramps may arise during chemotherapy with 5-fluorouracil. See Abdominal pain and Hand-and-foot syndrome.

Pain during therapy that involves radiation implants may occur. Ask for pain medication immediately if the implants or the position you must hold cause pain. Report any unusual symptoms such as burning or sweating.

Many other examples could be listed, as pain is a symptom of many aberrant physical processes. The best treatment depends on a correct diagnosis. Consult your doctor or a pain management specialist to find the best treatment for your pain.

A discussion group for those suffering from cancer pain exists on the Internet. Visit *http://www.acor.org* to enroll in the Cancer-Pain discussion group.

Palmar-plantar erythrodysesthesia

See Hand-and-foot syndrome.

Pancytopenia

Pancytopenia is a lowering of all blood cells counts. It's treated with transfusions of red cells, platelets, or irradiated whole blood. See Infection for additional information.

Peripheral neuropathy

See Numbness and tingling.

Poor wound healing

Some treatment regimens call for chemotherapy, radiotherapy, or both before surgery in order to reduce the size of the tumor, thus enhancing the chance of a more successful surgical removal.

Both chemotherapy and radiotherapy can cause delays in wound healing by compromising the ability of healthy tissues to multiply and form scar tissue. Speak with your doctor as soon as possible if you suspect your healing is not progressing as it should.

Postsurgical confusion

Mild confusion to frank psychotic behavior occurs in some people following general anesthesia, especially in those over age 50. Although time is the best cure, a change in pain medication or room location might also help.

Pulmonary thrombosis

See Blood clots.

Radiation enteritis and proctitis (RASBI)

Radiotherapy targeted to the abdomen or pelvis can cause abdominal or rectal pain, diarrhea, bloody stools, or mucus in stools, also called radiation-associated small-bowel injury (RASBI). It may be a short-term effect that fades in four to eight weeks after treatment ends, or, in 5 to 15 percent of patients, it may become a long-term chronic problem.

Interference with the absorption of nutrients is one of the chief concerns. Enteritis is treated by controlling diarrhea with Kaopectate, Lomotil, Paregoric, Cholestyramine, Donnatal, Immodium, or narcotics. Steroid foam may be prescribed if the rectum is quite sore.

For some people, a change in diet might alleviate symptoms. Avoidance of lactose, fats, wheat gluten, and high carbohydrates reportedly help some colorectal cancer survivors with RASBI.

See also Abdominal pain and Diarrhea.

Recall sensitivities

Radiation therapy may damage tissue in a way that leaves it reactive to further treatment for months or years afterward. Radiation to an area can cause tissue in that area to react with pain and dysfunction when chemotherapy is administered afterward.

Rectal perforation

Radiotherapy for rectal cancer can weaken healthy tissue such that it may rupture. This is more often a late effect of radiotherapy, but may occur more quickly in certain people.

If you have unusual rectal or pelvic pain, fever, unusual odor of bowel movements, passage of feces from the vagina, contact your doctor immediately.

Runny nose

Administration of the drug CPT-11 (irinotecan) can cause production of excess bodily fluids in some cases. Addition of atropine offsets these symptoms.

Sexual problems

A variety of problems with sexual performance and enjoyment can arise after surgery or radiotherapy for colorectal cancer. These problems are discussed in Chapter 18, *Sexuality, Fertility, and Pregnancy*.

A discussion group for those dealing with issues of sexuality following cancer treatment exists on the Internet. Visit *http://www.acor.org* to enroll in the Cancer-Sexuality discussion group.

Skin problems

A variety of skin problems—pain, burning, discoloration, scaling, wrinkling, dryness, rash, hives, redness, peeling, sun sensitivity—are associated with some treatments for colorectal cancer. Radiation therapy and certain chemotherapies used for colorectal cancers, such as fluorouracil and irinotecan (CPT-11), can cause skin problems.

Ask your doctor for help before tackling this on your own, because dermatology problems can be complex and hard to diagnose, and because certain skin symptoms, such as itching, may be a sign of an allergic response, or of serious changes such as relapse in the liver. Common remedies, such as lotions that contain alcohol, may make the problem worse, especially if itching is your chief complaint or if radiotherapy is still underway.

> *Sitz baths, baby wipes, and Balmex are good for symptoms that follow radiation therapy. I might add that I switched around to A&D ointment here and there. My radiation therapists told me to tell them about any side effects and were a great help. They gave me a purified aloe vera gel to use (don't get it over the counter).*

> *The way I look at it is, some people will have greater problems than others. The main thing is speak up as soon as side effects show up, and the sooner relief will be attained!*

Sore throat

For several drugs used against colorectal cancer, sore throat is a known side effect that is generally bothersome but not always serious. Contact your doctor so that she can determine whether this side effect is serious in your case, especially if sore throat is accompanied by other symptoms of allergic reaction or by fever.

Stomatitis

See Mouth or rectal pain.

Sun sensitivity

See Skin problems.

Sweating

Administration of the drug CPT-11 (irinotecan) can cause profuse sweating in some cases. Addition of atropine offsets these symptoms.

Tumor lysis syndrome

The waste products of a tumor as it dies may disrupt natural levels of body substances such as electrolytes or antidiuretic hormone.

Tumor lysis syndrome, arising from the death of large tumors, may arise shortly after chemotherapy is started. Symptoms of kidney failure owing to excessive amounts of calcium, phosphate, and potassium being released by dying tumors are noteworthy, and can be offset with oral or IV hydration, careful monitoring of electrolytes, and use of diuretics.

If you or your loved ones notice any unusual symptoms, especially excessive thirst, unusually high or low levels of urination, swollen limbs, yellowing skin, decreased sweat, abdominal pain, or heart or circulatory symptoms, call the doctor.

Ulceration

Following radiation therapy, healthy skin that was in the path of the radiation beam might ulcerate. The condition might become chronic.

See Poor wound healing for more information.

Urinary problems

Radical pelvic surgery may affect urination by damaging tissue or nerves, or by causing adhesions—stringlike scar tissue—to develop and constrict the bladder or ureters.

Radiation therapy that cannot avoid the bladder may cause temporary or permanent changes in bladder function. The bladder may become less elastic, and the urge to urinate may become more frequent.

Urinary problems should be reported to your doctor promptly, as tumor pressure upon the bladder, or upon ureters that drain the kidneys into the bladder, also can cause urinary problems.

Water retention

See Urinary problems, Kidney damage, and Heart damage.

Weight loss

Most chemotherapies as well as radiotherapy for colorectal cancer cause rapidly dividing cells to die more frequently than other cells. As the cells lining the gastrointestinal tract are rapidly dividing cells, when these are exposed to anticancer drugs, they die sooner than their natural cycle would dictate. As a result, it may become difficult to absorb nutrients during treatment for colorectal cancer; the effect is made worse if nausea and diarrhea are present.

If you are losing weight during treatment, notify your doctor.

See the suggestions included under Appetite or taste changes, Diarrhea, and Nausea and vomiting.

Summary

Many cancer survivors expect that treatment will make them feel bad, but they're not sure exactly what to expect. Some are delighted to find that they experience very few side effects of treatment, or none at all.

This chapter may serve as a reference for you as treatment unfolds. Knowing which effects of treatment are temporary, which are harmless, and what to do about those that are not, is a useful beginning to dealing with treatment.

Some side effects linger, and can be classified as late effects. Some effects that usually do not emerge until months after treatment may emerge sooner in some patients. Late effects are described more fully in Chapter 17, *Late Effects, Late Complications*.

See the bibliography for a selection of excellent books that describe side effects, and how to deal with them, in greater depth.

Points to remember:

- The most common side effects of therapy for colorectal cancer are fatigue, nausea, diarrhea, and mouth sores.

- Contact your doctor if you experience unpleasant side effects. Almost all can be treated successfully.

Stress and the Immune System

*A good laugh and a long sleep are
the best cures in the doctor's book.*

—Irish proverb

SOME PEOPLE BELIEVE THAT THEIR COLORECTAL CANCER was caused by stress, or that it will be made worse by stress, or that perhaps they have a cancer-prone personality. Many research studies have attempted to discover links between cancer, stress, depression, personality, and coping skills. The connections are complex:

- First, there is no consistent evidence that stress causes or worsens cancer. Studies done using animals and humans do not consistently show a positive association between stress and cancer, not even when underlying disease already exists. In fact, in some animals, some forms of stress cause tumors to shrink. More details are provided later in this chapter, under "Stress and cancer?".

- Second, the few studies that hint at a link between personality and cancer are not conclusive for various reasons, such as the design of the study. Details are discussed in the section entitled "A cancer personality?", which appears later in this chapter.

This chapter will describe the known associations—or the lack of them—between stress, the immune system, illness, and cancer. A definition of stress is offered, then physical and emotional responses to stress are described, followed by a discussion of the evidence, or the lack of it, regarding stress and cancer. This chapter concludes with ways you can minimize stress or make stress a useful experience.

What is stress?

Experts in various fields of medicine and psychology recognize many different circumstances and events as stressful. Depending on the circumstances or point of view, stress could be viewed as a threatening object or the event itself, the physical reaction within our bodies to the threat, or the state of mind that precedes our taking some action in response to the threat.

To the psychiatrist studying brain chemistry, our awakening in the morning and the corresponding rise or fall in levels of several hormones may be viewed as a stressful event for the constantly adapting brain. For the psychologist, overcrowding of humans in urban areas can be viewed as a stressful event. For an orthopedic surgeon, the impact sustained by cartilage within the knee when one runs on concrete is viewed as stress.

The psychoneuroimmunologist, however, views the interaction of the immune system with the central nervous system as an adaptation to stress. This interpretation, which can accommodate both physical and emotional stress, will be the chief focus of this chapter.

For the sake of readability, we won't differentiate between responses and reactions, nor between anxiety and worry. We will assume that the stress of a cancer diagnosis causes distress, although some authorities maintain that not all stressors cause distress.

Responses to stress

Our bodies and minds respond to stress in many ways. These adaptations may change with the type and intensity of the stressor, with the amount of time we have been exposed to it, with our previous experiences trying to adapt to similar stressful events, with the person experiencing stress, and his or her physical and emotional state at the time.

Although many emotional responses to stress are possible, such as anger and withdrawal, the responses most often reported by cancer survivors are fear, anxiety, and depression. The National Cancer Institute reports that during and after diagnosis and treatment, almost 50 percent of cancer patients report anxiety and about 25 percent report significant anxiety; 20 percent experience transient or long-term depression; and 15 percent are diagnosed with post-traumatic stress disorder. Estimates by other researchers are sometimes much higher.

Fear is sometimes useful

Several bodily changes occur as a reaction to a fearful event. During fear, hormones that prepare us to adapt to stress are released in a chain reaction, first from the brain, which trigger in turn the release of antistress hormones from the adrenal glands. Our heart rate increases, blood is redirected to body parts associated with fight or flight, and extra sugar is made available in the bloodstream via the liver.

Fear can be a useful, goal-oriented reaction to a stressor. Each of these physical changes is aimed either at our fleeing from danger or conquering it bodily.

Fascinating research into brain structure and function has shown that the amygdala, part of the "old brain" conserved in most creatures from reptiles up through the primates, including humans, is the brain organ responsible for finding safety quickly when fear arises. Direct connections between the amygdala and our sensory organs bypass the higher brain centers of decision-making, allowing us to react very quickly to threats, sometimes without our being aware that we have perceived them. For instance, if you hike in the woods, have you ever stopped abruptly after sensing just a muted change of color or pattern, and upon closer inspection realize that subtle difference is a snake? This brain connection is probably responsible for the immediate, calm, highly effective, goal-oriented behavior that some people exhibit in unbelievably horrifying situations.

Although fear doesn't feel good, it can be a useful, goal-oriented reaction to a stressor. It galvanizes us and prepares us for action. The extreme and immediate physical reaction to fear, however, does little or nothing to prepare us to deal intellectually with a fearful situation that requires extensive analysis, planning, and decision-making, such as absorbing the technical medical information about our cancer diagnosis. On the contrary, research has shown that both very low and very high levels of the antistress hormones from the adrenal gland interfere with learning new tasks. Short of our ability to jump up and flee the doctor's office, or our sudden acquisition of strength to throttle the bearer of bad news, we have been poorly prepared by evolution for dealing with cancer as a stressful event. As a result, an out-of-phase mismatch of events is what many of us experience when being told of the cancer diagnosis—with a strong likelihood that we will remember forever and with great acuity the perceptual cues that were present, instead of the key points that the doctor attempted to relay.

Anxiety is unhealthy

Most adults have experienced the difference between fear and anxiety. Fear is an acute, strong, visceral response to stress. Anxiety is a nagging, chronic, or generalized fear response. Although some would choose the chronic physical distress of anxiety over the pronounced physical distress of fear, anxiety may be the more physically harmful of the two experiences.

Unresolved fear may convert to anxiety as we begin to grow accustomed to a threat. When we're anxious, the same physical changes that accompany fear occur at lower levels, with deleterious effects on our body. Sustained increased heart output and constriction of blood vessels to rechannel blood to certain organs can contribute to the development of high blood pressure and cardiovascular disease. Altered sugar metabolism can worsen diabetes. The tendency for digestive activity to increase in times of stress can exacerbate underlying gastric ulcers.

Worry and anxiety involve recycling the same fear, repeatedly examining the outcomes and evaluating interventions. We sometimes use this activity to justify worry, assuming that repeated scrutiny will result in knowing what to do if worse comes to worst, but this continual rehearsal of negative events in search of solutions may not benefit us should danger actually arise. The two thought processes, worry and planning, center in different parts of the brain. On magnetic resonance imaging, those who worry show activity in the emotional part of the brain, whereas those who plan show activity in the opposite hemisphere, the so-called logical half of the brain. This may mean that, from the standpoint of providing a good solution in the face of danger, worry is not the best strategy. Worry does not determine the best solution and move on to the next problem. It prevents us from detecting and dealing with new problems in a timely and effective way.

Physical symptoms of anxiety may include any of these: shortness of breath, sigh breathing, dry mouth, inability to swallow, trembling, weakness, incessant crying, circular or obsessive thoughts, inability to concentrate, paralytic or manic movements, insomnia, headache, recurrent nightmares, or extreme fatigue.

What feels like anxiety is not always caused by worry. Sometimes it can have physical causes. In some cases, symptoms that are indistinguishable from anxiety can be caused by the tumor itself:

- Colorectal cancer tumors in the lung can cause shortness of breath.

- Tumors in parts of the kidney can stimulate the adrenal gland to over-produce cortisol, a hormone released during fearful episodes.

- Tumors of the brain near or in the pituitary can stimulate hormones that in turn stimulate the adrenals to overproduce cortisol.

These medications also can cause anxiety:

- Corticosteroids such as prednisone

- Bronchodilators and certain other drugs used for asthma

- The newer antidepressant drugs to control nausea and pain, such as Prozac

- Cessation of the use of the quick-acting anti-anxiety drugs, such as Valium or Ativan

Certain physical changes that accompany incipient medical conditions are heralded by feelings of anxiety:

- Pneumonia

- Heart attack

- Electrolyte imbalance

- Angina

But the chief cause of anxiety among cancer survivors is worry and sustained, unresolved fear. Fear of pain, of abandonment, of dependency; fear of financial ruin, of professional ruin, of relapse, of death.

> *The day following the end of treatment, I got what I can only describe as a feeling of food stuck in my esophagus mid-chest area. For the next 72 hours I could not keep any food or even sips of water down without promptly vomiting them back up. I finally called the doctor Monday morning and he suggested I take Maalox and ordered Compazine suppositories.*
>
> *I wasn't nauseated at all, and thought, "How is this going to help?" But after reading the insert that came with the Compazine prescription, I discovered that it also is good for anxiety. I don't know how exactly it works, but I guess it relaxed the spasm enough that I was finally able to eat something and keep it down, for a day anyway.*

When we worry for a long time about one problem, new electrical circuitry is laid in our brains. Sometimes conditions resembling or related to our problem will trigger anxiety symptoms, or symptoms of physical distress. Many cancer survivors report anticipatory nausea just smelling the rubbing alcohol used to clean the skin over a vein before chemotherapy is administered. Studies have shown that this response can cause their blood counts to drop—even if they are not given chemotherapy in that session.

Obviously this reaction, called a conditioned response, can have a direct impact on the immune system, as has been demonstrated many times in animals. For example, when rats in one experiment were fed a combination of immune suppressant and saccharine dissolved in water, their white blood cell counts dropped afterward, as expected. When the experiment was repeated using only saccharine in water, white blood cell counts still dropped. This demonstrates that the association of event and outcome does not require knowing, for example, what chemotherapy is intended to do. Physiological cause and effect can occur absent the cognitive processes as we know them today.

This does not imply, of course, that you can skip chemotherapy because just thinking about it may have some of the same effects. There's no evidence that a conditioned drop in blood counts coincides with an attack by the immune system on tumor cells.

Depression

Research has shown that those who are depressed often have suboptimal immune system function.

Most cases of depression that coincide with cancer are called situational depressive episodes, directly related to the stress of adjusting to cancer. These depressive episodes differ from organic disturbances such as manic depression or unipolar depression, unless the person has had episodes of these diseases in the past, well before the cancer diagnosis.

Depression may be diagnosed if one or more of the following symptoms persist for more than two weeks:

- Despair
- Excessive sleepiness
- Insomnia

- Appetite disturbance

- Irritability

- Inability to function

- Loss of interest in sex and other pleasurable activities

- Thoughts of suicide

Cancer-related problems that seem to have no solution can cause depression. When we experience repeatedly that our efforts to solve problems don't work, or are punished, we cease trying. Experts call this "learned helplessness," but we know it as despair, and it is linked to depression. Subsequently, when new problems arise that we could indeed solve, or when new methods of dealing with old problems emerge, those exhibiting learned helplessness fail to act. A therapist trained to deal with depression can help overcome learned helplessness and despair.

In addition to the psychological factors surrounding cancer that can cause depression, chemical treatments for cancer that are neurotoxic or toxic to the thyroid, such as Taxol, prednisone, interferon alfa, or interleukin-2 can cause chemically induced depression. Please note, though, that these possible side effects do not necessarily occur in every person.

The effect of stress on the immune system

The stress hormones released by the adrenals during episodes of fear and anxiety also affect white blood cells, the infection-fighting army within our blood. Initially, the surge of brain and adrenal hormones that accompanies stress causes an increase in circulating white blood cells. When cortisol remains high, however, white blood cell numbers are reduced. As stress, anxiety, or depression continue unabated over weeks or months, output of the adrenal hormone cortisol is consistently high and white blood cell numbers remain reduced.

Stress and cancer?

If prolonged stress and resulting anxiety affect the number of white blood cells in our body, does this mean that cancer can be caused or made worse by stress? The answer, based on animal and human research, is unclear.

Animal studies support what many recognize intuitively: if stress had an unequivocal link to the development of cancer, just about every one of us would develop cancer. If stressful life events within the last three years were responsible for the emergence of cancer, then everyone who survived imprisonment in Auschwitz and other Nazi annihilation camps ought to have been diagnosed with cancer soon after being freed by the Allies. Continuing with the same analogy, all people who are diagnosed with cancer should either develop a second cancer triggered by the stress of the first diagnosis, or should never be able to recover from the first cancer. Likewise, all loved ones of those diagnosed with cancer should then develop a cancer from dealing with the stress of their loved ones' suffering.

In fact, animal studies show a very wide range of tumor response to stress, depending on the type of stressor used, the ability of the animal to modify or escape the stressor, the species being tested, the gender, the animal's previous experience with this stress, whether the tumor was chemically induced or transplanted, whether the tumor is primary or a metastasis, and so on. In some cases, stress causes animal tumors to shrink.

Human studies to date have been somewhat less direct in measuring stress and tumor response, because few humans would tolerate having tumors chemically induced or transplanted, or being deliberately subjected to stress. The best study design would follow cancer-free people for years, recording stressful events and subsequent cancer diagnoses.

Most human studies so far have relied on retrospective self-reports of stress levels prior to the cancer diagnosis. This method of collecting information is often criticized as of dubious reliability. For instance, a person who has just been diagnosed with cancer and who has agreed to fill out a questionnaire on life factors may report that other recent stressful life events were not very stressful. Compared to this newest problem, cancer, indeed these events may, in retrospect, seem not to be. Yet at the time the previous stressful events occurred, they may have been perceived and reacted to as very stressful events.

In short, while stress has been undeniably linked, over and over, to increased rates of some illness such as upper respiratory infection and certain autoimmune disease, there is no clear causative link between stress and cancer. Three excellent texts on the topic of stress, the immune system, and cancer are listed in Appendix A, *Resources*.

A cancer personality?

If stress causes both emotional and physical changes, but does not consistently have a part in the development of cancer, what other factors might be responsible? Can the ways a person adapts to stress affect his or her health? Do habitual ways of adapting hint at a "cancer personality"? The evidence, based on animal and human research, is conflicting.

Obviously, animal studies on this topic are difficult to perform because we can't know with certainty what animals are feeling, so most studies are done on humans. Often, the design of these studies has been criticized.

For instance, melancholia, or what we would call depression today, received attention in the past as a personality trait possibly linked to cancer, but we know today that depression is less a personality trait or coping mechanism than an imbalance in brain chemistry with many different causes, including genetics, situational adjustment, influenza, and stroke.

One study of breast cancer survivors assessed personality and coping styles, using a questionnaire and interview the day before breast biopsy. The study concluded that women who were stoical and "psychologically morbid" rather than expressive and emotional were more likely to have malignant findings in biopsied tissue. Here are some reasons why the design of studies of this kind are criticized:

- Those of us who have had biopsies know that this is often a stressful experience, likely to derail our responses, if we are able at all to take such an interview seriously in this very emotionally charged setting.

- Suppose those found to have a malignancy already had a good idea what their diagnosis might be? Suppose this idea had time to develop for a week or two while they waited for the surgery? Would the women questioned be likely to display more evolved, thought-out, stoical coping styles, perhaps not consistent with their usual more spontaneous reactions? In fact, some of the women in this study indeed had been informed by their radiologists that the lesions appearing on mammography were most likely malignant.

- How can we know that the answers on a questionnaire, even when the anxiety surrounding a biopsy is not an issue, reflect how someone really behaves?

- Suppose coping styles early in life predispose us to breast cancer, but our coping styles at maturity are what is measured by these questionnaires?

- What kind of person volunteers to fill out a questionnaire? (Questionnaire studies always face this criticism.) Would emotional women be more likely to decline, and stoical women more likely to comply? Or, if a small honorarium is offered, say about thirty dollars, as is common for many psychological studies, will less affluent women be over-represented because, for an affluent women, the invasion of privacy and the time lost isn't worth thirty dollars? If so, do less affluent women have other life conditions that would predispose them to breast cancer, such as living in an air-polluted neighborhood?

- Suppose the behavior described as stoical is an artifact of some other circumstance, such as working long, exhausting hours under artificial light for several years? Other, equally plausible theories suggest that the increasing rate of breast cancer is linked to increasing lifetime estrogen exposure. Studies have demonstrated that estrogen exposure begins earlier now, for the age of first menstruation has steadily decreased in industrialized countries since the use of electric light became widespread in the twentieth century.

- And finally, if this study had been designed in an era when being stoical was admired, and being expressive was considered "psychologically morbid," would the researchers have attempted to prove that *expressive* women were more likely to develop breast cancer?

> *In my family, we have had five cancers: one male denier who has survived eight years, a female outspoken fighter who has died, an emotional, expressive man who has died, an introverted female who has died, and an outspoken, complaining female who has survived twenty years. In each case, type of cancer—lymphoma, colorectal, prostate, and breast cancers—and stage of disease at diagnosis were far more meaningful to survival than personality type.*

No doubt each of us can think of similar cases within our own experience, in spite of the findings of studies published on this topic. Indeed, some studies have found no association between personality, coping style, and breast cancer.[1]

As you can see, the supposed link between personality and the development of cancer is a tenuous one.

What can we do?

If fear is not very useful in dealing with cancer, and anxiety and depression pose risks for long-term health problems, what reactions and responses deal effectively with cancer-related stress? And if stress is not linked conclusively to the inception or growth of tumors, and may in fact shrink tumors in some cases, why attempt to reduce the stress that is associated with the cancer experience?

First, most people prefer feeling good to feeling bad. Stress reduction techniques can help you feel better.

Second, increased levels of stress clearly are tied to the worsening of certain illnesses such as upper respiratory infections. If you've decided on a course of chemotherapy or radiation therapy, your immune system may be compromised for a few days or a week during each cycle. It's best to avoid infections, and to minimize those that may arise, during these troughs. Stress reduction techniques may help you keep secondary health problems at a minimum while undergoing anticancer therapy.

Third, high levels of stress for long periods of time can contribute to the development of high blood pressure, gastric ulcers, migraine headaches, certain autoimmune diseases, and other stress-related illnesses.

Fourth, stress may upset the balance you're trying to maintain between constipation and diarrhea.

Behavioral and medical ways to interrupt the worry cycle are discussed next.

Stress reduction techniques

A chapter of this length cannot do justice to the history of theories of stress and stress reduction, and the ways of life that arose to accomplish this. Nonetheless, stress reduction has always been of interest to humans albeit under different names, and has received close scrutiny in the twentieth century after the chemical link between stress and hormones was delineated. Thus, various ways to reduce stress have been discovered or rediscovered.

Listed below in alphabetic order are techniques that many have found useful for reducing stress. Not all of these will work for any one person; in fact, it's possible that none of these will work for you during particularly stressful times such as during periodic checkups, or if you have a symptom that causes fear of relapse. It is hoped, though, that the following ideas will help you discover your own ways to unwind.

Acupuncture

Acupuncture is a versatile way to reduce stress and pain, and is particularly good at relieving certain kinds of pain.

The ancient Chinese mapped the flow of energy in our bodies through pathways called meridians. These pathways are thought by Western medicine to be neuroelectric, although there continues to be discussion about the exact nature of these meridians. Eastern medicine believes that the stalled or misdirected flow of energy through these meridians accounts for most of the imbalances that occur within our bodies, and that these imbalances cause illness, and can be detected in twelve pulses.

The central nervous system produces hormones for which receptors exist on the surfaces of white blood cells. Recent gains in knowledge regarding this interaction of the central nervous system and the immune system may explain more fully some of acupuncture's mode of action.

An experienced acupuncturist will spend at least an hour taking a comprehensive medical and emotional history; will use few needles, perhaps no more than six; may prefer Japanese to Chinese needles because they're thinner; and will be skilled at using the needles in a way that is not perceptible, or barely perceptible.

The needles come in packets for single use only. You'll be able to see your practitioner opening these packets, which is reassuring if you have well-justified doubts about the reuse of needles. All body surfaces on which needles are used are cleaned first with rubbing alcohol.

If you have asthma or hyper-reactive airway, tell the practitioner. Certain acupuncture treatments call for the burning of an herb called moxa that may irritate your breathing. When moxa is used, only a sensation of warmth is felt on the skin.

Shoes should come off last and go on first. The easiest and most regrettable way to find a tiny, thin, lost acupuncture needle on the floor is with your bare foot.

It's becoming increasingly common for health insurance companies to pay for part or most of acupuncture treatment, although they generally pay less for psychological diagnoses such as stress than they do for medical diagnoses such as migraine or endometriosis.

In some states, an acupuncture practice must be supervised by a medical doctor. Verify the licensing and credentials of your practitioner with your state health department.

Additional resources for information about acupuncture are listed in Appendix A.

Biofeedback

Biofeedback is a way to relearn how to relax, usually monitored by a psychiatrist or psychologist.

During initial biofeedback sessions, sticky sensors are attached to various muscle groups on the part of your body that seems tense or is in pain, and a graph of muscle tension is displayed on a screen that is similar to a home computer screen. Relaxation tapes or the guiding voice of a therapist are used to establish a calm atmosphere.

When you have relaxed these muscle groups, you can tell you've succeeded because the indicators on the screen have changed.

After a few sessions with the sensors and the screen, you no longer need them for echoing success, and you switch to doing relaxation exercises on your own. It is important to rehearse this stage of independence over and over with a therapist so that soon you can do the exercises independently in any setting.

As with acupuncture, it's becoming increasingly common for health insurance companies to pay for part or most of biofeedback treatment, although they generally pay less for psychological diagnoses such as stress headache than they do for medical diagnoses such as migraine.

Counseling

Counseling sessions with a mediator or therapist who is experienced in cancer survivorship issues have proven very helpful to many people. Three randomized studies, including Dr. David Spiegel's work with breast cancer survivors, have shown increased survival among melanoma, colorectal cancer, and breast cancer survivors who received counseling.

Counselors might be a psychiatrist, a psychologist with a PhD or a master's degree, or a licensed social worker. Some insurance companies pay a larger percentage of the cost for sessions with a psychiatrist or psychologist, but often social workers charge less to begin with.

Group counseling or support with other cancer survivors is a wonderful way to reduce stress. The group generates camaraderie, reduces feelings of isolation, offers practical as well as sympathetic support, and can become the source of many new friendships.

See Support groups for more information.

Exercise

Modest regular exercise is a wonderful, well-documented way to reduce stress as well as improve overall health. Exercise also generates endorphins, the body's natural opiates, which reduce pain and ease depression.

Be careful, though, not to be too strenuous, for very strenuous exercise, such as training for a marathon, can lower white blood cell counts for about 24 to 48 hours. Do only what feels good, stopping before the point of exhaustion. Check first with your oncologist before starting a new exercise regimen, especially if you have had radiation therapy in the chest area. This treatment, if given in high doses, entails a risk of cardiac damage. The same is true for very high doses of 5-FU.

Family

Of all social support factors that appear to contribute to the positive outcome of an illness, including cancer, the support of family or very close friends appears to be highest. This effect has been shown most clearly in studies of white males recovering from heart conditions. The beneficial effect is less clear when other illnesses, females, and members of non-white ethnic groups are studied.

> I am blessed to have a wonderful supportive family with the most positive outlook. That is the advice my surgeon gave me, "Surround yourself with positive people, just walk away from the negative ones, they'll only drag you down."

Most people are both blessed and cursed with family. Cancer survivors report family members who range from saintly, indispensable soulmates to those seemingly hatched by Fate as an example of how not to behave. Nonetheless, at times, there's something uniquely comforting about being surrounded by those who resemble you, share your body language and your mother tongue, regardless of their inclination, or lack of inclination, to offer support. If nothing else, the less helpful ones can unintentionally provide wry entertainment.

Occasionally people have family members who need more support than the cancer survivor does, or who are tooth-grindingly insensitive to what they're going through. And once in a while, stories surface about family members who actually blame the cancer survivor, or family "rivals" such as a daughter-in-law, for the cancer.

Don't berate yourself if you find you frequently need a vacation from family members who put themselves first at all costs. Often these unhealthy imbalances in family dynamics were present all along, but remained subtle and bearable until the cancer experience highlighted them.

Friends

Few other stress reducers are as good as having sympathetic, listening friends.

When friends offer to help, don't be too noble to say yes. Keep in mind that often they don't know quite what to say when they learn of your cancer, especially at first, so they may prefer to act instead.

> *The journey isn't over yet, but I have so many delightful friends to help me along the way. I have to say I have never been happier in my life. I have learned not to sweat the small stuff, to embrace life and enjoy every minute of it.*

If they're good listeners, let them know if you do, or do not, feel like talking about cancer today—and that tomorrow might be different. Undoubtedly there will be days when reducing stress means talking about cancer, and other days when one more word about cancer will make you want to run for cover. Try to sense or ask if *they* feel like listening, too.

Far too many cancer survivors report that friends, even very good friends, disappear when cancer appears. These friends are speechless, sad, frightened, or guilty that they're healthy—never mind that perhaps we're much more sad and frightened than they are.

Each of us has to decide on a way to handle this abandonment that meshes with our system of ethics. Many cancer survivors say that they just don't need additional sources of sadness and stress in their life, and they move on to find new friends, often in cancer support groups. Other cancer survivors try to keep their old friends by never talking about cancer. Bear in mind, though, that for those who are very fearful about cancer, just being around someone with cancer might be frightening.

If you have healthy friends who have remained a presence in spite of cancer—lawn-mowing, grocery-buying, baby-sitting friends, friends who have listened to you when you're scared, or friends who have just spent time with you if talking about cancer is not your style, you're very lucky. Show them that you're glad they're around. The harmony that results is a guaranteed stress-reducer.

Take solace, too, in the goodwill of those you may never meet. The daffodils that appear in hospitals during the American Cancer Society's Daffodil Days in March, for instance, are from someone who wants you to feel better.

Gaining knowledge

Not surprisingly, a book such as this supports the belief that gaining knowledge about your cancer, and thus gaining some control over your cancer experience, is an excellent coping mechanism. Learning about your illness and your options has been proven to reduce anxiety and stress, and may be the crucial factor in your illness and its outcome. Not only can obtaining a correct diagnosis and learning about new, more effective treatments result in sound choices, but animal studies have shown that those who perceive that they have a means to escape stressful situations maintain higher white blood cell counts than those who perceive otherwise. Bear in mind as well that, while our doctors often must master information about a broad variety of cancers, or are immersed deeply in their own research projects, we have the luxury of going narrow and deep, learning a great deal about our own illness.

If your doctor seems unreceptive about things you've learned, seek a second opinion or consider changing doctors. An excellent book on this topic, *Working with Your Doctor*, by Nancy Keene, is available.

Worthy of mention is the observation that some doctors react badly to the idea that their patients find information on the Internet, because the information available on the Net ranges from abysmal to superb. If you use the Internet to research your illness (see Chapter 24, *Researching Your Illness*), avoid using the word "Internet" when discussing your findings with your oncologist. Instead, use terminology that credits the sources on which your findings are based: Medline, the PDQ database of the National Cancer Institute, Cancerlit, certain reputable medical journals, and so on.

Hobbies, volunteer work

As a form of healthy denial and, in some cases, a form of exercise, hobbies are an excellent stress reducer. Immersed in an activity you enjoy, you're likely to forget cancer, breathe and laugh more easily, and feel capable. Hobbies are especially important for reducing the stress that may be linked to the lowered self-esteem of those who are temporarily or permanently unable to return to work.

Laughter

In his book *Anatomy of an Illness as Perceived by the Patient*, Norman Cousins says we should take humor seriously. Cousins was diagnosed in 1964 with ankylosing spondylitis, a degenerative disease of the connective tissue that causes disability and pain. He undertook to improve or cure his condition by focusing on positive, happy thinking, and he believes he succeeded.

Funny friends, books, and movies are good ways to forget about cancer for a while, and can invoke some of the healthy bodily changes that come about when we laugh and relax. Two studies have found that mirthful laughter reduces blood levels of the hormones associated with stress.

Sue Browne shares a way she and her sisters used humor and distraction to ease her husband's worry while he was hospitalized:

> To help ease some of the stress of this nightmare and hopefully cheer Steve up a bit, my sisters and I put on a little performance for him. Since he is an avid fisherman, we each picked out a fishing hat and made up our own words to, "Row, Row, Row Your Boat," singing it in a round harmony. The poor guy had to hold his pillow tight to his stomach to laugh— we about busted his stitches wide open! We even made the surly old man in the bed next to him smile for a brief second.

The humor we have been able to share also has a lot to do with our faith. Friends ask us how we can be so calm and joke around about this, and we just tell them that humor has replaced the anger and fear that would be there in its place. We used to always tell our kids, "You can do this hard, or you can do this easy," meaning that you have choices in how you deal with life's situations. Keeping busy also helps especially when you are waiting for the next milestone.

Massage therapy

The back-rubs and neck-rubs given to you by loved ones will release endorphins that reduce pain and depression.

The lymphatic strokes practiced by massage therapists, on the other hand, are location-specific and utilize a lot of pressure. Always check with your doctor before having deep massage therapy, because massage may hasten the spread of colorectal cancer through lymphatic vessels.

Your doctor may determine that professional therapeutic massage of certain parts of the body, those that appear unaffected by colorectal cancer, is acceptable.

Massage therapy is licensed by some states, and recognized by a national organization, the American Massage Therapy Association (AMTA). In some states, massage therapy can be performed only under the supervision of a doctor, nurse, physical therapist, or chiropractor. Your local phone book will list the nearest chapter of the AMTA for verifying your practitioner's credentials, or you can contact the national office at (847) 864-0123 or *http://www. amtamassage.org*.

Meditation

Meditation is a way to interrupt negative, cyclic thinking by focusing on one soothing word or peaceful scene. Those who practice meditation regularly eventually are able to lower their blood pressure and levels of stress hormones. These reductions persist beyond the end of the meditation session, and sometimes well beyond.

Lowering of blood pressure is beneficial for those who have cardiac or vascular damage following radiation therapies.

One study has shown that those who meditate have higher levels of melatonin in their urine, and another study has shown that higher levels of melatonin are found naturally in those with certain cancers. The significance of higher levels of naturally produced melatonin, or melatonin supplements, on colorectal cancer survivors is not fully understood, but a few studies have shown that melatonin can increase the growth of myeloma cells in the test tube. (Myeloma is a cancer of the blood and bone marrow related to leukemia.)

Owing to this unquantified risk, the FDA requires a warning on melatonin dietary supplements made or distributed in the US about possible health risks for those with white blood cell disorders such as ulcerative colitis or Crohn's disease.

It is likely that naturally elevated levels of melatonin associated with meditation do not have an undesirable effect on tumor growth, and that only the higher doses associated with dietary supplements do. It is also possible that all relaxation efforts, not just meditation, increase urinary levels of melatonin, and that future studies will demonstrate this—or that blood levels, not urinary levels, are significant for an effect on cancer. Clearly, more research on melatonin's effects on the colorectal cancers is needed, but it's not likely that meditation will harm you.

Mini-vacations, healthy denial, and escapism

Denial is a healthy coping mechanism as long as is doesn't cause us to neglect the care we need for cancer. Some healthy ways to take a mini-vacation from cancer are:

- Drive to work along a prettier route.

- Schedule day trips away from daily stress.

- Buy your favorite author's latest hardcover edition instead of waiting for the paperback or library version.

- Grant yourself permission not to worry for one hour, one day, one week, and so on.

- Take a nap on your lunch hour.

- Buy a pair of wild golf pants, or lipstick that "isn't your color" and wear it anyway.

- Spend all day Saturday in your bathrobe reading old *New Yorker* cartoons.

- Write a limerick and mail it anonymously to a friend.

- Odd as it may sound, you might enjoy celebrating the parts of your body that still work. Most of them still do work, of course, and rejoicing in this and using our bodies may have healing effects as yet unknown to medicine.

> *One of the highlights of my day is to gaze out the patio window at my lovely flowers, hummingbirds, butterflies, and many birds and squirrels. God has created such a beautiful world for us, we often forget to stop and savor it.*

Music, song, and dance

Dr. Albert Schweitzer once said that he couldn't imagine life without music or cats. Schweitzer was an extremely productive, altruistic, humorous man who lived and worked in a difficult setting well into old age. He was a strong believer in the doctor within each of us, and thought of himself as only the facilitator of his patients' own healing processes.

Music can lower stress and enhance emotions. You can experiment with music to see which type suits your needs at different times. Some people find the relaxing or soul-thrilling effects of classical music best; others find that loud pop or rock music numbs pain, and that its relatively simple, repetitive rhythms and singable melodies interrupt incessant worries. Still others enjoy rediscovering the ethnic music they may have abandoned in the past. Listening to a type of music we've never heard before, such as the Australian didjeridu or Tibetan chord-singing, might distract us from the worries of cancer.

Singing can release cares from your soul, and may realign anxious breathing. Singing out loud in the car when you're alone, like screaming, can lower tension levels.

Classes in dance for people of all ages and both genders are available in many community centers. If you feel that you need greater control in your life, ballet's discipline, controlled breathing, and classic beauty may make you feel better. If, on the other hand, you feel there's too much control in your life, jazz dance or aerobics may allow you to set free some inhibitions.

Flamenco might help you rediscover the sexuality that may have gone to sleep when you heard the word "cancer." Yoga, t'ai chi (an Asian discipline), and Feldenkrais movement, all of which span the disciplines of exercise and dance, are fine ways to stretch and relax.

Nutrition

In general, the diet that is recommended for those without cancer—a diet high in vegetables, fruit and grains—remains the best diet for those with cancer, although those who are losing weight, suffering from loss of appetite, or recently recovering from colon surgery should consult their oncologists before substituting vegetables for meat.

A few nutritional factors seem to have some effect on mood:

- A diet high in animal protein has been linked to anxiety and panic attacks. Other studies have found that certain flavonoids, compounds found in plant but not animal tissue, are similar to Valium in their relaxing action. This might mean that it's not reducing meat intake, but increasing vegetable intake, that lowers anxious episodes in some people. If you're suffering from severe anxiety symptoms related to your cancer diagnosis, you might try modifying your diet to contain more vegetables and grains—but check first with your oncologist.

- Drinking milk at bedtime, or eating turkey for dinner are known to help with relaxation. These foods are high in tryptophan, an amino acid that aids sleep. Tryptophan is used by the body to make serotonin, a neurotransmitter that affects mood and is the target of many of the newer antidepressants.

- Low blood levels of zinc have been correlated to treatment-resistant depression, and to an increase in the undesirable immune system inflammatory response sometimes seen in depressive patients.

- Cachexia, the weight loss experienced by some cancer patients, has been linked to depression, which is thought to be triggered by nutritional deficits, or by the tumor's commandeering of dietary substances otherwise needed for the manufacture of brain neurotransmitters.

Always verify a change in diet first with your oncologist.

Pets

You may find that your pets, considered family members by some, are a unique solace to you through the cancer experience. Animals seem to have a knack for knowing when we need help, and they don't care if we smell funny or if our hair is missing. They don't become instantly bashful because of our diagnosis, and they aren't afraid they'll catch cancer from us. How many humans will sit by us for an hour in the bathroom while we're sick, as our dogs will? And who's funnier than the cat who thinks the bathtub filling with water must be a sign from the gods? Or the puppy who barks at the wig on the dresser?

Positive thinking and visualization

Positive thinking and visualization have been shown to increase immune system function in some studies. Oddly, one study has shown that when cancer survivors visualize an immune system attack on the tumor, using attack images that are incorrect according to what is known today about immune system function, immune system parameters still improve. This may reflect the "taking charge" phenomenon: the belief that you can escape stress tends to lessen the effect of stress on the immune system.

Visualization can be used as described above, to attempt to direct inner forces against the cancer, or to relax by calling to mind pleasant experiences, places or dreams. Initially it might be useful to practice visualization in a quiet, relaxed atmosphere, but eventually you can do it anywhere.

Reading

As a form of escapism, reading is a good way to reduce stress.

As a means of learning more about your illness, reading may make you feel more stressed temporarily, but this may be offset by long stretches of peace of mind after you're able to make better medical decisions based on what you've learned by reading.

If you have a personal computer, reading from and writing to the various cancer discussion groups on the Internet can provide a cathartic outlet for you.

See Support groups.

Relaxation training

This technique is similar to Biofeedback, described earlier, and incorporates visualization techniques, described previously under Positive thinking and visualization.

Sleep

Research shows that even one night of missed sleep lowers levels of natural killer (NK) white blood cells that attack tumors. Although NK counts recover quickly once sleep is restored, persistent lack of sleep is an opportunity for illness.

Animal research on the artificial shifting of the phases of light and darkness shows that the immune system is depressed by the shifting. Fish that occupy parts of the ocean that receive low light in winter experience an additional breeding cycle if artificial light is increased, and simultaneously their white blood cell counts decrease.

Snuggles and smooches

Being kissed, hugged, and patted by people who love you causes endorphins to be released within the central nervous system. Endorphins are natural opiates produced by our bodies, capable of reducing pain and depression, and producing feelings of well-being.

Hugging, kissing, snuggling, and giggling with a child who has cancer has been shown in several nursing studies to lower the child's pain and anxiety levels.

Hugging and kissing your partner can be enjoyable and healthy, even if you're feeling too tired at the moment to enjoy all of the sexual activities you enjoyed before diagnosis.

Spirituality, religious beliefs

Your religious beliefs may provide comfort when little else is making sense. Some people find that their spiritual beliefs sustain them in spite of a seemingly arbitrary infliction of suffering, either because their religion provides answers for the question of human suffering, or owing to theological beliefs they have developed independently.

I am 48 years old—too young to have this disease. I know I cannot control the cancer. I can just fight it, but that's me. There are times when I need my faith to carry me through. We are all different, and we find what we need—and maybe that's a doctor telling us everything will be all right (just like our moms used to when we were little).

Other cancer survivors, however, experience a crisis of faith after their cancer diagnosis. They find it difficult, for instance, to reconcile the emergence of a seemingly undeserved, life-threatening illness with their belief in a kind, nonpunitive deity.

On a more human level, the support that fellow church or temple members furnish to those who need help is clearly an asset in stress reduction. Support might take the form of emotional support (cards, calls, hugs, visits), prayer, practical support (drives to and from the doctor, or casseroles for supper), or financial support for someone who is underinsured.

The May 1995 issue of the *Journal of the American Medical Association* contains an article showing a correlation between religious practice and prayer and increased good health. At least one other study has shown that a person who is prayed for improves when ill, even if he or she is not aware that prayers are being said.

Sue Browne describes her reliance on faith to keep her and her husband on an even keel:

Without our faith, I don't believe that we would be at peace with all that this disease has thrown at us. You go through lessons in humility you never would have had to go through, or at least not until you were very old and senile. As a relatively young man, Steve has been poked, prodded, and shaved by good-looking, young-sweetie nurses, had his wastes monitored, and his hair fall out. We pray all these are "costs" for his survival.

Support groups

For some of us, support groups can be the difference, literally, between life and death. The opportunity to exchange information with those who have already weathered colorectal cancer can provide you with everything from emotional support to knowing when to question your treatment and seek medical help elsewhere. Support groups are an immeasurably useful way to do this, bringing together a variety of skills, sometimes including medical and legal knowledge.

Moreover, Dr. David Spiegel's work with breast cancer survivors shows longer survival among those who are part of support groups, a serendipitous finding from a study intending to highlight other aspects of survival.

Support groups are offered locally in many areas by organizations such as the American Cancer Society, the Wellness Community, or local hospitals.

If you have Internet access, support groups are also available on the Internet. See Chapter 14, *Getting Support*, for instructions about subscribing to these groups.

Water

In the 1930s, marine biologist Sir Alister Hardy noted that humans have features in common with water mammals, features not found in any other primates, such as a subcutaneous layer of body fat, hair that grows in one direction to reduce water resistance, a protective dive reflex within the respiratory system, a nose that blocks water during a dive, residual webbed toes, and fully webbed toes in 7 percent of humans. He argues that we humans may have spent a period of our evolution in water.

Anthropologists may settle this point eventually, but for our immediate use, it means that, for some of us, water is a wonderful way to relax. A good swim or a warm tub with salts and a good book can make you briefly more than just human.

Discuss swimming or bathing first with your oncologist if you have an ostomy. Some water activities might entail a risk of introducing bacteria at the stoma.

Writing

If you have an urge to write, you'll be encouraged to know that those who write very honestly and emotionally about their frightening, negative experiences increase the function of their white blood cells. Writing can be in a range of formats. You can write for yourself in a journal, write letters to friends, write letters for your children to be read when they're older, or write email to cancer discussion groups on the Internet.

Stress medications

Stress associated with cancer responds well to anti-anxiety and antidepressant medication. Research has shown, though, that these medications are most effective when used in combination with counseling and behavior modification training.

There are many drugs to choose from to ease anxiety or depression, or to aid sleep. The newer drugs available today have fewer side effects, and are less likely to be addictive than drugs used just a few years ago.

All mediations prescribed by any physician, including a psychiatrist, should be reviewed first by your oncologist for their effect on your digestive system.

Anti-anxiety medication

Anti-anxiety drugs (anxiolytics) fall broadly into two groups, the fast-acting drugs and the slower-acting drugs. The fast-acting benzodiazepine drugs such as Valium, Ativan, or Xanax are potentially addictive, and can cause rebound anxiety when they're stopped. The newer anti-anxiety drugs such as Buspar (buspirone) cross the boundary between anti-anxiety and antidepressive drugs, are not addictive, and can be stopped abruptly with no ill effect. They take two to three weeks to work.

The mood change following use of the older anti-anxiety drugs in the Valium family is pronounced and rapid, similar to the effect of alcohol. It's unwise to drive or operate heavy machinery when using drugs in the benzodiazepine family.

The mood change following use of newer anti-anxiety drugs such as Buspar is more subtle and gradual, and sleepiness, if present, is less pronounced than with the benzodiazepines.

The anti-anxiety drug Ativan, a benzodiazepine, is often used just prior to chemotherapy to control nausea.

Antidepressant medication

The availability of today's more effective, safer antidepressants is a blessing for those coping with cancer. Unlike the antidepressants of a few years ago, which caused sleepiness, weight gain or other undesirable side effects, today's antidepressant medications are far safer and less disruptive of weight and sleep patterns.

Some of the newer antidepressants can cause restlessness and insomnia for the first two or three weeks they are used. You might discuss with your doctor the temporary use of a sleeping pill until your body has adjusted to the antidepressant.

Antidepressants are also good pain relievers, although their mechanism as such is not entirely clear.

Improvement in mood is gradual with most of the antidepressants used today, changing slowly over a few weeks or months. The fullest effect is gained if the drugs are used continuously for months. Always check with your doctor before stopping an antidepressant lest gains in improved mood be lost.

The best source for antidepressant medication is a psychiatrist. This specialist is the one most likely to be familiar with all antidepressants and their side effects, and can rotate you through several until the best one for you is apparent.

Sleep medications

Sleep medications range from the very mildest, including over-the-counter antihistamines and Tylenol, to the stronger medications necessary for those using prednisone, or those coping with moderate to severe anxiety.

The anti-anxiety drugs in the benzodiazepine family, such as Ativan, are also used as sleep aids. See "Anti-anxiety medication," earlier in this chapter, for cautions about these drugs.

One of the newest sleeping pills available is Ambien, a drug that aids those who have trouble falling asleep. It's cleared very rapidly from the body, so it's less useful for those having trouble staying asleep. When Ambien first was approved by the FDA, it was marketed as a nonaddictive sleeping pill, but post-market experience has shown that, for at least some people, it may be addictive.

Drugs prescribed for severe pain, such as codeine and morphine, also induce sleep.

Some people use melatonin, a substance marketed as a food supplement, to aid sleep. Melatonin has been shown to increase the quantity of white blood cells. This is a risky phenomenon for a person with a gastrointestinal cancer linked to an autoimmune disorder such as ulcerative colitis, because the white blood cells increased by melatonin or another immune-system enhancer could stimulate undesirable gastrointestinal activity. Accordingly, the FDA requires a warning on melatonin dietary supplements made or distributed in the US about possible health risks for those with white blood cell disorders. Always consult your oncologist before using any drug, whether prescription, nonprescription, or a "natural remedy" marketed as a food supplement.

Summary

The effects of stress and personality on the inception and growth of cancer are unclear, and are still being studied. Animal models indicate that a wide range of tumor responses to physical and emotional stress are possible, depending in some instances on species, gender, stressor, season, previous exposure to stress, and biological state.

Regardless of the effect of stress on cancer, there are good reasons to reduce stress. Your sense of well-being will improve, and you can lessen or prevent the chance of secondary illnesses.

Key points to remember:

- Your oncologist should be informed of, and approve, any change in diet, exercise, or medication that you might be considering to reduce stress.

- If you have an ostomy, exercise or relaxation that includes water activities may introduce pathogens into the stoma. Ask your oncologist or the rehab nurse how to avoid this.

- There are no proven links between cancer and stress, or cancer and personality types.

- Reducing stress can help you avoid stress-related illnesses such as upper respiratory infections, gastric ulcers, or the worsening of autoimmune diseases such as lupus, diabetes, or ulcerative colitis.

- Reducing stress can help you avoid digestive extremes of diarrhea and constipation, thus helping you maintain good absorption of nutrients through your digestive system.

CHAPTER 13

Interacting with Medical Personnel

How was it possible that he, a doctor, with his countless acquaintances, had never until this day come across anything so definite as this man's personality?

—Boris Pasternak
Doctor Zhivago

YOUR DOCTOR'S STAFF HAS PHONED LATE ON FRIDAY TO SAY that the doctor would like to meet with you to discuss your latest scan results. By the time you hear this cryptic message, it's too late to contact them for an appointment. On Monday, you're told that no appointments are available for two more days.

During your appointment on Wednesday, the doctor explains that the scan showed unusual shadows in the liver that may or may not be problematic, but additional tests are needed to clarify these results. He describes the purpose of the tests, but you don't hear much, because you're in shock. Your mind is tumbling with questions and doubts, and you find yourself losing track of what he's saying.

When you arrive home, you realize you forgot to set up the test appointments. You realize that you didn't write down the names of the tests—one of them sounded sort of like "pet"—nor did you ask what they'll entail or how to prepare for them.

Parts of this scenario and others like it unfold every day for colorectal cancer survivors, or we may have other experiences that are equally hapless and frustrating. In contrast to receiving caring, intelligent, concerned, and respectful treatment from our doctor, we may experience instead condescension, paternalism, coldness, impatience, or black humor. We may experience indifference at the hands of certain medical personnel—in each case a grotesque imbalance between some of society's most vulnerable and most privileged members.

The relationship you experience with your treatment team will play a critical part—indeed perhaps the most critical part—in your recovery from colorectal cancer. It's imperative that you communicate well with each other; that you, the patient, feel free to ask questions; that you become well-informed in order to make decisions; that there is enough mutual respect to disagree with each other amicably while adhering to a productive plan of treatment and care. This chapter will assist you with learning how to communicate with medical personnel, improving communication, handling problems that arise, and moving on to new and better patient/doctor relationships if improvements are not forthcoming.

What issues arise?

Oncology personnel are human. Because they are human, they will at times be tired; they may be less successful listeners on busy days; thoughts of problems at home may interrupt their concentration; they have likes and dislikes that may be irrational; and they'll experience treatment failures that make them sad and depressed. They are busy people who need to keep abreast of advances in care for many different types of cancer, not just colorectal cancer. Often these demands emerge in their dealings with us. Doctors and nurses may develop techniques for dealing with patients that are, in some measure, a defense against their own pain.

Unfortunately, outright rudeness, ineptitude, or blatant lack of concern may also manifest, and must be dealt with promptly before your health is placed in jeopardy.

Only you can define what matters in your relationship with your doctor. You may prefer to have your doctor make all decisions for you, shielding you from uncomfortable details; or you may prefer to be privy to both the worst and most minute details concerning your care. You may find that you occupy a somewhat passive patient role initially, but at some point you may evolve into a more proactive patient. You may enjoy a joking, casual relationship, or it may make you feel belittled.

Keep in mind that, in the absence of your forthright requests for a certain quality of interaction, a doctor's assumptions about your needs are likely to shape how she interacts with you. The colorectal cancer experience, like most cancer experiences, can be a volatile one, and thus your needs may change from day to day. You're entitled to say, for instance, that, for today only, you want your doctor to do your thinking for you, or that jocularity is not on the agenda today.

Keep in mind, too, that the medical staff deserve the same respect you do. If your oncologist was the first person to give you the bad news about your having cancer, for example, you may unknowingly harbor resentment and anger toward her, just because she was the bearer of bad news.

When should we raise our concerns?

It's ideal if you have developed the habit of clarifying your expectations at the inception of a medical relationship. Few people, however, do so—or need to—until serious illness entails complex long-term communication with the medical community.

If you're feeling disappointed with your care and haven't communicated your concerns to your oncologist, don't postpone doing so. Having an angry discussion regarding a long string of past disappointments is much less likely to succeed than realigning the relationship soon after you feel uncomfortable with it.

If you're the victim of blatant mistreatment or you sense an unacceptable lack of concern for your well-being, it's best to address the problem immediately. It may be an honest mistake, and if so, the doctor and staff will be grateful to you for bringing it to their attention. Conversely, rudeness or indifference may be a bad habit that other patients have been too intimidated to challenge. Delay won't make these problems go away.

Who are the players?

This chapter assumes that the most common failure of good communication arises between you and your oncologist or your surgeon. Nonetheless, most of the strategies and tactics that may work in improving patient/doctor communication also might prove useful if problems arise with an oncology nurse, a radiotherapy technician, a member of the clerical staff, or your HMO gatekeeper.

Doctors have different styles of interacting with patients. The best among them may vary this style based on the perceived needs of the patient, or by a patient's changing circumstances over time. A certain core style generally will emerge, though, and you may or may not be comfortable with it. The following sections discuss a few common styles found among doctors.

Paternalistic doctors

The paternalistic doctor is likely to be a fine, skilled practitioner who will provide you with excellent care. He views his responsibility to you as all-encompassing, and is likely to err on the side of total, but accurate, control. If you're in need of a doctor who will make all decisions for you—and this is not at all a criticism, if this is what you want and need at any point—you'll be very happy with this doctor.

Your first clash with the paternalistic doctor may arise if you want to understand everything about your illness, to ask many questions, and to receive patient, detailed answers. Sooner or later, he's likely to ask you if you'd like to have your very own medical degree. He may even suggest that you ought not to read articles from medical journals, perhaps saying, "They'll just frighten you."

These replies hint that the accrual of medical knowledge is the province only of the doctor, never of the patient, and are the hallmark of the paternalistic style.

Given that you may not be able to change doctors owing to certain constraints such as geography or insurance requirements, here are a few ideas for dealing with the paternalistic doctor.

- Do your homework carefully. Find information from the National Cancer Institute or from reputable medical journals. He may never respect your efforts as much as you would like, but it will be harder (not impossible) for him to argue with pedigreed medical facts in print.

- Be matter-of-fact and forthright; don't slouch; use appropriate eye contact. Note that if you use humor with this kind of person, unless it's terribly urbane, it's likely he'll decide you're someone that he doesn't need to take seriously.

- Be kind but overt. Subtleties may waft right past this ego.

- If you're really annoyed by a particular exchange, you might try saying in a level tone, "Please don't say that. It sounds condescending, although I realize you didn't intend to sound that way."

I found that you have to be a bit assertive when dealing with all these things. I asked them if they were going to do a delayed CT scan and they said no. I told them that a hemangioma was found in my liver at the last scan and that I wanted the scan done the same way so a true comparison could be made. They said that was a good idea and did it the same, but they wouldn't have if I had not asked them. I also asked if they were scanning my pelvis and they said no, that it wasn't on the slip. I knew my oncologist wanted both so I asked them to do that also. At the end, I asked the technician if they had done my pelvis. He said that they did once they looked at my diagnosis and since I was just lying there anyway! It is easy to become so compliant and let the "professionals" do their job. But there is a lot to be said for knowing something about your disease and what should be expected to be done. Don't be fearful of speaking up and questioning anyone.

The impatient, insensitive doctor

Any doctor can have a bad day, perhaps seeming impatient or even cruelly insensitive, but if it happens consistently, you should consider finding another doctor.

If you are unable to change doctors, you should discuss with her as soon as possible your unhappiness about being offended or hurt. You may have some success in being very forthright and firm with this sort of doctor, because when humane factors cease to be honored, what remains is a business relationship, and you're the paying customer.

Ironically, this doctor may be a very good and knowledgeable technician, but you're not likely to benefit fully from her expertise if she upsets you each time you see her. Moreover, the stress of having to deal continually with a vexatious person might reduce the ability of your immune system to fight off infection, might disincline you from adhering to a chemotherapy regimen, or might discourage you from phoning her if you notice unusual symptoms.

The aloof, guarded doctor

Some doctors seem to want to distance themselves from patients. It's diffi-cult to know if this person is cool by nature, or is suffering the pain and burnout of being overexposed to the bittersweet results of practicing oncol-ogy. More often they are genuinely concerned about you, as a patient and as a person, but momentarily lack the emotional wherewithal to express it.

You may find that this kind of doctor opens to you gradually, in response to certain aspects of your own attitude, your sense of humor, or to things you have in common, such as children. Many patients report finding a meeting ground with an aloof doctor gradually, as experiences are shared. To the extent that you warm to each other over time, you probably can expect expressions of compassion, support, and understanding from your doctor regarding your circumstances and the decisions you make.

The equitable doctor

This is the doctor that most people probably prefer. She's able to sense whether you'd like a little information or a lot, and when; she seems to know when you need help making a decision or just more time to think; doesn't react personally if you decide to learn as much as you can, or if you decide to get a second opinion. If you're having an especially bad day, she seems to understand and doesn't hold a grudge.

You can tell clearly that she hurts when you hurt, and she's happy to be able to help you. She rejoices when she sees you evolve through the cancer expe-rience into an informed patient, capable of making sound choices; and when she sees you succeed in finding a perspective that will give you some respite from worry.

The oncology nurse

The oncology nurse is the third most important person involved in your treatment, following only you and your doctor as key players.

Generally, oncology nurses are a uniquely loving breed. Not surprisingly, in some hospitals this specialty of nursing sees a high turnover of personnel owing to feelings of vulnerability and burnout. They care deeply for their patients, often thinking of their charges long after returning to their own homes and lives.

If you take the time to befriend the nurse, you'll have an intelligent, well-informed, soothing ally to help you deal with treatment and its side effects.

The HMO case manager

Cancer survivors report disparate degrees of satisfaction with their health maintenance organizations (HMOs). Often the case manager is the pivotal factor.

The case manager's role is to streamline your treatment approval process, to keep costs down by eliminating redundant tests and treatments, to review your proposed care plan to ensure it meets certain standards, and to intercede for you to bend rules when your care must deviate from the standards of the HMO.

Some, but by no means all, HMOs use registered nurses or physician's assistants to oversee the approval of your care. When this is not the case, it means that decisions about your care might be made by someone with no medical training at all, who is simply basing decisions on rules provided by his superiors.

It's to your advantage to get to know your case manager well, and to communicate as thoroughly as possible. If you feel you are not being fairly treated, however, do not hesitate to ask to speak with a superior, or to have the case reviewed by the HMO's medical doctor. HMOs often keep doctors on retainer for this purpose. At times, just the suggestion of a review by an MD is enough to cause the HMO to bend rules in your favor.

Family members

Family members and others intimately involved in the patient's care may find that they are in an awkward position when dealing with a loved one's doctor. Some oncologists cleave to the concept that their relationship is with the patient alone, and, without instructions to the contrary, all communications are considered the patient's privilege. If you sense this, while in the doctor's presence clarify your wishes regarding your doctor's sharing information with your loved ones.

Sue Browne describes how she and her husband act on treatment decisions:

> Steve has taken a fairly passive role in his illness, depending on the
> doctors and me for his treatment protocol. He is thankful that I have the

desire to learn as much as I can and have learned. (I have subscribed to a colon cancer discussion group on the Internet to learn as much as I can about colon cancer.) He focuses on work and projects around the house to keep him feeling that he is needed and has some semblance of control in our lives and with this whole experience.

General suggestions for interacting successfully

Now that the players and the circumstances have been defined, specific ideas for improving communication are discussed.

In general, the more you communicate, the better your chances of getting good care, even if the exchanges are not always smooth. Many patients make the mistake of not telling their doctors enough, perhaps because they feel intimidated or feel they'll be perceived as whining, or because they suspect they're wasting the doctor's time. Here are a few tips to facilitate communication:

- Keep a journal between appointments of things that you notice and questions that arise.

- Before each visit, make a list of all your concerns, side effects, unusual happenings, and so on, and number them in order of priority—but be sure to relay all of them. What seems insignificant to you may be quite meaningful to your doctor.

- Allow the doctor to distract you only briefly. If she interrupts, be sure to get back to your list after answering her question. If she interrupts often, say calmly that you want to finish this thought before moving to another topic.

- Between appointments, do not hesitate to call your doctor about anything unusual that arises. At your next meeting, remind the doctor of these calls and reiterate your understanding of the content of her replies.

- Use a tape recorder to capture the doctor's wisdom. If he seems uncomfortable with this, you might offer a non-threatening explanation, such as the well-documented fact that one's memory doesn't work well when under stress. After the meeting, review the recording with a friend or caregiver.

- If you don't have a recorder, ask your friend or caregiver to accompany you as an advocate. Lowell S. Levin, a professor at the Yale School of Public Health and Chairman of the People's Medical Society, says you should take along a family member or friend who is assertive but diplomatic. You're likely to feel more relaxed and focused; you'll be perceived as wanting to be on top of your own issues. Your friend may remember issues you'd discussed but forgotten, or may think of things that neither you nor your doctor had considered. Make it clear that you want the medical staff to communicate as fully with your advocate as they do with you.

- In Chapter 15, *Insurance, Finances, Employment, Record-keeping,* we mention how important it is to get copies of all of your medical records and acquaint yourself with them.

- If you have many questions, offer to make an appointment just for this purpose. It's unfair to the doctor and to other patients if your 15-minute follow-up exam turns into a 90-minute discussion.

- If your doctor is willing to have a phone consultation to answer many questions, offer to pay for her time.

- Tell your doctor's staff whether it's okay to phone you at your work. Clarify whether they may leave detailed messages on your answering machine without concern for violating your privacy. Make these arrangements in advance.

- If waiting over a weekend for clarification of disturbing news is unacceptable to you, tell your doctor, and find out her policy about being paged on weekends and holidays.

- Ask how you can reach the doctor or his staff during off hours.

- If you have a complaint, voice it first in a calm, objective way, and suggest possible solutions. Explain that you understand the stress many oncologists face, but that this problem has caused you considerable distress. This leaves you with the option of being increasingly strident later if necessary, and reassures the medical staff that they're dealing with a reasonable, tactful person who understands compromise and human error.

- Keep written details of complaints you've expressed: when and how often.

- Above all, strive to have good relations with all of the medical staff by remembering to say thanks, telling them if you're feeling especially stressed, giving them an idea of how much information you're comfortable hearing, and by treating all people with whom you come in contact with kindness, as if they're facing the same problems you're facing—because in fact, they may be.

Second and subsequent opinions

A second opinion is always in order if you have any concerns at all about the decisions made for your care. While you may have to justify getting a second opinion to your insurance company, and while you should tell your doctor you want a second opinion, you do not have to apologize to your doctor for doing so. In fact, the Hippocratic Oath requires your doctor to seek outside advice when your well-being is in question.

The National Cancer Institute or the nearest medical school can supply you with the names of oncologists available for consultation. See Chapter 2, *Finding the Right Treatment Team*, for more information.

Conflict resolution

Occasionally problems arise between the patient and medical personnel that require more than tact and compromise.

Negotiation

If your concerns evolve around occasional mishaps and miscommunication rather than grossly inadequate care, trying to work through the problem with your doctor may be worthwhile. Schedule an appointment just for discussion, write down your main points and examples, and, unless you have had a great deal of experience negotiating, rehearse what you'll say first:

- Use "I" phrases, or neutral phrases, instead of accusations. "I felt belittled when you joked about my question on infertility," or "I'm afraid that kind of answer about my questions seems condescending," rather than "You like making your patients feel stupid, don't you?"

- Use a level, calm tone and appropriate eye contact. Getting angry will be a less useful tool in achieving good care than an honest attempt to communicate. Either staring down the other party or avoiding eye contact entirely are often interpreted as hostile, obstructive body language.

- Make it clear that your purpose is a permanent, workable solution, not revenge.

- Be specific. For example, don't say, "Whenever I..., you always..." Say instead, "When I needed your help last week with understanding side effects, you looked at your watch and told me to just stop worrying."

- Don't repeat gossip heard from other patients, no matter the volume or apparent accuracy of such third-hand information.

- Recognize that anything perceived by the doctor as an insult is not likely to advance your chief goal of receiving good care. If, in order to satisfy your pain, you corner the doctor into admitting that she learned virtually no social skills in medical school or in life, plan to find a new doctor, because you'll almost certainly be punished for this victory later if you continue in her care.

- Demonstrate calmly that you understand occasional mistakes or that miscommunications may occur, but that you expect them to be fixed promptly and tactfully, and ask how you can help make this easier.

- Don't threaten to change doctors unless you mean it. If your doctor feels defensive, your care may suffer instead of improve.

Third-party intervention

The medical community is a rigid hierarchy: use this to your advantage. If the doctor's staff continually disappoints you in spite of your tactful efforts to get satisfaction, tell the doctor. If a specialist to whom you were referred was unkind, tell the doctor. If the doctor repeatedly mishandles your concerns, say so. Unlike many relationships in life that require a great deal of subtlety and finesse, in this instance you can be quite overt as long as you're not cruel, incorrect, or unfair. Altruism and humanity aside, you are a paying customer. While tact is usually fruitful, superhuman efforts to be tactful, far exceeding those of the medical staff, for example, are not called for. It's your *life* at stake, not your reputation.

If you feel you have a problem with your current or previous doctor that you cannot resolve, you might contact your state health commission, the administrators or social workers at the hospital where the doctor treats you, or the local chapter of the Medical and Chirurgical (MEDCHI) Society, a group that acts as arbiters in disputes between doctors and patients.

Changing doctors

The decision to change oncologists is a wrenching one for many colorectal cancer survivors, but it need not be. If you believe you've done everything you can to resolve difficulties with your doctor or his staff, and if your medical insurance allows, a clean break and a new start may be the best option.

It isn't absolutely necessary to tell your doctor you're leaving—the fact will become obvious soon enough when your new doctor requests information from your former doctor—but you might feel better if you handle this transition courteously, and certainly it will facilitate the pragmatic aspects of changing doctors, such as getting timely copies of medical records and doctor-to-doctor communication.

All states have laws providing for transfer of records, accomplished by sending the records either directly to the new doctor or to you. Expect to pay photocopy and shipment fees for this service.

Summary

Successful communication with medical personnel, especially with doctors, may require a variety of tactics. A combination of skills—language skills, listening skills, body language, assertiveness, diligent checking of facts, tenacity, compassion, and tact—is required.

If a doctor is not inclined by nature or training to accord you kindness and respect, it will be up to you to attempt to level the playing field. If your needs for care, information, or emotional support from your doctor are continually unmet, however, or are met with hostility, do your best to discuss this with your doctor, or consider finding a new oncologist.

Key points to remember:

- Be assertive but diplomatic. You have a right to good medical care, both by virtue of the doctor's Hippocratic oath and the fact that you're a paying customer.

- Get the facts before communicating: keep good records, and take your notes with you to appointments.

- Do not remain in the care of a doctor in whom you no longer have confidence or with whom you have a serious conflict regarding communication style. A second opinion or a change of doctors is neither selfish nor out of the ordinary.

- Be respectful to all medical personnel. They're human, too, and some of them may be facing problems that are just as serious as yours.

- If you have a serious problem with a doctor or with HMO personnel, contact your state health department or state insurance commissioner for options open to you.

CHAPTER 14

Getting Support

Falling down you can do alone, but it
takes helping hands to get back up.

—Yiddish proverb

COLORECTAL CANCER CAN BE A TERRIBLE BURDEN in its physical aspects alone, but to face any cancer without support can be far worse. Cancer can be an isolating experience for the patient, because for others, it calls to mind issues that many people dread, such as chronic pain and the surrender of physical independence. Many people, especially younger people, have never experienced any form of long-term illness in their families, much less the chronic and very serious aspects of cancer or cancer treatment.

This entire book is, of course, about getting you the support you need. Support can take many forms: emotional, practical, legal, financial, professional, and medical. Detailed legal and financial support are dealt with in Chapter 15, *Insurance, Finances, Employment, Record-keeping.* Various organizations offer an almost staggering variety of services to colorectal cancer survivors, most of them free, and Appendix A, *Resources,* contains a full list of such services, including emotional, informational, medical, financial, travel, research, and legal services. Still other forms of institutional support are discussed in Chapter 21, *Traveling for Care* and Chapter 24, *Researching Your Illness.*

The goal of this chapter is to get you the help you need by priming you to anticipate difficulties in communication, by offering tips on articulating needs in a reasonable way and on re-evaluating your expectations of others. How can you ask for what you need, and how can you reconcile yourself to being disappointed or to seeking help elsewhere if support is lacking? How do you keep the physical problem of facing colorectal cancer from growing into additional emotional and social problems if you have a misunderstanding with someone who tries to help you? The support you ultimately receive from others is, in some measure, a result of how good you are at asking for help and at thanking others.

This chapter first details specific issues that may require the help of others: the emotional and practical support needed to deal with everyday issues such as ostomy care, keeping positive, transportation, child care, house-cleaning, medical care within the home, workplace issues, and so on. Next, a few general aspects of communication and support are addressed, such as some typical reactions that the "healthy unaware" have to serious illness.

We'll examine in detail the groups of people from whom you might ask support. We'll work outward from the circle of intimacy, first discussing your strongest, most abiding relationships with family members and loved ones; then friends, support groups, coworkers, and social contacts. Please note that emotional issues specific to the end of treatment and the beginning of remission are discussed in Chapter 16, *After Treatment Ends*.

Cancer counselor and cancer survivor Nan Suhadolc points out that those you must deal with for support tend to fall into three categories—nurturing, supportive, and toxic—whether they're family, friends, or acquaintances. In other words, your closest family members, upon whom you may hope to rely, might be negative and unsupportive, emotionally toxic to you. Those who are less close actually may be more nurturing than family members. In the discussions that follow, the term "loved ones" implies those who are nurturing, even if they are not related to you by blood or marriage.

The chapter ends with some examples of challenging moments in communication, and how you might handle them.

Specific needs

The word "support" means different things to different people, or different things on different days, depending on what you're dealing with at the moment.

First, there are very tangible, instrumental ways that others can support you, such as:

- Offering to locate and interpret medical information about your illness (for which see Chapter 24)

- Offering their points of view for your decision-making process

- Organizing blood donor drives

- Helping you move about at home after surgery

- Offering to do some of your cooking, cleaning, laundry, or shopping

- Driving you to and from treatment visits

- Acting as an advocate for you when you're not well enough to express your needs or demand better care

- Keeping track of medications you must take if you're too groggy to do so on your own

- Monitoring your reactions to specific medications and your health in general

- Helping you with ostomy care when you're unable to do it alone, or buying supplies for you

- Organizing fund-raisers

- Calling insurance companies, medical offices, or employers to iron out misunderstandings

- Being a surrogate parent to your children or grandchildren

- Offering to stay overnight with you if you need nursing care

- Offering to assume temporarily some or all of your workplace responsibilities

- Understanding that fatigue is the most common long-term effect faced by cancer survivors, often lasting for years, and by remaining constant in their efforts to help and understand as time unfolds

> *Fatigue can be a big issue. I have learned I must pace myself, take a nap if I feel I need it, accept offers of help from family and friends. It makes them feel good that they're able to do something to help, too. Don't be afraid to ask for help.*

Next, there are ways that others can provide emotional support:

- Empathizing, at least in principle, with the terror of facing a life-threatening illness. Attempting to understand how you feel, however alien it may seem to them, while avoiding assuming that they know how you feel.

- Avoiding making inaccurate, frightening, and frustrating comparisons of colorectal cancer to other cancers.

- Just being around when you want company.

- Sending gifts and cards if you're housebound or hospitalized.

- Attending to your children's or grandchildren's emotional needs.

- Avoiding asking nosy or inappropriate questions, offering instead to listen when you're ready to talk.

- Saying, "I'm sorry this happened to you. Please let me know what I can do for you."

> *I am observing people paying more attention to me than they did before I was diagnosed. Strange, huh? I shouldn't complain, though. There is even good that comes with cancer.*

Almost all cancer survivors face the issues just listed. There are also several issues colorectal cancer survivors face that other cancer survivors may not face:

- The financial devastation that may accompany the long-term course of some colorectal cancers. Metastases or second colonic tumors may require re-treatment, entailing additional recovery, fatigue, side effects, and long-term effects that impede your ability to work.

- The loss of support over time. Some healthy people get tired of hearing about illness as time goes by.

- Lack of understanding about stable metastases in the liver or other organs. Because you may look and act healthy while knowing these metastases will require treatment soon, others might think you're lying to them or deceiving yourself.

- Lack of understanding about ostomy and its care. Others may assume your activities are more restricted than they are, for example, or they might be uncomfortable around you if they fear odors or sounds will escape. They might fail to understand that your specific circumstances require fairly rigid care such as irrigation.

- Lack of understanding about the abdominal pain that may persist after surgery, chemotherapy, or radiotherapy.

> *I think that the people who come to my ostomy group are the ones who need help. One woman who had a colostomy and urostomy was very sensitive to the whole issue and didn't date at all for a number of years, but now has a boyfriend (non-ostomate) who's very supportive of her. Another guy who's had problems on and off recently got married. Her*

reaction was, "Whether you've got that on your side or not, I'm not inter-ested in that. I'm interested in you. The fact that you come along with this appliance doesn't make any difference."

Communicate these details

Those who have no experience with colorectal cancer seldom can under-stand intuitively what you're facing. You should consider communicating very clearly about the following issues.

They need to be told that:

- Your illness may recur years later if any colonic tissue remains. This is considered a second cancer, often treatable, not a terminal spread of disease.

- For some people diagnosed at any stage, but especially in stages II, III, and IV, the path is an uncertain one regarding recurrence of disease and the success of treatment.

- You may look and seem healthy even while harboring stable disease or a progression of disease.

- Colorectal cancer may travel to the liver, but this is not necessarily a hopeless circumstance. Surgery may effect a cure. For detailed informa-tion about this issue, see Chapter 4, *Prognosis*.

- Repeated treatment, and the fatigue that may follow, may leave you unable to work for long periods of time.

- The course of this illness and its long-term effects may be lengthy, per-haps requiring their patience and understanding for many years.

- Ostomy products today are reliable, not likely to leak or cause other embarrassing problems.

- Permanent abdominal pain requiring strong painkillers may result after surgery, chemotherapy, or radiotherapy.

Shelly describes his ambiguous feelings when trying to balance his quality of life with his treatment and its side effects:

Today is another chemotherapy infusion. Right now I'm struggling with whether I should ask the doctor to cut the dosage this week so I have a better week. On one hand, I want the dosage cut so I can enjoy life a lit-

tle more this week; on the other hand, the chemo is working, so I guess I should go for the full shot. Oh well, I will leave the final decision until later when I'm in the doctor's office.

I'm still trying not to let the negative feelings I'm having overcome my desire to do whatever I can to fight this disease. Every day is a new adventure for me and a new struggle. Some days are definitely tougher than others. Hope this one is one of the better days.

I am flabbergasted hearing some people say they don't want chemo. Hell, I will be the first to admit that chemo sucks, but I would never refuse the treatment, knowing it gives me a few more days, at least, of life.

Typical reactions

In an ideal world, you would be surrounded by people who come forward as soon as you need help. They would know what you need before you need it, would give lovingly and unselfishly, and would never become exhausted. Money would flow without a second thought, and those who help you would expect nothing in return.

Sue Browne describes the wonderful support she and her husband received when he was diagnosed:

The doctors' faces were anything but encouraging. Yes, it was cancer. My knees buckled slightly, and our family doctor that assisted in the surgery held on to me and we went into a quiet room. I barely remember anything that was said after the word "cancer" except that it had spread to his lymph nodes and his liver, classifying it as the most severe grade or stage of cancer. I just bawled my eyes out, and the doctor called the hospital chaplain to come and talk with me. While we waited for her to come, the doctor talked to me about God, but I knew that God was already with me. God helped me call my sisters, and He helped make a way for them to come out to be with me.

I was devastated when I woke up the next morning and knew it wasn't all a bad dream. My sisters arrived the next day, and none too soon! We hugged and cried, and talked and cried, and I felt so relieved to have them there. They were my elephants. (When an elephant is sick, two other elephants get on either side of it to help hold it up so that it will not fall, because their organs cannot handle the tremendous weight and they can die.) I knew this whole nightmare was just beginning, but I also knew that I would get through this now that my sisters were here with me.

In reality, it's not always that way. Often others are only partially aware of what you're going through. Nausea? Fatigue? While they may have had nausea and fatigue in the past, it's likely that they were quickly remedied. They may not realize what it's like to experience nausea for days each week, even before the chemotherapy treatment has begun. They don't truly understand what it's like to be tired all day, every day, as soon as they wake in the morning. Most people may have considered their own mortality, but seldom have they done so with the sense of immediacy that a cancer diagnosis entails.

I had my chemotherapy dosage cut because of my complaints about diarrhea coupled with fatigue and nausea. My wife actually gave me a dirty look when I asked the doctor to cut the dosage, but she knows that at this time it's what is best for me. I don't think I could tolerate another week like the last one without going a bit nuts.

The doctor asked my wife if she noticed any changes in my personality in the last week. She said, "He's still nuts." The doctor smiled and said, "Well, great! At least he's still himself." Well, here's one case where being a bit off the wall is good.

If I ever lose my sense of humor, call 1-800-Kevork for me.

At times, others would like to offer support, but don't know what to do or say. They may say the wrong thing. In some instances, others find it easier just to avoid discussing the issue of your illness. They hope—it is presumed—that if they dwell on other topics, you (and they) will feel normal again.

In very rare cases, the motives of others are not at all honorable, and they may say or do things that are despicable.

Frequently there are good explanations for what you may perceive as the failure of others to provide adequate support. Other people, being mortal, have finite logistic, emotional, and financial resources. They still have their own responsibilities and needs to address.

If they are loved ones, they may have assumed some of your responsibilities as well. They might be attempting to manage this on a reduced income if the colorectal cancer survivor is unable to contribute financially. They may be concerned that the time they're missing from work to provide care will jeopardize the family's only remaining source of income. The thought of losing a loved one is probably highly threatening to them, perhaps causing anger, terror, sadness, and a host of other debilitating feelings. None of these issues justifies unkind behavior, of course, but hidden concerns might cause loved ones to seem withdrawn, distracted, inattentive, overly controlling, or insensitive.

> *I know how hard it is to be a caregiver. Some days we never seem to do anything right. My husband wanted to go away recently and we did. He said, "I just want to go somewhere and not be a patient for a while." He seemed to be so tired of talking every day about his cancer and what was going on, and so on. If we don't have to talk about his health he would rather we ignored it.*

> *Over the past week my husband has been very angry with me. I just try to do the best I can to make him happy. As hard as it is for us caregivers, I can't imagine what it must be like to be walking in their shoes. It must be so frightening, and they must be so angry at the cancer and how it has changed their lives.*

Fortunately, it appears that many colorectal cancer survivors receive most of the support they need, when they need it, with just an occasional bump along the way—if they make their needs known.

How to communicate about needs

There's no one way to communicate successfully with others about your needs. Even among people who believe they know each other well, misunderstandings and hurt feelings arise because of daily variations in mood or because of circumstances of which they're unaware. Your own skills in dealing with colorectal cancer come into play, too, when what was not upsetting yesterday may be upsetting today if you're sick, tired, and discouraged.

> *Part of the reason I don't have problems getting support is because I'm not easily offended. I told anyone who was interested about my ostomy for the first year or so when I guess it was still a significant emotional issue for me. If they so much as looked at me like they might be interested I told them as much as I wanted them to know. One of the guys*

I worked with once called me an asshole. "Nope," I said. "You can't call
me that anymore. I don't have one." He turned about four shades of red.
It was quite amusing.

Despite these ups and downs, many colorectal cancer survivors have learned by experience about communicating with others. Details regarding how to discuss your illness will be touched on in each section below, but some very general guidelines are:

- With your closest loved ones, be as honest as possible, as gently as possible.

- With those to whom you're not very close, use your judgment about what, and how much, to say in order to protect yourself and them from undesirable consequences until you can assess the quality of their responses. You may choose, for example, to tell some family members, social acquaintances, and coworkers a few things about your treatment while avoiding lengthy, painful discussions, or topics they're likely to misunderstand.

- For that group in the middle comprising good friends and perhaps some other family members, try to sense the boundary. Just as you have limits to what you can bear, few friends are able to absorb all of your pain all of the time. Asking, "Are you in the mood to listen to this today?" or "Do you have the time and energy to be my sounding board?" are two possible approaches. And the reverse is true: you need to be clear but tactful if you don't feel like discussing your circumstances, for instance, or if you aren't feeling sturdy enough to have visitors, or if caring for your ostomy is still challenging.

Exceptions to the rule

The previous general suggestions are probably no surprise to you. Nor will be the fact that there are exceptions to every rule.

The general guidelines of telling your closest loved ones the most, with greatest honesty, may not hold. For example, you may have a close relative who handles bad news better if you joke about it a little, but who will never be able to react appropriately to the rawer emotions. He or she may turn tail and run if you cry, for instance. Conversely, you may have a casual friend with a medical background who is a skilled listener, and who can at times provide you with more objective support than your family can. From such an interaction a very deep friendship may grow.

Although most loved ones will support you, it's not unheard of for some family members and friends to disappear when they discover you have cancer. There's no one solution to this very painful problem. Often, colorectal cancer survivors just move on to find new friends, but some cancer survivors justifiably neither forgive nor forget. Sometimes the absentee friend will reappear and apologize, perhaps not until years later.

Cultural and gender differences

Gender and cultural differences in communicating about illness can affect the outcome of asking for help, especially in the US, as our population is composed of so many cultural groups.

Insight into possible cultural and gender differences can help you understand how you're being perceived, how you react to others' responses, and can help you make corrections if needed. For instance, people who are less demonstrative may feel manipulated by people who are highly expressive of emotion; whereas those who are more emotionally demonstrative may feel that less expressive people are cold and uncaring.

Generally, the perception in our culture is that Black Americans, Native Americans, and those of Northern European extraction tend to "report" on their illnesses and feelings in a matter-of-fact tone, or not discuss them at all, rather than show emotion while discussing them. Americans from cultures of the Mediterranean or some Asian groups are reported as being more dramatic and forthright when talking about how they're feeling. Japanese and Japanese Americans, in contrast, often are reluctant to talk at all about disease.

Aside from differences in cultural backgrounds, there are perceptions, exhaustively discussed in the popular press, that females are more expressive of emotion than males.

In short, there can be obstructive differences in the styles of different groups of humans as they confront illness. Keep in mind that any method of expression is simply a style, not a fault or virtue: that is, each style is adaptive or maladaptive in different settings. For example, keeping a stiff upper lip and trying to be the strong, silent type might be maladaptive when you need to ask for help.

Loved ones

Some families work better as a team than others. It's rare for any team of people to respond perfectly when it comes to dealing with a crisis. You may observe these lapses often in the workplace, but it can be especially hurtful when one's family fails to respond appropriately.

Owing to the many variations in group behavior, it's not possible to cover in this section all family behaviors with which you might have to contend. Instead, the most common problems and solutions are discussed.

For many people of all ages, a new crisis tends to elicit behaviors that worked well in the past, especially at first. These reflexive behaviors might be arguing, escapism, intellectualizing the problem, or taking control. For children or grandchildren in crisis, we might see a return to the dependent behaviors they had outgrown. The overall impression in a crisis may be that those around you are reverting to immature, maladaptive behaviors. Keep in mind that colorectal cancer is a brand-new experience, and that learned coping behaviors can be hard habits to change, especially in a time of great stress.

Shelly describes his family's understanding of what he's going through:

> My wife always said, "Salt is no good for you." While she's a good cook, I found some of her offerings bland because she uses very little salt.
>
> Recently she put the salt shaker in front of me and said, "Enjoy." I guess she, too, is compensating for this disease.

It may be harder for your loved ones to help you if you don't communicate clearly about your circumstances. With this group, don't be shy or proud. Ask for all the help you need, even if it embarrasses you. Many family members express chagrin at the seeming reluctance of cancer patients to "trouble" them. They in turn hesitate to invade the patient's privacy by prying or being dominant. Consequently, the already upsetting cancer experience can transform into an even larger menace than it is, because nobody will talk about it.

On the other hand, if your family is closely knit, sharing and verbalizing just about everything, the stresses associated with colorectal cancer might *appear* to be taking a greater toll than one might see in a family with fewer emotional ties and more independent members. The telling point is the success of your family's long-term adaptation, not any temporary disequilibrium, emotional flotsam, or distancing you may experience. Shelly's remarks illustrate what works for him in the long term:

> Crying is a catharsis for me. I am not ashamed to show my feelings even with tears. It's who I am. I've always been a softy when it comes to emotions.

What you need from loved ones may change as your experiences evolve from diagnosis through treatment. Different relatives and loved ones may prove good at handling different things. Unlike coworkers and casual acquaintances, close family members and loved ones probably won't surprise you too often with their reactions, because it's likely you already know their weaknesses and strengths. You may find yourself occasionally disappointed, but perhaps not surprised.

Communicating needs to adults

Ideally, communicating with the loving adults in your life about your needs should be relatively easy. Honesty, gentleness, and especially gratitude should serve well. With a couple of exceptions, such as a relative who's mentally ill or physically frail, adults who are nearest and dearest should be trusted to handle every aspect, even the worst aspects, of your illness appropriately.

> My wife wanted to learn to take care of my ostomy in case I got really sick. In the last two years, though, I've never been sick enough to need help. No matter how lousy I feel, if I can get up and take a shower I can take care of it myself.

In reality, however, cancer might challenge a family's beliefs and myths about their family unit, and might alter the established dynamics of the family. If the father, mother, husband, or wife has always been a wise and strong provider, for example, the balance of power may shift temporarily during treatment for colorectal cancer. If the partner without colorectal cancer has developed an untoward reliance on the strong one, it may be a difficult transition to assume control for a while. The partner with colorectal cancer may suffer lowered self-esteem when roles shift. It's important to keep in mind that often these shifts are temporary. Older people with colorectal cancer may have adult children who want to return to their parent the nurturing they received when they were young.

Many colorectal cancer survivors note that their loved ones become ill, too, while trying to help them deal with treatment and emotional issues. Upper respiratory infections such as sore throats, persistent GI tract problems such as diarrhea, emergence of autoimmune disorders, and worsening of certain other chronic illnesses such as herpes, diabetes, or heart disease often go hand-in-hand with the extreme emotional stress associated with a loved one's having cancer. At times, though, colorectal cancer survivors report that a relative seems to want to be sicker than the person with cancer. This does indeed happen in some families, and if it happens in yours, chances are you've seen this kind of behavior before from that individual. The deciding factor is whether the ostensibly ill person continues to provide help to the best of his or her ability, or uses the illness as an excuse not to help—or even to punish you.

If you find that the adult loved ones in your life are reacting to your needs in unhelpful ways, do ask why. It may be a simple thing to put right. If they seem angry, of course you needn't apologize for having cancer, but it's likely some older, unresolved issues are being forced to the fore by the stress of dealing with colorectal cancer. They may feel, for instance, that they owe you little because in the past you were not supportive of them when they needed help. Communication, humility, and open-mindedness may work to break the impasse.

If attempts to communicate don't make much difference, it may be a disappointment to realize that the strength you thought existed in the relationship does not exist—or at least not for this set of circumstances. Perhaps you could rely on someone else temporarily for what you need. Sometimes loved ones just need some time to settle down and get used to the changes and increased responsibilities that cancer brings.

Avoid asking a third family member to intervene if you have difficulty getting along with a loved one. Triangles such as this seldom succeed because they hint at two-against-one and talking behind each others' backs.

If reasonable attempts to get the help you need fail, you might discuss attending family counseling with the person who seems to be acting out of character.

If none of these attempts works, then finding alternate support or finding ways to live without such people, temporarily or permanently, is in your best interest. Because of the seriousness of colorectal cancer, your concerns must be put first, at least for the time being. You may be surprised to find that, in spite of colorectal cancer, your life is more serene and enjoyable in the absence of such difficult people. A decision not to deal with someone is also a means of dealing with him.

One survivor describes her experiences with being nurtured by her mother in a way she finds less than ideal, and how she and her sisters are handling it:

> Four years ago, when it looked like my colon cancer had returned, I busily planned my "last Thanksgiving." I've managed three more Thanksgivings without being poisoned by my mother's turkey.
>
> Luckily, we evaded her kitchen again this year. My sister cooked the turkey. It was delicious and didn't have pink bones. Mom, in her own bizarre way, has managed to cook turkey in cool ovens and hot ovens, always leaving it a bit underdone or vastly overcooked. If you think the colon cancer drug CPT-11 is powerful, you should taste Mom's turkey.
>
> I'm approaching a new Christmas this year where I hope to avoid being poisoned by Mom's roast beef. Some lady down the street—it's always a lady down the street—gave her a recipe for cooking roast beef by putting it in a 500-degree oven, posting a sign on the oven door that says DO NOT OPEN, turning off the oven, and waiting until everyone is starving.
>
> For those of us with challenged colons, this holiday cooking is the pits!
>
> Each year one of my four sisters gently undertakes the cooking of the meals, keeping Typhoid Mother as far away from the kitchen as possible.

Another survivor, an ostomate, describes problems he's heard about from other ostomates:

> One of the people in our ostomy support group commented that her husband couldn't deal with her ostomy. Somebody else who had had a colostomy for 11 years can't really talk to her husband about how it sticks, how it works, how it makes her feel. Her husband just can't deal with it. It also took her daughter 10 years to talk about it—she's in college now. She said, "Mom, I hope you don't mind I told my friends in college, and they thought it was really cool that you had this, that you live

well with this." It was the first time her daughter acknowledged it in a positive way. One woman who was at the meeting never changed her own appliance; her daughter did it for her. This meant she couldn't go anywhere without her daughter. The woman was in her forties, the daughter in her twenties—both quite capable physically of moving on and taking care of things on their own.

Communicating with children

Communicating with young children has different goals than communicating with adults. While it's true that children sometimes provide major instrumental support if no other family members are available, generally it isn't necessary or fair to expect a great deal of help from children. More often, they can be asked to help with small, safe chores in order to make them feel part of the solution, and to reinforce the honest relationship they've grown accustomed to.

Human children are inclined by biology to think the world revolves around them. Very young infants do not understand, for instance, that Mommy is a separate person who can leave them with Daddy and go grocery shopping, and they may become quite upset when they discover that Mommy is gone. This bonding trait is probably essential to survival for a species whose young have a long and vulnerable nurturing period such as humans and some other mammals have.

This egocentric thought process lingers well throughout childhood, though, and causes children to think that bad things that happen are their fault. They may think that you developed cancer because they were very angry with you when you once punished them, for example. They may even have wished you were dead, and now it appears to be coming true. Depending on their religious upbringing, they may believe that God saw them misbehave and is punishing them.

For many reasons, children see us differently from our view of ourselves. Lack of experience with emotions, fear of abandonment, or just plain being shorter than adults means their perspective is truly different. Often small children can't distinguish a sad or aging adult face from a grouchy one, for example, and because adults are all-powerful from their perspective, unconsciously they hedge their bets by tailoring their actions to forestall anger instead of sadness, which from their perspective is the worse of these two in terms of the consequences for the child.

This difference of perspective may also cause efforts to explain colorectal cancer to backfire. If you try to compare colorectal cancer to any illness they've had, it may create an extreme fear that becomes obvious when the next normal childhood illness strikes them.

For these and other reasons, honesty with children about colorectal cancer is essential.

Communicating needs to teenagers

This is a topic on which an entire book could be written.

An adolescent trying to break away from the family and become independent is likely to experience quite ambivalent feelings if a parent or grandparent is diagnosed with cancer. Just at the time in his life when he'd rather avoid talking to any adult, circumstances may force him to become very intimate and empathic with an older person viewed as powerful. He must be patient and caring toward one of the people most likely to make him angry by holding him to high standards, enforcing rules, denying him privileges, or restricting his freedom. Some find that teens turn surly, or run amok, when faced with the physical, emotional, and financial hardships associated with cancer. Some experts say that boys are more likely to act out anger and grief in violent ways than girls are.

Nonetheless, some people find that their adolescent children or grandchildren are extraordinary in their ability to comprehend what's needed, and that they follow through with a maturity that's well beyond their years.

But, even more so than younger children, teens can appear to be knowledgeable and well adjusted when in fact they are not. This group may have an intellectual maturity that is beyond their level of emotional maturity. A willingness to overlook unexplainable lapses, a keen awareness of dangerous symptoms such as excessive silence, and an honesty that is geared to their level of understanding are wise. Frequent offers to chat candidly are a good tactic. These offers confirm their belief that they can approach you about difficult subjects.

If you have a teen who's developing behaviors that are a danger to herself or others, such as acting out rage, violating laws, or considering dropping out of school, find a counselor who specializes in the adaptation of children to serious illness. Attempts to handle these problems by yourself may risk compounding your health problems, may make you a psychologically abused parent or grandparent—and they may fail anyway. A teen may carry "cancer anger" formed during these especially rebellious years well into adulthood.

If you have a teen who's doing housework and assisting with medical care while continuing to carry his academic responsibilities, thank him at least daily.

> *I have a ninth grader, a boy. It is such a hard time for someone that age to begin with, trying to deal with both adolescence and cancer. My son has been handling my having cancer pretty well, but he is very sensitive and even though I appear to be fine (I haven't lost any hair, and actually gained quite a bit of weight since my diagnosis), when I wasn't doing as well after my last operation, Joe was constantly being sent home from school with stomach problems.*

> *I think it is important for us to be honest with our children concerning our cancer, but I always try to be positive and upbeat, and by being so, I feel it puts my sons more at ease. Since I am now on disability, at times I feel I am able to help my sons even more because I am there more for them.*

Good friends

You expect your good friends to stand by you while you're facing serious problems. Close friends can offer you help such as emotional support, occasional running of errands, some cooking, household chores, baby-sitting, or an escapist night on the town. As with loved ones, you may occasionally be disappointed or surprised if they fail to live up to your opinions of them. On the other hand, many colorectal cancer survivors have discovered that good friends earn their wings in heaven by way of loyalty and selflessness, and that some come to mean as much to them as their family members.

Because they usually have a lower emotional investment in the relationship than family members, good friends can be easier to deal with at times. They can be more objective about some of your problems.

This objectivity is purchased with their relative distance. Good friends, in order to remain good friends, may need an occasional vacation from you and your problems. If you give them space to refresh themselves, they are able to return to you with more emotional vigor.

Most people will find that at least some friends or acquaintances will have responses that are disappointing, but you can't control how other people react to cancer.

Support groups

It would be difficult to say too many good things about the effect of a support group on a colorectal cancer survivor. In addition to the personal testimonials from people who feel they found sanity, love, and knowledge from the members of their support groups, research by Dr. David Spiegel has shown that emotional support can extend the lives of some cancer survivors.

Support groups are the one place outside of your inner circle of loved ones where you can ask or say just about anything. In some cases, you can ask help of support group members that you would be afraid to ask of family for fear of overburdening or frightening them. Moreover, the setting is some times freer than the family setting regarding candid speech, because everyone present understands all too clearly what you're going through.

For some, support groups can be the difference, literally, between life and death. The opportunity to exchange information with those who have already weathered colorectal cancer can provide you with the knowledge to question your treatment and seek medical help elsewhere. Support groups are an immeasurably useful way to do this, bringing together a variety of skills, including medical and legal knowledge.

Support groups are offered locally in many areas by groups such as the American Cancer Society, the Wellness Community, the United Ostomy Association, or local hospitals. Telephone support groups are overseen by several of the nonprofits dedicated to curing cancer. If you have a personal computer (PC), support groups are also available on the Internet.

Local, telephone, and Internet support groups have their advantages and disadvantages. Many people use several.

Local support groups

Local support groups are useful for those who are able to get about easily, have access to a car, and enjoy face-to-face discussion, even about topics that might be upsetting. If you're in a local support group, you're likely to have a stream of visitors if you're hospitalized, and friends to offer you instrumental support such as help with groceries or baby-sitting. Often, members trade phone numbers and form deep friendships.

The disadvantages of local support groups are that they usually contain only a small number of people, perhaps ten or less, and only meet at certain times of the week or month. The smallness of the group can affect the quality of the information shared. For example, if no group member has traveled for care, you'll have to make your travel plans with less foreknowledge. Some members of local support groups report that they feel excluded when things take a turn for the worse, as if some group members want to shield themselves from the possibility that similar bad things may happen to them, too. This is less likely to happen if the group is moderated by a trained therapist.

Internet support

Internet support groups offer several hundred friends available at all times of the day. You can communicate at 3:00 AM when you have insomnia, and you can communicate with other survivors even if you have trouble getting around for various reasons. The people you meet will be from all over the country, and in some cases, all over the world, and represent a tremendous amount of experience. Furthermore, if you're a little shy about expressing emotion in front of other people, an Internet group is a good choice because you can write a message and read what you plan to say before you decide to send it. If you need to cry, you can do so without feeling conflicted about crying in front of other people.

Many of the Internet support groups schedule in-person reunions and gatherings. Often, members form personal friendships and write private email, or trade phone numbers to form even closer friendships. Sometimes members discover that they're living quite close by, and become very good friends.

> Thankfully, I quickly learned the ropes from many people on the Internet discussion group I joined. Knowledge is power. If I hadn't searched the Web first for information on colorectal cancer, I think I would have been shocked to hear I would have part of my colon removed. At least I learned that only about 5 percent of patients these days wind up with a colostomy. Whew! That was encouraging. Sure was glad I knew what to expect when I saw my surgeon for the first time. It gave me the tools to ask intelligent questions. While it may have been possible to have the surgery done laparoscopically, from what I learned, I opted for the big

incision so he could really look around and see what's what, and have the Life Port implanted, and oophorectomy, as radiation would cause menopause anyway.

The Association of Cancer Online Resources (ACOR) has pointers to many cancer email discussion groups. ACOR (*http://www.acor.org*) offers a handy automatic subscription feature for these and other discussion mailing lists.

A list of ACOR and non-ACOR colorectal cancer-related Internet support groups follows. Because the Internet is a dynamic resource, this list may not be comprehensive. The number of subscribers given was approximate at the time of writing and will vary over time:

- COLON, an ACOR discussion group for those with colorectal cancer and other diseases of the colon. This group was started by Marshall Kragen, a long time survivor of colorectal cancer and fierce defender of the rights of cancer survivors. Marshall was a member of the National Coalition for Cancer Survivorship who designed and developed the original NCCS Internet site, and was the original author of CanSearch, Internet software that helps Web users find cancer resources. Marshall died in 1998 of heart failure. About 600 colorectal cancer survivors and their loved ones take part in the COLON group discussions. See ACOR's site, *http://www.acor.org*.

- SICKKIDS, a discussion group just for children, but supervised by adults. See *http://tile.net/listserv/sickkids.html*.

- YAP, a discussion group for young adults age 18–25 dealing with their own illness or that of a loved one. This list was formed in late 1998. See ACOR's site, *http://www.acor.org*.

- Cancer-Pain, Cancer-Sexuality, and Cancer-Fatigue are ACOR discussion groups for those with cancer-related side effects and long-term effects. These groups were formed in early 1999. See ACOR's site, *http://www.acor.org*.

The chief disadvantage of an Internet support group is that the loss of a friend can be very difficult when you cannot say good-bye in person, when you have no photographs to remind you of them, and no grave to visit. Sometimes group members simply will never hear again from another member, and they never learn what really happened. Some group members deal with their grief by creating a memorial web page dedicated to a lost friend, containing photos and examples of wisdom learned about living with colorectal cancer.

Other disadvantages of Internet support groups include cultural differences that cause mistaken communication and needless arguments, heavy mail volumes about topics that you may feel don't pertain to your circumstances, incorrect medical information, a range of social and communication skills, and, of course, the cost of a personal computer and access to the Internet.

A recent survey has shown that the over-65 age group is among the most active and fastest growing groups on the Internet, seemingly not reluctant to acquire the new skills needed to use a PC.

Coworkers

What you can ask of your coworkers depends on the structure and size of your workforce, the level of competitiveness your profession experiences, and the degree to which your work relationships drift into friendships. The minimum you can ask of coworkers is patience and discretion, but frequently they give you much more. Often the feelings your coworkers express and the support they offer are a tremendous reinforcement for your well-being. To know you are needed and missed can be uplifting.

In general, though, exercise some caution asking favors of coworkers who are not also friends, because the request may seem out of bounds, or may backfire if you're deemed too sick to perform well after revealing a weakness or need. As with some friends, coworkers may want to know everything about your illness, nothing, or some intermediate subset of information that's hard to define and may change daily.

The good news is that many colorectal cancer survivors report that coworkers pitch in and offer assistance without being asked: blood donations, bake sales, shopping, baby-sitting, cheering visits, and so on may materialize without your having to ask. Many colorectal cancer survivors report that coworkers donate unused sick days to them, or pinch-hit for them if they miss work or feel sick or tired.

Shelly found that his perspective on work changed:

> Since I have been having such a bad time in the last few weeks, the oncologist decided to give me next week off from chemotherapy. I welcomed the rest. To me it's almost like looking forward to a vacation. God, how my life and outlook has changed in the past few months. A rest from chemo is now considered a "vacation."

I used to be jealous of people who had off the day after Thanksgiving. Working in a bank, the bank was open the Friday after Thanksgiving. Look at another bonus from cancer: to be so fatigued I had to retire, and now have as many days off as I want. Don't know if I want to laugh at the irony or cry.

On the other hand, if some coworkers are reluctant to recognize your illness owing to their own fears or lack of social skills, they might never refer to it, not even to wish you well. You can feel free to say nothing to the potentially unsympathetic coworker if you choose, but there are disadvantages in not keeping your immediate supervisor informed about your health status. For example, if your supervisor is unaware of problems you're experiencing as a result of your illness or its treatment, you may have difficulty winning a favorable decision if a dispute about your performance arises.

Remember that cancer is considered a disability under the Americans with Disabilities Act (ADA), so negative reactions in the workplace that result in demonstrable emotional or professional harm to you, such as denial of a promotion or censure for using earned sick time, don't have to be endured without legal recourse.

Employee assistance programs (EAP)

Increasingly, employers are finding that it's to everyone's benefit if they offer formal assistance to employees who have special needs at difficult times. Employee assistance programs are designed to help the employee weather life changes and become happy and productive again. If your employer has an EAP, you should ask what it has to offer.

You should be aware, however, that if a health-related dispute over job performance goes to court, employers can subpoena any doctor's records, and so are given access to records that accumulate when you use an EAP. This includes material that most people assume is confidential, such as the notes a psychologist or social worker takes during a therapy session, even if they don't bear directly on your job performance.

If you're seeing a psychologist privately, your employer may not know that you are, or whom you're seeing. Clearly, this makes serving a subpoena more difficult. But if you use an EAP, the wolf is guarding the chickens, so to speak. In spite of safeguards that supposedly shield irrelevant material from nonprivileged eyes, your employer may become privy to information, for example, about a dependent child or a grandchild who began using drugs after your diagnosis. These confidential documents also may be admitted as evidence into the permanent and public legal record should you have a workplace dispute that is settled in court.

Moreover, the *Wall Street Journal* reported on May 26, 1994, in its "Your Money Matters" column that some less ethical managers put pressure on EAP personnel to open files they have no right to see, in the absence of any dispute in court.[1]

Social acquaintances

Social acquaintances comprise a wide variety of people, some of whom, such as church or temple members, expect to be asked for help, and others, such as the spouses of coworkers, touch on your life only briefly or occasionally, and probably don't expect to be asked to help. Many colorectal cancer survivors are pleasantly surprised, though, to find that people they thought were practically strangers pitch in and help without being asked.

Unlike your family, friends, and coworkers, social acquaintances don't usually have the opportunity to see you doing everyday things, and consequently they may have more misunderstandings about what you're going through. On the other hand, people you choose to see socially may have more in common with you than, for instance, those you have no choice but to work with.

In general, what you can ask of social acquaintances depends on the context in which you know them. If they're fellow Junior Leaguers or Jaycees, you might expect help, as these groups specialize in helping others. If they're the friendly couple with season tickets next to yours at the theater, perhaps not.

Organizations that focus on help

Your church, local chapters of the Elks, Rotary, or Shriners, or other civic groups may be able to offer you help ranging from transportation for treatment, to financial assistance, to pitch-in efforts for lawn care and cooking. Moreover, an enormous collection of nonprofit organizations exists to help you in various ways. Groups for general needs, children's aid, young adults' aid, home care or temporary hospice care, and pain management can be found in Appendix A.

Challenging moments

Almost every cancer survivor has had a verbal exchange with one of the "healthy unaware" that has left him angry, hurt, or speechless.

One colorectal survivor reports an unpleasant incident:

> We had had a lovely summer day and for once I felt good enough to spend a large portion of it doing some much needed yard work. I suddenly realized it was getting late and I had forgotten I needed a couple of things from the grocery store. Taking just a few minutes to wash my hands and face and run a brush through my hair, I took off, dirty clothes and all.
>
> As I stood in the express lane clutching a quart of milk, I became aware of a woman in the lane next to me who was talking in a very loud voice to the two teenagers who were with her. "Look, you see, that's a perfect example of what drugs will do to you. It's so obvious: the red eyes, the runny nose, and see how skinny she is. You see, that's what will happen if you start using those hateful drugs..." On and on she went, as others began to turn and look.
>
> I have so often wondered how she would have responded had I informed her that these were side effects of chemotherapy.

What you choose to do or say to remarks like these depends on what consequences you're willing to endure. In most cases, the classic reply from Judith Martin (also known as Miss Manners), "Now, why would anyone say such a rude thing?" is right on the mark, but not always socially adroit.

In instances where consequences do matter, you might want to try one of the following replies. These responses are listed only as suggestions; there are no answers that are right for all settings and all personalities. Your style might be completely different, but it's sometimes helpful to know that these kinds of rude questions have been asked of others, and that a few people have found comebacks that were satisfying to them. If someone asks you a rude or outlandish question, there's no rule that says you must be serious in return. Nor do you have to stretch, in your reply, to soothe and comfort the person who asks it, as if his discomfort with your illness was the most important issue:

- The Profound Thought. A deliberately obtuse reply, perhaps quoting something in a foreign language that sounds impressive, but is meaningless. Latin is a good choice because so few people speak it anymore. How many people know, for instance, the CIA's motto, "Veritas vos liberabit"? ("The truth shall set you free"). They needn't know you're having fun at their expense. They'll just think that cancer has made you a better person, a deep thinker. And they're right, aren't they?

- The Escape. "Gotta go! Time for my bungee-jumping lesson." You can, of course, substitute basket-weaving or yodeling lessons if you think this person might actually *be* a bungee-jumper.

- The Sympathetic Noise. Neutral replies, used by therapists. You can say, for example, "That's an interesting point of view," or "You appear to have given this a lot of thought." These replies give the other party the attention he's trying to get, without committing you to agreement, continued dialog, or revealing intimacy. They're also good transitional phrases for shifting the conversation to a less offensive subject.

If you prefer the head-on approach, here are a few of the most disturbing and least informed reactions that some colorectal cancer survivors have encountered, and a few suggested replies, both factual and humorous:

Q: *What did you do to deserve this cancer? (Variation: "Why did you want this cancer?" based on the philosophy of a popular self-help book.)*

A: Maybe because I once ran with scissors? Or because I tore those "do not remove under penalty of law" tags from my pillows?

Q: *They say you develop cancer because of negative thoughts.*

A: That's interesting. Actually, I'm having homicidal thoughts right now, but many studies have shown no link between negative thoughts, stress, and colorectal cancer.

Q: *How long does your doctor say you have?*

A: Why?

A: She says I'm still safe buying green bananas.

A: How long does your doctor say *you* have?

Q: *You look so bad/thin/pale/et cetera.*

A: Actually, I've regained ten pounds, my blood pressure is down fifteen points, and last weekend I walked in a 6-kilometer race.

A: My, what a lovely smile you have! Are those your own teeth?

Q: *What happened to your beautiful hair?*

A: Oh, *this* hair. I borrowed it from a friend.

Q: *You don't look like you have cancer.*

A: Hey, better living through chemistry!

A: Neither do you.

Q: *God doesn't give us anything we can't handle.*

A: My God is too kind to be that petty.

Q: *God must be punishing you for something. (This is a particularly painful comment if it's your child who has cancer.)*

A: Fifty percent of men and thirty-three percent of women will get cancer. That's a lot of people to punish.

Q: *It seems like it always comes back.*

A: It's not possible to make accurate generalizations about colorectal cancers.

Summary

Your experience with colorectal cancer may be the most vulnerable, powerless experience of your life. Getting the support you need is critical to adequate recovery, especially during and after surgery, chemotherapy, or radiotherapy.

We humans are imperfect. It's unfortunate but true that if we don't communicate clearly, if old resentments linger, or if altruism dries up, the formidable single problem of facing colorectal cancer might evolve into six or seven additional problems.

This chapter attempts to help you get the support you need. While nobody knows better than you how to interact with your family, acquaintances, and coworkers, the past experiences of other colorectal cancer survivors may help you spot problems before they arise or view old problems in a new way.

The unique characteristics of colorectal cancer, and the problems you may face because of them, are discussed in this chapter. Others need to be told of these differences in order to do their best for you.

Key points to remember:

- The American Cancer Society, the Wellness Community, and the United Ostomy Association offer various forms of support for colorectal cancer survivors, including support group meetings, buddy systems, wigs, and ostomy supplies.

- Ask for help when you need help. Often, others want to help but don't know what to offer or say.

- Various studies have shown that anxiety and depression are common among cancer survivors. Consider seeking help from a cancer counselor if you're having trouble with incessant crying, loss of appetite, insomnia, or other symptoms of anxiety and depression.

CHAPTER 15

Insurance, Finances, Employment, Record-keeping

*Financial ruin from medical bills is almost
exclusively an American disease.*

—Roul Turley

RECOVERING YOUR HEALTH SHOULD BE ALL THAT REQUIRES your stamina and concentration after being diagnosed with and treated for colorectal cancer. Unfortunately, the side effects of cancer go beyond the physical, impacting your social, professional, and financial well-being. If you're an American with colorectal cancer, you're likely to become an instant but unwilling expert on finances, insurance, and workplace issues.

You can ease the nonmedical aspects of your cancer experience in some ways. By becoming familiar with the somewhat harsh business side of cancer, keeping careful records, and anticipating problems, you may avoid hospital billing convolutions, insurance payment denials, employment pitfalls, and financial degradation.

This chapter discusses some of the more common problems you may encounter, gives tips to avoid problems, and steers you to up-to-date resources that provide detailed solutions to these problems.

It is not the intent of this chapter to address in detail all issues concerning health insurance benefits, federal legislation such as ERISA, Medicare and Medicaid coverage, unemployment insurance, and financial issues. In the bibliography and in Appendix A, *Resources,* are many excellent books and other resources which explore much more thoroughly each of these topics. Some issues covered in this chapter, such as estate planning or declaring bankruptcy to protect your house and car, clearly require the aid of professionals such as financial planners or tax attorneys.

Insurance issues

For colorectal cancer survivors, problems may arise with health insurance, unemployment insurance, or life insurance. Of these, health insurance is the most likely to cause heartache, frustration, and anger, but first, we'll discuss the main impediment to purchasing all kinds of health, life, disability, and care insurance: medical underwriting.

Restrictive medical underwriting

State and federal authorities have begun to address the problem of health insurance being denied to those with serious illnesses (for which see COBRA and HIPAA, discussed later in this section), but purchases of life, long-term care, and other insurance policies are still impossible or expensive purchases for those with a cancer diagnosis.

The impediment is the medical examination or medical history questionnaire. If the policy is indeed offered to you after the actuaries have examined the statistics for your illness, it may be offered only with very high premiums. Moreover, employers who have no annual open enrollment period may refuse to ever insure you if you did not elect certain insurance options at time of hire, which is their only open enrollment period.

> When my husband changed jobs, we decided to just add his name to my employer's medical policy in order to save money and have one provider. What we didn't realize is that his employer did not have annual open enrollment—the only time he wouldn't be asked about his health was when he was hired.

> After he was diagnosed with cancer, I wanted to change jobs. By then, I'd heard horror stories about changing jobs and losing coverage because pre-existing conditions were excluded. I asked him to follow up with his employer to see if he could enroll for their medical insurance. They referred him to the policy's underwriters. (That should have given us a hint of what was to come.) "We will never insure you," they said. This meant I could never leave my job.

> Since then, his employer's policy has been renegotiated for more leniency, and federal laws have been passed to look after the medical insurance needs of people like us. But it was a bitter experience.

If your insurance needs are unmet, you should consider any offer that states that medical underwriting—insurance jargon for a close scrutiny of your health—is not necessary. Some advertisements state very clearly that a medical exam isn't necessary, or that pre-existing conditions will not result in refusal.

Note that some medical questionnaires for insurance enrollment ask health questions but do not mention cancer, not even in the section titled "Other." It's always worthwhile to ask for an application form to see just how rigorous the medical scrutiny may be.

Of course, while most of these offers may be aboveboard, a proportion of these policies may be very expensive. The usual considerations for shopping wisely still apply, but if your insurance needs are great, or your estate planning justifies purchasing a whole-life policy that might bypass estate and inheritance taxes, for example, the additional cost may be worth it.

Insurance companies are evaluated by A.M. Best, Moody's, and Standard and Poor. Choose only those with top ratings.

Health insurance

Cancer survivors in the US complain about health insurance problems more than any other issue except cancer itself. The delays and denials of managed care are the most common complaint, but other insurance issues also arise.

> I have battled with insurance companies and won. I start at the top when things don't go my way. I call the state insurance commissioner. That office can make a difference. My next call is to the state attorney general's office.

> I had one doctor who failed to respond when I asked for a copy of my records. After three phone calls, I wrote him a letter. The records were in the return mail. You can even pose more of a threat to them by sending it by certified mail, signature required. This way you will know who picked up the piece of mail.

> Back in 1997 I wanted to sell a small business, but since I had a group policy, I had to keep the business until the Kennedy-Kautzenbaum bill that protects the portability of an employee's health insurance passed and became law. Maine had no problem giving me insurance; however, Florida thought they found a loophole and would not provide insurance to

my ex-wife due to pre-existing conditions. I ended up writing to the insurance commissioner and then emailed my state senator. It took us a while, but we did prevail, and got the insurance.

If your medical insurance plan is in some way lacking, find out if your employer:

- Offers more than one medical insurance plan.

- Holds an open enrollment each year. Open enrollment is the time period during which you may change plans without a medical examination or questionnaire, that is, without having your pre-existing health conditions held against you.

If so, use the open enrollment period to upgrade to a better policy. Examine all plans closely for what they cover, especially for coverage of care given under the auspices of a clinical trial. Weigh an indemnity or preferred-provider plan, which may trade higher convenience for lower coverage, against a high-coverage HMO requiring referrals and gatekeepers. The indemnity plan may cost more per doctor visit, but may provide you with the freedom to get care wherever *you* think best, without the delay of preapproval, including out-of-state care within a clinical trial, or at a distant but excellent cancer center.

If you have been approved for Social Security Disability Income (SSDI, discussed under "Disability income," later in this chapter) you'll be automatically enrolled in Medicare after getting disability benefits for two years. Moreover, Medicare coverage is free for 39 months after returning to work if you're still disabled. If your income is low, your state may pay your Medicare premiums as part of Medicaid benefits. Contact your local Social Security Administration office for more information.

Losing medical insurance coverage if you change or lose jobs is still a problem, but less of a problem than before. In addition to various state laws, two federal laws exist to help you retain coverage:

- HIPAA, the Health Insurance Portability and Accountability Act of 1996, is a federal law intended to prohibit the permanent denial of medical coverage based on pre-existing conditions. HIPAA covers only employers with 20 or more employees. In general, it states that if you have had continuous medical insurance coverage for more than 12 months, your new medical insurance company cannot refuse to pay for medical care for your previous health problems. If your previous health coverage was for less than 12 months, each month you were covered reduces by one month the amount of time your new medical insurance company can refuse to pay for your previous health problems. No medical insurance company, however, can refuse to pay for your previous health problems for more than 12 months. There are loopholes in this law, though, that medical insurance companies might exploit. Some companies define a change of coverage from husband-and-wife to family coverage, for example, as a switch to a new plan, which could, in theory, restart the 12-month clock. In July 1998, President Clinton issued a warning to insurance companies covering federal employees, stating that such denials of payment will not be tolerated.

- COBRA, the Consolidated Omnibus Budget Reconciliation Act of 1985, provides for a continuation of your old employer's medical insurance coverage for a temporary amount of time—from 18 to 39 months, depending on your circumstances. Always elect COBRA continuation coverage if you lose or change jobs, until you're certain that your new employer's policy will cover expenses associated with your care. HIPAA, discussed above, does not always provide the continuous coverage the law intended, owing to its design and various loopholes.

Some states have older, stricter laws that resemble HIPAA but provide better coverage. Call your state insurance commissioner for details, but note that self-insured employers, which generally include very large businesses, are governed by the federal Employee Retirement Income Security Act of 1974 (ERISA) laws that override state laws.

Self-insured employers may hire a medical insurance company, such as Blue Cross, to administer their plan. The insurance information you receive, such as explanations of benefits, may contain the insurance company's letterhead, but your employer is bearing the exact and full cost of your care at the time it is incurred, instead of paying large indemnity premiums in advance.

ERISA was a piece of legislation intended to safeguard employee pension rights, but it has impacted employee health insurance as well, and in confusing ways. For example, owing to the overlap of state and ERISA regulations, self-insured employers cannot be sued in state courts for failing to pay claims. For this and other reasons, disputes about health insurance claims can become very complex and may require the assistance of an attorney.

Shelly describes his unhappiness with his HMO:

> I'm on the Freedom Plan, which is a misnomer. Here Zofran is about $25 or so a pill—wonder what they will think if my oncologist gives me a month's supply? I can almost see the rejection and frustration now. I am going to ask for a prescription tomorrow because Zofran so far is helping me.
>
> I had a major problem with my HMO not wanting to pay for Prilosec that I must take on a daily basis to prevent acid reflux. They wanted me to buy the over-the-counter Zantac tablets. Finally I got my oncologist to write them a letter and they agreed to continue paying for my prescription Prilosec.
>
> If not for the HMOs in this country, a lot of us would have a better chance of living longer. The doctor said I should avoid stress. How can I when my HMO drives me nuts at least once a month by refusing to pay a bill?

Medicare and Medicaid

Medicare is not just government-supplied medical insurance for those over age 65. If you have been entitled to Social Security Disability (SSDI) benefits for the past two years, you are eligible for Medicare.

Most frequently we hear of Medicare Parts A and B, but much fuller (and more expensive) coverage may be provided by purchasing Medicare Supplemental Insurance, often called MediGap insurance. Ten versions of MediGap insurance are available, identified as A through J, with J providing the highest coverage.

Medicaid is a health payment program for the financially needy that is run jointly by the federal government and each state government. As such, its rules and benefits vary greatly depending on where you live. Examples of those who may qualify are recipients of Aid to Families with Dependent Children (AFDC), those receiving the Social Security's Administration's Supplemental Security Income (SSI), or certain nursing home patients.

For more information on either Medicare or Medicaid, see the Mercer Guide, which is published yearly and is readily accessible in libraries and bookstores.

Unemployment insurance

Always apply for unemployment insurance if you lose your job, are laid off, or if your hours are substantially reduced. Never assume that you're not eligible. Apply even if you have a suit pending for wrongful discharge.

Unemployment law and the granting and calculation of benefits are very complex, and vary from state to state. In order to find information that's appropriate for your circumstances, you'll need to research the laws for your state, either on your own or with an attorney who specializes in these cases.

Life insurance

Life insurance that you buy as an individual is likely to be terribly expensive, if at all available, once you have had cancer. As mentioned in the section called "Restrictive medical underwriting," if you have an opportunity to buy a good life insurance policy at a reasonable rate without a qualifying medical examination or other penalty for having a cancer diagnosis, consider the opportunity carefully.

Some employers offer life insurance policies requiring no medical exam with face values in multiples of one's annual salary. Although this usually is term coverage instead of whole life coverage, it may meet your family's needs very well. Some such policies can be kept even if you leave the company.

Whole-life policies often can be borrowed against, or sold in a viatical arrangement to a company that will buy your policy from you at less than its face value in order to provide you with money now. This is a useful option if your heirs don't need your money, but you do, in order to pay current bills. Generally, viatical settlements require proof of terminal illness.

Check your existing life insurance policies for a clause that states you needn't pay premiums if you're receiving disability benefits.

Long-term care insurance

Now more than ever, you should consider a long-term care policy as a safeguard against financially crippling nursing-home or nursing-care costs. As with life insurance policies previously discussed, however, you're not likely to be able to find or afford a long-term care policy once having had a cancer diagnosis, unless one is offered at group rates with no medical examination required.

One very good option is to ask your children and their spouses if their employers offer such a policy for parents or in-laws as well as employees. This recent trend in employment benefits offerings is an attempt to recognize the increasing responsibilities that families face in caring for their older relatives while trying to work outside the home.

Many long-term care policies are eventually dropped by the client because they are so expensive, and the probability of needing long-term care seems so far away. If expense is an issue for you, you might choose a policy that has a clause that allows you to stop paying premiums after a number of years in return for lower benefits or payments over a shorter time. This compromise, while not ideal, will afford you at least some protection against potentially devastating long-term care costs.

Long-term disability insurance

Employers often offer long-term disability insurance at reduced rates or for free. If you can elect or purchase such a policy, do so. Although the Social Security Administration can pay you long-term disability under some conditions, often it's temporary, and frequently policies available in the private sector pay a better monthly benefit.

Note that most long-term disability policies encourage you to apply for SSDI, and then pay you only the difference between SSA's monthly benefit and the higher benefit your policy authorizes.

Some long-term disability policies can be taken with you if you leave your employer. Choose only a policy marked *guaranteed renewable*, so that your policy cannot be canceled if your health gets worse.

Financial issues

In general, financial issues cannot be addressed adequately in one chapter of a medical consumer's book. Nonetheless, a few issues are discussed in this section to inform you, rather than advise you, regarding problems you may encounter.

Major points

Here's an encapsulation of some fairly prominent issues:

- It may be worthwhile to refinance your home mortgage for a lower interest rate. If the current market rate for mortgages is significantly lower than yours, refinancing may reduce monthly payments, increase equity more rapidly, and ultimately reduce debt.

- Contact the Social Security Administration to see if you, your spouse, or your children are eligible for Supplemental Security Income: *http://www.ssa.gov* or call (800) 772-1213. (SSI differs from SSDI, Social Security Disability Income.)

- Fundraising in your community or your place of employment can be a very effective way to address debts related to medical care. The Organ Transplant Fund, for example, provides sound help with raising funds for liver transplantation. See Appendix A, *Resources*, for a list of other organizations that can help with financial issues such as fundraising.

- Estate planning should always be considered, even for seemingly small estates. Some options, such as a supportive care trust or purchase of a whole-life insurance policy, may preserve some assets for yourself, your spouse, or your children—but may interfere seriously with your eligibility for Medicare. Estate planning is especially important if your spouse or a child has serious health problems of his own, requiring long-term financial support.

- A debt consolidation or home equity loan may be a useful device for reducing debt.

Bankruptcy

The two leading reasons for declaring bankruptcy are excessive medical expenses and credit card debt.

Declaring bankruptcy has changed from a last-ditch, unethical, and humiliating way to escape obligation to an honorable if humble effort to restructure or reschedule debt payment. Of the three forms of bankruptcy that individuals (as opposed to businesses and farmers) may use, only one, Chapter 7, discharges the debtor of most debt (there are a number of statutory exceptions). The others, Chapters 11 and 13, provide for a repayment plan in a hierarchical and agreed-upon way, eliminating or postponing foreclosure on your home or repossession of your car. Once you have declared bankruptcy, your creditors are forbidden by law from harassing or suing you.

Declaring bankruptcy still should be close to your last resort for solving financial problems, and should always be done under the guidance of a professional financial advisor or bankruptcy attorney.

Disability income

Several means are available to replace your income while you are disabled.

Social Security Disability Income (SSDI)

The Social Security Administration may grant disability benefits under the Social Security Disability Income (SSDI) plan to replace lost income for an adult or to provide assistance with caring for a child with colorectal cancer.

To smooth the process of applying for Social Security Disability Income, bring all medical records with you, and let your doctors know you're applying, as they will need to give evidence.

If SSDI is denied—and frequently it is denied on the first application—ask for Publication No. 05-10041, "The Appeals Process." Sometimes just a request to have your case reviewed by the SSA's physicians will speed an approval.

In some cases, it's possible to return to work and continue to collect SSDI benefits. This is possible owing to special incentives the SSA provides to rehabilitate the disabled. The formula used to compute disability benefits while working is complex, but in general, you may attempt a trial work period of nine months, not necessarily consecutively, during which benefits are unchanged. If the trial does not succeed, benefits may continue. Ask the SSA for the publication called, "Working While Disabled...How We Can Help" (Publication No. 05-10095).

Private long-term disability income

If you don't have a long-term disability insurance policy, it's wise to consider buying one. For those under age 65, the likelihood of long-term or permanent disability is far greater than the risk of death, especially for cancer survivors who, owing to improvements in treatment, now face an illness that is shifting from a fatal to a chronic illness. For colorectal cancer survivors who face repeated treatment and aftercare, disability insurance is an emerging need for times when treatment leaves you unable to work. See "Long-term disability insurance," described under "Insurance issues," earlier in this chapter.

Note that almost all private long-term disability policies will reduce your monthly benefits if you receive other income, including disability benefits from the Social Security Administration.

Employment issues

Having and being treated for colorectal cancer can disrupt your job attendance and performance. If you're very lucky, you'll have managers and coworkers who accommodate your ups and downs, perhaps holding fundraisers for you, or donating their own unused sick or vacation time for your use. Many of us are not this fortunate.

As with finance and insurance issues, you have certain protections under the law. Verify the details of these laws, as they may change over time.

- The Americans with Disabilities Act (ADA) recognizes cancer as a temporary or permanent disability for which you cannot be penalized by demotion or dismissal. It's also illegal to deny a qualified candidate a job simply because of a disability, but it's difficult to prove this kind of discrimination unless you know intimately every other job applicant and all of their qualifications.

- The Family and Medical Leave Act (FMLA) guarantees you 12 weeks of leave annually for your own healthcare or to attend to a sick family member. During these 12 weeks, your job or a very similar one must be held open for you, and your benefits must be maintained. The FMLA applies only to companies with 50 or more employees within a 75-mile radius. Violations of this law should be reported to the US Department of Labor.

Some employers sponsor Employee Assistance Programs (EAP) to counsel employees who are having problems that affect their job performance. A subset of these employers may require participation in their EAP in order to approve payment for benefits for counseling. Please see Chapter 14, *Getting Support*, for the possible drawbacks associated with using EAPs.

Record-keeping

The value of record-keeping cannot be overemphasized. Having evidence in writing of your position is indispensable should disputes or questions arise. Records should be obtained for all treatment, employment, and financial circumstances, and should be kept in some organized way, in a place safe from fire, theft, or flood.

Biopsy samples

A new and very important concern you should address is the permanent storage of your biopsy tissue samples. Owing to the development of new treatment technologies, such as monoclonal antibodies and tumor-derived vaccines, your biopsy samples may be needed years after they are removed from your body.

Yet some hospitals limit storage time for such samples because their storage resources are finite. This means that, lacking instructions otherwise, they may discard your tissue samples after a number of years.

Ask the hospital to keep your samples forever. If they are not able to do so, make arrangements to store the samples elsewhere.

Establish a record trail

Simple though it may sound, getting copies of all medical information, including films, and getting written copies of all tangential records related to employment, insurance, and finance are sometimes overlooked. Here are some tips for obtaining records:

- Request and keep copies of all medical records and bills as you go through diagnosis and treatment. This will establish with the doctor's staff your expectations and set a tone of efficiency, and will permit you instant access to material if you need it for second opinions. Having copies made and mailed after the fact can add five or more days, even weeks, to the time you need to collect records.

- If you're requesting records that must in turn be forwarded to another health center, make a copy for yourself before forwarding the material.

- When you're hospitalized, or if your treatments are done in the hospital on an outpatient basis, ask for *itemized* copies of bills. General or summarized hospital bills can be astonishingly obtuse, and even an itemized bill can be unclear. Most errors in hospital billing are found only by using an itemized bill's relative clarity.

- Always address financial, employment, or insurance disputes in writing, and keep a copy of what you've written.

- Keep a detailed phone log of all calls made to insurance companies, mortgage companies, and so on.

- Any decision reached verbally to correct errors should be followed by a written confirmation from the company. Ask for this, and if they won't furnish a written reply, write your own reply, stating, "Based on our phone conversation, it is my understanding that the following will happen," listing what you perceive to be true.

- Keep a calendar of appointments. Do not discard it at the end of the year. Keep it as a permanent part of your medical and financial files.

- If space permits, your calendar can double as a log for phone calls, changes in medications or symptoms, blood results, and so on. Otherwise, school exercise books or blank journals, the kind from which pages cannot easily be torn, may serve well.

- Record outgoing correspondence. Send all correspondence that's even remotely important by certified mail, using the return receipt option. Unlike registered mail, which is logged at each stop in the postal system, certified mail does not travel more slowly than regular mail, and isn't much more expensive than regular mail. When the return receipt arrives, staple it to your copy of the correspondence: it is your proof that the mail arrived at its destination. Use fax transmission for speed when needed, but follow up with certified mail. An example of an appropriate use for certified mail is correspondence with an insurance company that requires 30 days' advance notice in order to review and approve treatment plans.

- Have copies of all original colonoscopy, CT, or MRI films made for your own files. While copies of the reports that describe and analyze these films are useful, access to films is mandatory for certain kinds of review and decision-making.

- If the original colonoscopy, CT, or MRI films are loaned to other doctors for second opinions, follow up to be sure they are returned to the central film library or original office.

I have been to four cancer centers and I have records from each one. I actually have a copy of all records from before my surgery to present time. I check each record and file it by date.

Organizing the record trail

How little or how much you choose to organize will depend in some measure on how much energy you have, and on your record-keeping habits. Don't be surprised if you find yourself, normally a well-organized person, suddenly without energy to file medical reimbursement forms. Others, though, may find that they become more organized as a coping mechanism.

You may find that record-keeping is a task you can delegate to a family member, friend, or neighbor who would love to help you, but doesn't know quite what to offer. Although you may not care to have someone outside your family making phone calls to correct billing mistakes, having someone sort and file bills and receipts on a weekly basis may help you. Sorting mail into stacks for filing is a task that a child might enjoy; scanning and storing documents on a PC might be something that a computer-literate relative can do.

Whatever method suits your current needs, do attempt at the very least to store medical and payment records in some way. A minimal technique is to put all records in one place, such as in one or more grocery bags, in case you need access to them in a hurry. If you or your volunteers have the time and energy to do so, you may lean toward a fairly elaborate system of organization that gives you instant access to items by topic, health center, or date.

Summary

There may be the rare person with colorectal cancer who relishes a payment challenge from stubborn insurance companies, or the character-building experience of financial hardship, but most of us facing these issues along with poor health may begin to feel overwhelmed.

This chapter attempts to highlight the most important, most potentially damaging of these issues, and supplies many references for finding the best and most current information.

Before making irrevocable decisions or expensive purchases, please consider consulting professionals who are familiar with recent changes in the various laws that govern insurance, employment, and finances.

CHAPTER 16

After Treatment Ends

*Remember to cure the patient
as well as the disease.*

—Alvan Barach

THE END OF TREATMENT BRINGS A VARIETY OF NEW CONCERNS and plans for cancer survivors. A contradictory mixture of feelings, a changed relationship with the oncologist, perhaps a renewed immersion in one's job, a reassessment of long-range plans, a different physical self—temporarily or permanently—and different behaviors on the part of friends and loved ones all may come about. Your cancer experience doesn't end as the door closes behind you when you leave the clinic: normalcy creeps up on you in the months that follow.

This chapter will discuss the emotional and practical aspects of the end of treatment. We will share with you what others have found difficult, surprising, or exhilarating. First, the physical and medical aspects related to facing ahead at the end of treatment will be outlined, followed by the emotional aspects, and finishing with the social and professional aspects of adjusting after treatment ends.

In some cases, of course, these concerns overlap. For example, it's difficult not to have an emotional reaction to either upsetting or loving things that happen in the workplace, or to ambiguous test results.

Medical monitoring

Fifteen or twenty years ago, doctors and patients had few choices for verifying that cancer had gone away and was staying away. Now, we have blood tests and imaging tools that allow a view—often just a glimpse—of what's going on inside our bodies.

These testing tools are both a blessing and a curse. While it's true that now we can track progression and regression of tumors much more clearly, there are, for example, instances of both false positives and false negatives from imaging studies that can only be evaluated accurately within the framework provided by additional testing or a second biopsy.

Follow-up tests

As you finish your treatment, your doctor will discuss when to return for follow-up visits. All patients treated for colon or rectal cancer need follow-up surveillance for recurrent disease or the development of second cancers. Ask your doctor about the timing of these tests, which vary depending on individual factors. Follow-up visits most likely will include a physical examination, a discussion period for you and your doctor to share concerns, and a series of tests to confirm that you are disease-free.

In Chapter 6 of the 1997 text *Surgery for Gastrointestinal Cancer*, Paul Sugarbaker, MD, recommends these tests after treatment for colorectal cancer:

- Physical examination and assessment of symptoms
- CEA and CA19-9 blood tests
- Colonoscopy or barium enema (contrast radiographic studies)
- Laboratory tests for blood counts, liver, and kidney function
- Chest radiographic studies (x-rays)
- CT of the abdomen and pelvis, if specific symptoms warrant
- PSA blood test
- Rectal examination
- Mammogram and breast check
- Pelvic examination and cervical cytology (Pap smear)
- Radioimmunoscintigraphy (OncoScint is a commonly used agent)

In the 1995 text *Cancer of the Colon, Rectum, and Anus*, Drs. Parikh and Attiyeh suggest the following tests:

- Physical examination and assessment of history and symptoms
- Examination of pelvis and groin
- Occult fecal blood test
- CEA blood tests

- Colonoscopy or barium enema (contrast radiographic studies)
- Chest radiographic studies (x-rays)
- CT, MRI or ultrasound, if specific symptoms warrant
- Rectal examination

More reliable blood markers for colorectal cancer are constantly being sought, which means that your blood may be tested for substances not mentioned in this book.

It's usual to delay tests and imaging studies until a few months after the end of treatment, as radiotherapy and many anticancer agents continue to have a tumor-killing effect for several months after they're used. Thereafter, imaging studies, x-rays, and blood tests may be repeated every three months for a number of years, then every six months for a number of years, then once a year for a number of years, then every few years.

It's possible to have questionable liver lesions appear after certain chemotherapies that are channeled directly into the liver, or to have suspicious lung spots appear after irradiation of the chest. These phenomena can mimic relapse or spread of disease (metastasis), but PET scanning or biopsy may prove otherwise.

Regardless of the schedule of your follow-up visits, new or returning symptoms must be taken seriously and reported to your doctor immediately. Never assume that they'll think you're worrying too much. It's always better to err by communicating too much instead of too little when it comes to aftercare.

Regression of symptoms and side effects

In general, the lingering side effects and delayed effects you may have experienced during treatment should fade away in the months following treatment.

Certain side effects may take much longer to regress. Fertility may improve slowly over months or years following treatment, or it may never recover. Bowel cramping and intestinal blockages may recede or diminish for some people, but may persist for others. Pain, burning, weakness, or numbness in the hands or feet may linger for weeks, months, or—following platinum-based therapy—years. Dry or watery eyes may continue to be a nuisance;

fatigue may continue for years after treatment. Blood counts can remain low, or low-normal, for months or years afterward.

When your hair regrows, you may notice that it's a different color, a different texture, thicker, thinner, curlier, or straighter than it was before treatment. These changes are temporary. If you received radiotherapy to the pelvis for rectal cancer, pubic or perineal hair lost might not regrow.

You might also notice that food allergies are better or worse, or that you now seem allergic to foods you were never allergic to before.

For information about delayed effects that drift into long-term effects, see Chapter 17, *Late Effects, Late Complications*.

Venous catheter removal

Many people can't wait to have their central venous catheter removed; others prefer to keep it for a while as a talisman against relapse. If your stage and type of colorectal cancer entail an increased risk of recurrence of disease, it might be wise to consider keeping your catheter, especially if additional surgeries with general anesthesia are required to remove it and reinstall it. The wisdom of keeping it to avoid extra surgery should it need to be reimplanted must be weighed against the inconvenience of keeping it clean, and the increased risk of infection it may entail.

Emotional responses

Almost everyone looks forward to finishing treatment with feelings of joy, relief, and celebration. Indeed, there are reasons to feel joyous and celebratory. Side effects will diminish, energy will return, expectations of freedom from disease are realistic, and life will begin to return to normal.

Shelly Weiler expressed the energy and insight he felt he could share when his treatment ended:

> With my sharing myself with my family and friends I feel like I'm accomplishing something with my life, more so than I did when I worked in the real world. I'm finally making a contribution. Even when my time is up I will be remembered for what I accomplished during this time in my life. I don't ask for more. I hope that while I gain support, my sharing also gives support, and nobody suffering from this disease, be it caregivers or victims, ever feels they are alone in this world.

However, many people also report at least some ambivalence at the end of treatment. Side by side with the expected good feelings can be other, more painful feelings.

The remainder of this section talks about feelings that might unexpectedly arise at the end of treatment. These feelings, and all of the feelings described in this chapter, are completely normal. Some of them may not strike you as useful reactions, but they are nonetheless normal reactions for the circumstances surrounding cancer survivorship, and should be honored as such. If you decide to join a support group, for example, you'll likely hear many people describing these kinds of reactions, and offering very good ways to turn reactions into useful acts.

Keep in mind as well that many colorectal cancer survivors have long periods of feeling happy, sound, capable, productive, and blessed. For many, the positives outnumber the negatives:

> All in all, my treatments went very well and I am in remission! I had my last CT scan in late February that looks pretty good—just a few spots they will watch. Also had a colonoscopy where they did a biopsy that was not cancer. I will now be followed very closely by the surgeon with sigmoidoscopy every three months, and blood work, and CT scans. Oh yes, I nearly forgot to say that treatment put me in menopause. This has been quite a year, but the Lord has been my best friend and I am a survivor!

The following are loosely defined categories that describe the different kinds of feelings, fears, and reactions experienced by colorectal cancer survivors.

Moving on

Almost everyone who has had colorectal cancer wants to leave cancer behind and move on to normal living. Some people succeed well with this. Many of us, however, are not that lucky, or blessed with the right genes, or able to force this difficult mental shift.

Some people succeed in blocking the experience entirely and immediately submerge themselves in their old life, which is a very healthy and useful form of denial (as long as they don't skip follow-up medical appointments). Some people succeed well in readjusting after their course of treatment, but cannot recapture this serenity if disease recurs and they face more treatment—even if their odds of survival after retreatment are promising.

Many people feel almost like their old selves until it's time for their periodic testing, and then very strong fears resurface.

> It's taken me a while to realize I had cancer. I guess if I had known before surgery that there was a tumor, I would have gotten around to thinking about this profound issue sooner. A few months ago, my boss, who was also my good friend and six years younger than I, died of bone cancer. I am lucky to have not dragged my feet more than I did. It reminds me of a discussion I had when I was trying to decide if I should have the surgery. A friend's wife who is a pathologist said, "If you don't do it (the surgery), you either have a death wish or like playing Russian roulette."

> I am glad I had time to prepare myself for the surgery. I am grateful that I have survived. Seeing my boss try to find his problem for at least a year before they discovered the cancer makes me feel luckier. It would have been my stupidity and stubbornness if I had more trouble than I did. My feeling was that he never had a chance. He tried. His death really confirmed the conclusions I was slowly coming to: time is precious, my relationships are important, there is a lot more to my life than work, there has to be balance in all the areas of life. I find now that my feelings vary from day to day about being a cancer survivor, but I'm not really worrying about having had cancer or having it return.

Abandonment

Some people fear the end of treatment because they feel that medical intervention and care are all that's standing between them and cancer. Often people secretly feel abandoned by their surgeon, oncologists, or the medical staff at the end of treatment. To the emotionally charged survivor, the medical personnel's behavior during a normal wrap-up appointment may seem brusque or emotionally flat. Where are the trumpets, the pat on the back, the teary eyes?

If, on the other hand, the staff was loving and helpful throughout treatment and congratulatory at the end, afterward you may miss the all-pull-together camaraderie that was shared, and the special kindness you received.

You may fear the absence of regular and close physical scrutiny given by the doctor. The thought of waiting two or three months to the next blood test, scan, or other reassessment may seem like forever.

Absence of feeling

Sometimes colorectal cancer survivors report feeling nothing at all when their treatment ends and their doctor says their chances are good that their survival will be a long one. This numbness may come about as a protective mechanism, or from burnout. Most often, feeling will return with the passing of time.

Fear of relapse

Nobody can guarantee that you won't experience a relapse of colorectal cancer or develop a second cancer. In spite of many reassurances, it's human to be afraid. Most cancer survivors have fears of relapse that range from occasional to paralytic. Often the fears can be put to bed for months at a time, but they may resurface when it's time for a checkup, or when an odd pain manifests.

Fear of relapse is normal. Several good ways to diminish these negative feelings are by:

- Learning all you can about your type and stage of colorectal cancer
- Keeping abreast of improvements in treatment
- Retraining your thinking to focus on the positive
- Maintaining reasonably healthy diet and exercise habits
- Attempting to enjoy the small, free joys offered by each new day

Vigilance

Many people experience pronounced, abiding concern about relapse when a new ache or odd body trait is noticed. Fears of relapse are, of course, perfectly normal, and you're to be commended for monitoring your body's reactions and status. You're not a hypochondriac.

Randall feels his best course of action is action:

> I want to be very aggressive about my cancer follow-up. I am told that I won't need a colonoscopy until next March. No other tests or follow-ups are scheduled. However, I know I can push my doctors to recommend any tests and feel pretty confident that anything will be covered by my health insurance at this point.

Battle fatigue (post-traumatic stress reaction)

Some people may experience insomnia, nightmares about their cancer, fear and avoidance of doctors and hospitals, jumpiness or lack of trust during commonplace interactions with medical personnel such as annual influenza vaccination, or extreme anger or sadness when hearing of someone else with cancer.

Ruminations, doubts

Once the heat of the battle is past, some people may begin to recall survival statistics they've seen. You might become less than happy with what you perceive your odds of surviving to be. You might begin to second-guess whether what you went through was worth it, whether it was the right treatment choice, whether you'll ever be physically adept again, whether anything else in life is worth doing in comparison to battling cancer.

Diminished coping skills

For such a long time, all that was expected of you was to focus on beating cancer. Now it may seem that the rest of the world expects you simply to pick up where you left off with your normal responsibilities. For those who were not able to continue working throughout treatment and who have not retired, the thought of returning to a full workload of regular responsibilities can be overwhelming.

As you attempt to re-enter your wider world, you may notice that things that you used to be able to ignore may annoy you, things that used to annoy you may anger you.

Anger

Now that the time- and energy-consuming process of being treated is behind you, you may find that you're feeling angry about having cancer. You may find that you want to learn all you can about what causes colorectal cancer, or that you want to become politically involved to force legislation that favors cancer research or cleanses the environment of carcinogens.

Longing for the past

Some people expect and hope that they'll feel and perform exactly as they did before cancer became a problem, and are disappointed if they cannot. Sometimes the recovery of physical and intellectual stamina is a slow process. If you have an ostomy, you may have periods during which you're convinced life will never be the same. At times, you might perceive that all changes or a diminution of performance are cancer-related, when in fact they might be attributable to a number of other things.

> Cancer takes over your entire world for a while. I have been off chemotherapy for only three months and I am just starting to win a little bit back. My husband and I are both nurses, so our understanding of the situation seemed to be high. What we didn't take into account was that you still have to run the emotional gamut. One thing I longed for was one day where everything did not revolve around colon cancer. Where when people asked, "How are you?" you could answer "Fine," and mean it. Where the world doesn't revolve by the number of pills you take or the number of times you went to the bathroom today. Where every time you had a bump or an ache you wouldn't worry if some errant cancer cell is setting up housekeeping in a new spot.

> I told my husband that I didn't want him to be my nurse, that I needed him to be my husband. I needed to be responsible for myself. It forced me to acknowledge for the first time that I had to take an active role in my treatment and recovery. It wasn't his fault I have cancer, and he couldn't make me better. It gave me back some power that I thought was all gone.

Excessive caution

Some people feel that the gods would frown on pride if one celebrates at the end of treatment, so they avoid jinxing themselves by celebrating. They may spend years not allowing themselves to enjoy a return of reasonably good health.

Alienation and loneliness

People who haven't had to deal with cancer may strike you now as insensitive or shallow. The vacuous things others say about your cancer experience, or their inappropriate curiosity about your ostomy may leave you astonished or hurt. The everyday topics they want to discuss may bore you. The issues that they view as problematic you may find trivial. You may feel you no longer have anything in common with old friends, nor even with loved ones. You may begin to consider a job change or a divorce.

Altogether, you may feel out of phase with the rest of the world—until you meet a fellow colorectal cancer survivor, and a long, intense conversation follows, during which you're impervious to your surroundings, perhaps sharing funny stories about your experiences that healthy people would find morbid. Suddenly you're aware you're not alone, and that cancer support groups may be a good choice for you.

Watch and wait

Those with ambiguous test results have special considerations when treatment ends, as retesting at some future date will be necessary for clarification. The intervening time may be filled with unbearably obsessive worry about the possible failure of treatment, sleeplessness, crying, lack of concentration, and other extremely uncomfortable feelings.

Anxiety and depression

All of the above, combined with the physical toll of treatment, can result in anxiety or depression for certain people. Anxiety and depression are discussed more fully in Chapter 12, *Stress and the Immune System* and Chapter 17. A counselor who specializes in cancer survivorship can help you with these and other problems.

Chris tells of his paradoxical reaction to being disease-free:

> *This coming week marks the second anniversary of a doctor breaking the news to me that I had colon cancer. So far so good; in fact my biggest problem has been depression during year two. Seems odd as not reaching year two would have been much more depressing. I gather, however, that this is not all that unusual.*

Social and professional aftereffects

You may be quite surprised to discover that those around you who have never had cancer are totally unaware of the mixture of feelings you're experiencing—that, in fact, they may have a very full agenda of their own feelings, both happy and distressing, to sort out. Conversely, you may find that long-term cancer survivors are a tremendous resource to you in this stage of your adjustment.

Reactions of family and friends

Your closest family members and friends who have seen you throughout treatment have probably adjusted to your circumstances by the time your treatment ends, in a way that benefits all concerned. Nonetheless, you may find that some family members expect that, almost instantly, you'll be just as healthy and active as you were before, particularly if you're a young survivor of colorectal cancer. They may even become strident on this point, so strongly does human nature yearn for things to return to normal. You need to communicate clearly with them when you're feeling tired and under par, explaining that many cancer survivors experience long-term aftereffects such as fatigue.

Some family members and loved ones may have feelings of anger and frustration that they suppressed while you were being treated. They may now allow these feelings, as well as impatience, to emerge. Candid discussions may defuse these feelings, but if they are directed at you, family counseling may be a good choice.

In some cases, a spouse or partner may decide that this is a good time to end the relationship, now that it's "over," and you're "fine." This is more likely in relationships that were experiencing problems before the cancer diagnosis.

Your very young children or grandchildren, lacking adult coping skills, might still remain mired in the distress and terror they experienced during your diagnosis and treatment. They might need long-term therapy, or support with social and academic issues.

Getting out and about socially after treatment among those who know you less well can be glorious, fun and invigorating, or exhausting and disappointing. The reactions of coworkers, discussed later, mirror in some ways the responses that you're likely to encounter from the rest of society. Unlike coworkers and family members, though, social contacts may not usually have the benefit of seeing you performing and producing, so their reactions may be more skewed and less informed.

It might be wise to be prepared for a variety of reactions that range from loving and positive to very odd indeed, if you haven't already encountered the entire spectrum of these reactions in the course of being treated. Some colorectal cancer survivors report, for example, that others don't want the survivor to talk about their experiences at all. Others report that friends who avoided them during treatment relax and approach them again after treatment ends.

With a little forethought and practice, you can defuse negative reactions, reinforce your reputation for tenacity and positivity—or even wax a bit saucy if you're in the mood for humor and not concerned about the social consequences. Some of the negative reactions and questions you'll encounter are simply the result of ignorance or a lack of careful thought, or are a front for competitiveness, spite, or sadism. You're under no obligation to go along with agendas that are not in your best interest, nor to waste a lot of emotional energy answering seemingly serious questions that in fact haven't been carefully thought out.

Reentering the workplace

Resuming the full complement of professional responsibilities or volunteer commitments after cancer treatment has ended can be a wonderful experience, a way to occupy the mind with healthy things, a way to reinforce your belief in yourself and your re-emerging health with productivity and creativity.

Often the feelings your coworkers express are a tremendous reinforcement for your well-being. To know you were needed and missed can be uplifting; to be part of a team again can make you feel you've rejoined the human race. Many colorectal cancer survivors report that welcome-back parties are planned to greet them, and that coworkers pinch-hit for them if they continue to feel tired.

Occasionally the return to work is less rewarding. If you have been queried over and over throughout your treatment about when you will return, for example, you may feel that your employer thinks you're just a cog in the machinery rather than a human worthy of her concern. If some coworkers are reluctant to recognize your illness owing to their own fears or lack of social skills, they might never refer to it, not even to wish you well or to say they're glad you're back. Very rarely, a cancer survivor will experience horrible reactions from coworkers, such as discovering that, in one's absence, one's desk was sprayed with antiseptic "in case the cancer was contagious," but these extreme reactions from coworkers fortunately are rare.

More often, the hurtful reaction will be, "The treatment is over, so now you're fine, right? Ready for a full workload now, right?" If you're still feeling like something Jacques Cousteau would've thrown back, be sure to make it clear that you'll be phasing back in gradually, that you're not feeling up to working a full day or a full week for the first month or two.

Another fairly common reaction among the blissfully healthy is, "Why are you in such a pensive mood? Aren't you glad it's all over?" Your attitude about putting it behind you, or not putting it behind you, might be worth an explanation, but this explanation might meet with limited success with the less perceptive and empathic of your coworkers. American culture, like some other cultures, has a quick-fix or even a superstitious mentality toward many problems, including health problems.

In general, it's nobody else's business how you're coping with the detritus of treatment. You can feel free to say nothing to the potentially unsympathetic listener if you choose, but there are tradeoffs surrounding not keeping your immediate supervisor informed about ongoing problems you may be experiencing. For example, if she is unaware of continuing health problems you're experiencing as a result of your illness or its treatment, you may have difficulty winning a favorable decision if a dispute about your performance arises.

More subtle reactions from coworkers and employers are possible as well, such as denying a promotion to a person who had cancer several years ago, assuming she will never again be able to meet certain challenges.

Remember that cancer is considered a disability under the Americans with Disabilities Act, so the negative reactions that result in demonstrable harm to you, such as the denial of a promotion or censure for using earned sick time, don't have to be endured without legal recourse.

Unused drugs or equipment

Often at the end of treatment you may have drugs and equipment left over. There may be ways to pass these unused drugs along to those who cannot afford them. Although in general, federal law prohibits transferring drugs prescribed for one person to anyone else, you might ask your oncologist or veterinarian if there are exceptions to this law.

Nonpresciption drugs can be offered to fellow patients and veterinarians.

For donating drugs for use in developing countries with few health resources, contact International Aid Inc., in Spring Lake, Michigan, (616) 846-7490.

If you have equipment or supplies you no longer need, such as a wig, cleaning supplies for a catheter, or ostomy supplies that weren't suitable to your circumstances, many groups, such as the American Cancer Society, accept these as tax-deductible donations for helping patients who cannot afford to buy their own.

Summary

Earl Weaver, the long-time manager of the Baltimore Orioles baseball team, used to say, "It's not over until it's over." With colorectal cancer, sometimes it's not over *when* it's over. Certain physical, emotional, and social aspects may take longer to realign with the new you.

Most colorectal cancer survivors gradually see the cup as more than half full and experience increasingly good health, productivity, and a goodly measure of happiness. Many have occasional or ongoing fears and concerns that time, professional help, or support groups can alleviate.

Dr. Wendy Schlessel Harpham's book *After Cancer* is an excellent in-depth guide to meeting the challenges that face us after treatment ends.

CHAPTER 17

Late Effects, Late Complications

We don't consider a patient cured when
his sprain has healed or he's been restored
to a minimal level of functioning.
The patient is cured when he can
again do the things he loves to do.

—Stanley A. Herring

MOST DELAYED AND LONG-TERM EFFECTS and complications of colorectal cancer treatment are not common, but they can be serious. It's useful to be acquainted with them, particularly with those that can emerge years later with no warning, or those that can mimic a recurrence of colorectal cancer. Many, but not all, of these effects and complications can be corrected, stabilized, or lessened.

The likelihood is that undesirable long-term effects will become fewer as newer treatments are developed. The medical community is keenly aware that many cancer survivors pay a high price for their survival in reduced quality of life, and one goal among many in the development of new adjuvant therapies and surgical techniques is the reduction of toxicity and tissue damage.

Late effects are emerging phenomena

Until about 20 years ago, not enough cancer survivors treated with surgery, chemotherapy, and radiotherapy survived to characterize the lingering problems that are related to treatment or disease. The earliest cancer cures were affected with surgery only, and only for early-stage cancers. The introduction of multi-agent chemotherapy and combined chemotherapy and radiotherapy has saved enough people to make the pattern of late effects at least more obvious, while not yet fully understood. In some cases, combination treatments of surgery, chemotherapy, and radiotherapy make long-term effects more pronounced.

Terminology

What distinguishes the side effects of treatment from delayed or late effects and complications? The somewhat arbitrary definitions are that side effects of treatment are those that occur within days or weeks of treatment; delayed effects occur within weeks or months of cancer treatment; late effects occur months or years after treatment. Some side effects drift into becoming delayed or late effects, such as unremitting diarrhea induced by abdominal irradiation. The medical community distinguishes between effects and complications by defining effects as expected, and complications as somewhat unexpected.

Late surgical effects and complications

Before we discuss late effects and late complications in general, it's worthwhile to discuss separately those that are linked only to surgery.

Late complications and late effects arising from surgery vary enormously in type and frequency owing to the variety and complexity of colorectal surgeries, which are always tailored to the patient's specific circumstances. Your surgeon can and must inform you of all possible risks you might face as a result of the surgery planned for you, but it's unlikely that you'll experience many or most of these. Some of these complications, for example, are seen more often if surgery is preceded by radiotherapy, or only if radical pelvic surgery is performed for rectal cancer.

Nonetheless, a few late complications and effects of surgery are seen more often than others:

- Development of scar tissue called adhesions that immobilize or constrict bowels, causing pain
- Unavoidable damage to nerves causing pain, or sexual, urinary, or bowel dysfunction
- Urinary or fecal incontinence
- Difficult bowel movements

- Stretching, constricting, or weakening of abdominal or pelvic supportive tissues

- Abnormal tubelike formations that develop between two organs (fistulae)

- Formation of internal abscesses

- Herniation at incision sites

- Excess tissue protruding from the stoma (prolapse)

- Dysfunction of kidneys or ureters owing to blockages caused by adhesions

- Kidney infections

Randall is concerned about continued abdominal pain following surgery:

> The only complication is recent. I have an apparent "gas pocket" formed at the top of my newly shaped colon. We're working on it now first with upper and lower anti-gas medications. It's mostly an annoyance, causing distention, and it presses up against my abdomen which causes some shortness of breath. It feels like a gel sac in a pair of running shoes. My mother the RN said it looks like I'm in my "third month" and "carrying high." (And people wonder why I'm gay... sheesh!) Since my semicolon is now shaped like an isosceles triangle in my abdomen, rather than a rectangle, there is a sharp turn south at the top center of my belly. Apparently this is catching and trapping gas.

Ask your doctor about any symptoms you're having that you suspect may be related to prior surgery. Many of these can be repaired surgically or treated with medication.

Specific late effects

The following sections, listed alphabetically, discuss specific late effects and complications of surgery, chemotherapy, and radiotherapy. For a more detailed discussion of the late effects of cancer, see *Sexuality and Fertility After Cancer,* by Dr. Leslie Schover, and *After Cancer: A Guide to Your New Life,* by Dr. Wendy Schlessel Harpham, an internal medicine specialist who is a cancer survivor. The latter book contains excellent and detailed discussions of post-cancer fatigue and pain.

For all sections below that mention damage from radiotherapy, see the sections "Radiation enteritis" and "Radiation fibrosis" for more detail.

The most common late effects after treatment for colorectal cancer are diarrhea, abdominal pain, fatigue, and psychological issues such as anxiety and depression.

Abdominal pain and cramping

Abdominal pain that lingers months or years after treatment might be attributable to adhesions that form during healing from surgery, from organ surfaces affixed to the bowel by tumor activity, or from scarring (fibrosis) following radiation therapy.

While some adhesions can be surgically removed if not too numerous, there is currently no cure for radiation fibrosis.

See also Radiation enteritis and Radiation fibrosis.

Bowel obstruction

If you have abdominal pain and other symptoms of severe constipation such as sweating and fever, notify your doctor at once.

Painful or life-threatening bowel obstruction can occur after treatment for colorectal cancer when adhesions form or when disease recurs. Obstructions must be treated, and can be removed surgically.

Randall tells of his experience with intestinal blockage:

> I developed a small intestine blockage that, well, backed things up a bit with cramping, nausea, and vomiting... great stuff on a still-sutured abdomen (I blame Friday night's corn-on-the-cob). They put me back on that nose/throat/stomach tube thing (I hate that) to suck the acids up out of my stomach and relieve the pressure on the blockage, in hopes that the relief would allow the blockage to work itself out. It did. There was a telling moment when I called my boss to tell him that I would be out through Labor Day and the nose/throat/stomach pump thing just spewed acid.

Diarrhea

Persistent diarrhea after surgery and after adjuvant treatment with chemotherapy or radiotherapy is a well-known late effect for colon cancer survivors.

Those who have had the entire colon removed are more likely than others to have frequent and liquid bowel movements, as the colon is responsible for removing water from fecal material. For this subgroup of survivors, there is no cure for diarrhea, but modification of the diet may lessen the frequency or looseness of waste.

To control diarrhea that is not related to the absence of colonic tissue, tell your doctor that diarrhea is continuing, as prescription and over-the-counter medication may help.

See also Radiation enteritis.

Enteritis

See Abdominal pain and Radiation enteritis.

Eyes

Colorectal cancer survivors who remain immune-suppressed after chemotherapy may experience a reactivation of varicella zoster (herpes zoster or shingles, about which more is said in Shingles), which can affect eyesight permanently. If you experience eye pain or impaired vision accompanied by a rash on your face or scalp, contact your doctor. This infection must be treated promptly with antiviral drugs.

Fatigue

The National Cancer Institute reports long-term fatigue as one of the three most debilitating long-term symptoms associated with cancer treatment.

For far too long, many cancer survivors weren't believed when they reported fatigue that lasted for years following treatment. The opinion used to be that one should feel tired only while red blood cell counts remained in the abnormally low range.

Now, doctors are listening more carefully to what survivors are saying about fatigue. One study of survivors of Hodgkin's lymphoma has shown that 37 percent of about 400 people studied experienced fatigue for as long as nine years after treatment.

The remaining problem is that medicine often cannot tell us why long-term fatigue occurs, nor what to do about it, although fatigue seems to increase as the duration or intensity of treatment is increased. Other causes of fatigue include difficulty in breathing; cranial irradiation; chemotherapy-induced damage to the heart, liver, or kidneys; chronic pain; or the worry that accompanies cancer.

Currently, the only proposed solution for long-term fatigue not attributable to known causes such as low blood counts or organ damage is plenty of rest, good nutrition, a carefully balanced workload, and emotional support.

A web site staffed by oncology nurses for cancer survivors suffering from post-treatment fatigue can be found at *http://www.cancerfatigue.org*.

A discussion group for those suffering from cancer fatigue exists on the Internet. Visit the ACOR web site at *http://www.acor.org* to enroll in the Cancer-Fatigue discussion group.

Fistulae

Abnormal tubes called fistulae can form between two organs as a result of disease, or during healing following certain surgical procedures. For colorectal cancer survivors, a fistula can form between the vagina and the bowel, for instance, or the bowel and the ureter, or less often the vagina and the bladder.

If you notice urine leakage from the vagina or rectum, or feces or fecal odor in the vagina or in urine, notify your oncologist and your surgeon. Surgery usually is necessary to correct this problem.

Fluid retention

Fluid retention in the chest or abdomen may signal a recurrence of disease. Fluid retention elsewhere, especially in the legs, might signal lymphedema, or heart, liver, or kidney failure. If you have a swollen abdomen, swollen legs, or difficulty breathing, notify your doctor at once.

The swelling of body parts owing to lymphatic fluid that cannot move is called lymphedema, and can emerge as late as 15 or more years after cancer treatment. The lymphatic ducts are delicate vessels that collect fluid squeezed from veins during normal metabolism, and bring it back to the veins near the heart. When these vessels become damaged, lymphedema may occur.

If you had surgery or radiotherapy that might have affected lymph nodes or lymphatic ducts, and if you were given instructions to follow to reduce the chance of lymphedema, it's very important to follow these instructions for years afterward. Lymphedema can interfere with blood flow and wound healing.

> *From time to time I have had some swelling of the tissue of the colon. I asked my radiologist about this and he told me this was a permanent side effect of the radiation treatments. What I have found that helps are sitz baths with aloe. I am also on my feet during the day and I have found that this doesn't help, so I wear socks that have cushioning in them, and bought a very comfortable pair of shoes with plenty of support. I found this helps quite a bit—it didn't get rid of the edema, but it helps.*

Hair loss (alopecia)

While hair loss from chemotherapies commonly used for colorectal cancer will regrow, radiotherapy to any part of the body can result in the permanent loss of hair growing in that area. Sometimes the loss is not evident until months later when the existing hair is shed from the follicle, and the hair does not regrow.

There is no treatment yet for this disorder.

Heart and vascular damage

If you have any symptoms of heart disease, such as chest pain or tightness, swollen arms or legs, numbness in your arms or hands, difficulty breathing, unusual heart rhythms, or dizziness, see your doctor. Heart and vascular damage can emerge after treatment with no previous warning symptoms.

Fluorouracil (5-FU) is known to cause cardiovascular damage in some people when high doses are used.

An echocardiogram, a stress electrocardiogram, or MUGA testing can detect heart damage. In some cases, medication or surgery can help alleviate heart disease.

Hernia

Bulging of tissue beneath a section of skin on the abdomen or near an incision is possible after abdominal or perineal surgery. Contact your surgeon if you notice abnormal bulges beneath the skin of the abdomen or near any healed incision. While most hernias are not immediately dangerous, they can quickly turn life-threatening if a segment of bowel becomes entrapped, dies, and ruptures, spilling feces into the abdominal or pelvic cavity.

Herniation of intestinal tissue outward from the stoma might occur in some patients. This is easily corrected with surgery.

Randall describes knowing something isn't right:

> I want to know how come I have a deformed Frankenstein abdomen from my colon resection? I still look like I'm three months pregnant and carrying high, when I have been working this body at the gym for almost a year now. I still swear, in spite of what my surgeon told me, that he did not sew up all the muscle layers, particularly around my upper abdomen/diaphragm area where I can press my hand in all the way to my abdominal cavity and through which my stomach protrudes after I have eaten, then recedes as food is processed. I want a flat tummy! I just believe "in my gut" that my surgeon is wrong. This abdominal "ledge" isn't normal.

Randall, having found the answer, continues his story:

> I saw my primary care physician yesterday. He examined my abdomen, pulled in a colleague, they pressed, poked, conferred, and concurred: ventral hernia. Great. I've had it for a year. Surgeon couldn't see it on film last spring. I want to take care of this ASAP so I can walk in an upcoming cancer march and start a marathon training program I've signed up for. I'd say that we're talking about a distention along 12cm of my upper incision, just below the sternum.
>
> The good news: maybe I will regain my youthful profile after all.

Incontinence

Certain surgeries for colorectal cancer compromise the tissues and nerves that control bowel and bladder function. Ask your oncologist and your surgeon if there are any remedies that suit your specific circumstances. In some cases, a second surgery might be possible to free entrapped bladder or bowel tissue, or to provide better support for pelvic organs.

Infection

If you have a fever more than 1.5 degrees higher than your normal temperature, general malaise, severe chills, night sweats, burning or pain while urinating, headache, neck stiffness, coughing, or trouble breathing, phone your doctor without delay.

Late complications such as pneumonia can sometimes follow lung or liver surgery, especially in those over age 65. In any age group, formation of internal abscesses might occur well after surgery.

Kidney damage

If you have difficulty urinating, decreased urine flow, blood in the urine, back pain, pelvic pain, pain upon urination, or fever, notify your doctor at once.

The kidneys, ureters, and bladder can be affected in various ways by the course of tumor growth, by surgery, and by the healing that follows surgery. Surgeries to free blockages and to prop ureters open are possible, and antibiotics are available to control infections before kidney damage becomes permanent.

Liver damage

If you're tired, nauseated, or your skin seems yellow or suntanned, call your doctor.

Scarring called sclerosis may occur following liver surgery (resection) or chemotherapy directed into the liver via the hepatic artery. Blood tests can detect changes in liver function, and dietary changes or modification of medications and dosages may alleviate the problem.

Lymphedema

See Fluid retention.

Numbness, tingling, dizziness, deafness

Numbness, tingling, or pain in the hands or feet may persist for months following treatment with platinum-based drugs or 5-FU. There is no treatment yet for this disorder, although pain management techniques may help.

Treatment with the aminoglycoside antibiotics gentamycin, tobramycin, amikacin, or with vancomycin for infections that arise during cancer treatment can result in temporary or permanent hearing loss, vertigo, dizziness, or ringing in the ears. These disorders can be treated with surgery, drugs, rehabilitation exercises, or noise-blocking devices.

Pain

Unfortunately, pain is a common long-term effect of colorectal cancer and its treatment. Pain in various parts of the body can result from damage attributable to surgery, the healing following surgery, chemotherapy, or radiotherapy, or from the pressure of tumors on nerve pathways. Pain can affect the healing process, your overall health, your sense of well-being, and your ability to sleep. Moreover, chronic pain, even low-level pain, has an affect on mood and performance that you might not notice if pain gets gradually worse, or if you've been dealing with it for a long time.

If you have persistent pain of any magnitude, don't try to ignore it. There are ways to address pain so that it does not become worse or cause permanent damage. You might consider consulting a pain specialist or pain clinic for a multimodal approach to pain control that may include excellent long-acting pain medications; surgery; behavior modification; pain control devices such as implantable nonaddictive morphine pumps or electrical stimulators; ultrasound treatments; or relaxation training.

For pain associated with sexual activity, see Chapter 18, *Sexuality, Fertility, and Pregnancy*. For stress reduction to lessen pain, see Chapter 12, *Stress and the Immune System*.

All of the following groups offer support or referrals for pain management:

- American Academy of Pain Medicine, (708) 966-9510
- American Society of Clinical Hypnosis, (847) 297-3317
- American Pain Society, (847) 966-5595

- American Society of Anesthesiologists, (847) 825-5586

- National Chronic Pain Outreach Association, (301) 652-4948

- Agency for Health Care Policy and Research, (800) 358-9295

A discussion group for those suffering from cancer pain exists on the Internet. Visit the ACOR web site at *http://www.acor.org* to enroll in the Cancer-Pain discussion group.

Psychological damage

Post-traumatic stress disorder, depression, and anxiety are recognized as frequent long-term sequels to cancer's stress, and can be addressed by a professional experienced in handling the psychological issues of cancer survivorship. See Chapter 14, *Getting Support*.

Radiation enteritis

Long-term damage from chemotherapy or irradiation of the abdomen or pelvis may appear as malabsorption of nutrients, diarrhea, or constipation from narrowed, tightened intestines, rectal tissue, damage to the tissue lining the bowel, or damaged nerves. Medication or surgery may correct these problems.

> *We discovered what was causing at least some of my husband's cramping and diarrhea long after he finished his radiation and continuous 5-FU.*

> *He was diagnosed as stage III with two lymph nodes involved, and after surgery, he received 28 days of radiation and 5-FU continually by pump. Since then, he's been in the hospital twice for four days each with dehydration from diarrhea or vomiting. He had numerous tests and x-rays trying to find the cause. The doctors found no obstructions or bacterial causes. Since then, on three more occasions he has had severe abdominal pain, diarrhea, vomiting, etc., which caused him to not eat and to lose still more weight. The oncologist treats this by pain medication and one-liter saline/glucose injections for several days. The treatments always made him feel better and get back to eating. But the oncologist did not know what was causing the pain.*

A few days ago I found a discussion on Oncolink's web site: "Acute radiation enteritis," which (along with other useful information) said, "Damage to the intestinal villi from radiation therapy results in a reduction or loss of enzymes, one of the most important of these being lactase (...) a diet that is lactose free, low fat and low residue can be an effective modality in symptom management." This discussion can be found at http://cancer.med.upenn.edu/pdq_html/3/engl/304093-2.html.

I talked my husband into taking Lactaid, and 30 minutes after taking the first pill his intestinal cramping eased! He's been taking Lactaid for the past three days and has reduced the amount of milk he drinks. He has been able to quit most of his pain medication. We now have hopes of his recovery from radiation-caused stomach problems.

Radiation fibrosis

Radiation fibrosis is the formation of fibrous scar tissue within the body, caused by the immune system reacting to radiation. It develops over months or years.

This fibrous tissue is knotty and stiff, and interferes with an organ's ability to do its job. For example, fibrosis in the sexual organs can interfere with fertility or sexual pleasure.

There is some recent evidence that administering steroid drugs simultaneously with radiotherapy can reduce the body reaction that causes fibrosis, but it appears that not many doctors know of, or believe in, this circumvention yet. Administering steroids after radiation therapy must be done promptly upon noticing the onset of fibrosis, as delay causes steroid therapy to be ineffective.

Recent research with hyperbaric oxygen has shown some promise in reducing the negative effect of radiotherapy on certain tissues such as blood vessels in the brain.

Recall sensitivity

Certain body tissues are permanently affected by chemotherapy or radiation therapy, becoming indefinitely sensitized, and may react with swelling and soreness if chemotherapy is readministered months or years later. This is called recall sensitivity. It's a physical, not a psychological, phenomenon.

For instance, if chemotherapy happens to leak accidentally from an arm vein or central catheter (extravasation) during infusion, the skin into which it leaks may swell and hurt if chemotherapy is administered again—even if it's years later, and even if another infusion site is used.

In addition, when chemotherapy is administered following radiotherapy, previously irradiated tissue may become sore, even if it's nowhere near the injection site.

Ask your oncologist about precautions that can be used to avoid this problem.

Second cancers

One of the most serious risks associated with colorectal cancer is the risk of developing a second cancer.

Colon cancer survivors are at high risk for developing a second colonic tumor if any colonic tissue, including rectal tissue, remains. It is thought that the same environmental or genetic aberrations that triggered the first tumor remain to cause a second primary cancer—that is, a tumor whose development is distinct from a recurrence or metastasis of the first tumor. This risk is especially pronounced for those with hereditary nonpolyposis colon cancer (HNPCC), the Lynch syndromes, and multiple primary malignant neoplasia (MPMN).

Colorectal cancer survivors are more likely to develop second primary tumors in other organs than are the general population. Sites of second tumors are:

- Breast
- Kidney, after colon cancer only
- Bladder, after colon cancer only
- Prostate
- Ovary, chiefly after colon cancer
- Endometrium (uterus)
- Uterine cervix

Moreover, some studies have shown an increased risk of developing rectal cancer after colon cancer, and the reverse.

Those who have hereditary nonpolyposis colon cancer (HNPCC) face an increased risk of second cancers at these sites:

- Gastrointestinal tract
- Female genital tract
- Endometrium (uterus)
- Biliary tract (gallbladder, pancreas, and liver)
- Renal pelvis and ureter

Those with multiple primary malignant neoplasia (MPMN) face very high risks of multiple concurrent primary tumors at a variety of sites, of which colon cancer is always one.

Radiation therapy is linked to the development of second solid tumors. Second tumors that arise following radiotherapy almost always arise in or very near sites of previous irradiation, called radiation ports. The incidence of radiation-induced tumors begins to rise about fifteen years after treatment.

For all colorectal cancer survivors, regular surveillance with colonoscopy and other diagnostic aids such as chest x-rays and mammography is mandatory.

Sexuality and fertility

Long-term damage to sexuality and fertility is possible when colorectal cancer survivors are treated with surgery or with radiotherapy to the pelvic organs. Difficulties such as failed ovulation, failed conception, irregular menses, inability to achieve or maintain an erection, retrograde ejaculation of sperm into the bladder, and pain during intercourse are possible. These problems are discussed more fully in Chapter 18.

A discussion group for those dealing with sexuality issues following treatment for cancer exists on the Internet. Visit the ACOR web site at *http://www. acor.org* to enroll in the Cancer-Sexuality discussion group.

Shingles

All who had chicken pox as a child harbor within their nerve cells a herpesvirus called varicella zoster, the virus that causes chicken pox and shingles, two manifestations of the same illness.

There are many human herpesviruses; varicella zoster is just one. It should not be confused with the genital herpesvirus that is transmitted sexually.

When the immune system becomes suppressed or dysfunctional, varicella zoster may re-emerge from nerve endings, causing quite terrible pain and blisters called herpes zoster, or shingles. The virus can affect any or all nerve endings within the entire body, but it is most likely to appear along the side of the face, neck, arm, or side of the body. Although 10 to 20 percent of those with shingles may never produce blisters, they will still experience itching or pain, or both. The blisters tend to appear in a line, following the path of nerves.

Shingles that affect the eye can cause temporary or permanent blindness.

As soon as symptoms appear, call your doctor. An antiviral medication such as acyclovir, and perhaps pain medication as well, should be started promptly. It is not unusual to require codeine or even morphine briefly for severe shingles episodes.

Shingles normally heal within four to six weeks, but some patients experience lingering pain for years afterward. If this happens, a procedure called a nerve block or glycerine block can be performed by a neurosurgeon. It should alleviate pain for several months, and can be repeated if needed.

Shortness of breath

See Heart and vascular damage.

Skeletal damage

Radiation therapy can damage bone, particularly the spine, causing pain and fracture. There is no cure for this damage; see the section Pain for ways to deal with this long-term effect.

Summary

It is not surprising that surgery drastic enough or treatment strong enough to eliminate colorectal cancer would have an effect on normal, healthy tissue as well.

Many colorectal cancer survivors do not have long-term effects or complications after treatment, or at most they have just one or two lasting effects that may fade away to an inconvenience rather than a problem. A few people, however, have serious long-term effects. These differences among people and their reactions depend on what surgery was performed, how it was performed, what anticancer drugs were given, how and how long they were given, whether radiotherapy was used, what other health problems coexist with cancer, and so on.

Despite reluctance and fears, it's important to know at least a little about long-term effects, for they can be confused with a relapse or can of themselves be life-threatening. Often, they can be addressed and corrected.

CHAPTER 18

Sexuality, Fertility, and Pregnancy

*Any scientist who has ever been in love
knows that he may understand everything
about sex hormones, but the actual
experience is something quite different.*

—Dame Kathleen Lonsdale

COLORECTAL CANCER AND THE TREATMENTS USED FOR IT TODAY may affect male and female libido, fertility, and the success of pregnancy. For some of us, sexuality, fertility, and pregnancy take a back seat during the cancer experience, but for others, these are very emotional issues—almost as emotionally charged as cancer itself.

Ways to recognize, correct, or adjust to issues of sexuality and fertility are discussed in this chapter. Specific issues of sexuality are discussed first, then how chemotherapy, radiation, and surgery can impact fertility. Finally we discuss pregnancy during and after colorectal cancer.

Sources of information

A full discussion of techniques to enhance sexuality and fertility after treatment for colorectal cancer is beyond the scope of this book; only certain techniques are mentioned in the text that follows. References have been included in the bibliography and in Appendix A, *Resources,* so that you will be able to verify facts or do further reading, if you choose. Several sources of information are doctors, counselors, support groups, and books.

Doctors

Your oncologist or surgeon can be a source of basic information regarding how colorectal cancer and its treatment are affecting you physically, and how those physical changes are impacting your sexuality or fertility. Your doctors might not be able to address all of your concerns, though. They might lack knowledge in this specialty; they might have less time than you need for discussion; they may incorrectly interpret what's important to you unless you're very clear when communicating. They might feel uncomfortable discussing sexuality, or they may feel it's "just a psychological problem." The surgeon may disavow the fact that certain pelvic surgeries can cause problems with sexual functioning. Most doctors should be able to refer you to counselors or reproductive endocrinologists, however, who can guide you in separating the physical and psychological components.

Counselors

Psychological discomforts may be more difficult to address than overt physical problems, and success in this area may depend on one's access to good counselors. The best choice is a sexuality therapist who is familiar with both the physical and psychological effects of serious illnesses such as cancer. Large urban centers are more likely to have specialists in sexual counseling than rural areas.

Support groups

Support groups, either those focused on cancer or ostomy, or on the sexual problems following other illnesses, are an excellent way to discover common problems, useful tactics, insights, and clinical information regarding sexual problems after cancer.

The United Ostomy Association can recommend groups in your area that can help you with issues of sexuality and fertility associated with having had ostomy surgery.

A support group for those dealing with issues of sexuality after cancer therapy exists on the Internet. Visit *http://www.acor.org* to enroll in the Cancer-Sexuality discussion group.

Books

Two books about cancer in general that contain chapters on sexuality are *Everyone's Guide to Cancer Therapy*, edited by Dollinger, Rosenbaum, and Cable, and the American Cancer Society's *Informed Decisions*.

An extraordinarily good resource that deals with these issues specifically in a sensitive, fair way is Leslie Schover's 1997 book, *Sexuality and Fertility After Cancer*. Especially impressive is her sensitivity toward those over age 65, whose sexual needs sometimes are neglected by the medical community. As those over 65 are well aware, people remain sexual beings for their entire lives. Dr. Schover describes the techniques and technologies available for sustaining erection, reducing vaginal pain, getting pregnant, and many other problems that are all too often borne silently. She discusses sexual adaptation for those minus genitals or breasts, and those living with an ostomy or scarring. Childhood cancer survivors and their unique adaptations are covered. Her discussion of the possible differences in sexuality caused by cancer is grounded in a thorough introduction to sexual function in the absence of cancer.

For ostomates, both *The Ostomy Book*, by Barbara Mullen and Kerry McGinn, and *Coping with an Ostomy*, by Robert Phillips, contain chapters on ostomy and sexuality.

Sexuality

It's not at all unusual for cancer survivors to report decreased or frustrated sexual desire during, and months after, treatment. Indeed, some report these problems for many years following treatment, especially following surgery that results in nerve damage, or when fatigue becomes chronic.

> *Orgasms are anything but pleasurable. It might have been better to lose the desire. My doctor grinned and said keep trying. A urologist told me that surgery could not have caused it. I say bull----! I'm the one that knows the difference. It's been over a year since surgery, and no change for the better.*

Fortunately, an extraordinary array of medications and devices is available to help those with sexual side effects from cancer or its therapies, including various treatments to sustain erection or to relieve vaginal pain. If sexual hormones are out of balance, sexual pleasure and satisfaction may improve with hormone replacement therapy.

If you're unhappy with your sexuality, discuss with your oncologist a referral to a gynecologist, urologist, or andrologist who specializes in post-cancer care, and consider consulting a sexuality therapist if you feel it's warranted.

As a cancer survivor, you need to be aware, however, that separating the psychological effects of disease from the physiological effects of treatment may be difficult or impossible. It's important to bear in mind that most sources of support for sexuality after cancer deal with *all* cancers, and that subtle neuropathologic problems may remain after specific neurotoxic therapies for colorectal cancer, such as oxaliplatin, problems perhaps undetectable using the equipment available today.

Therefore, if you decide to seek help *only* from a sexuality counselor, it's possible for physical difficulties to be misdiagnosed as psychological problems. Medical history is full of such errors, such as the "Fakers' Disease" of the nineteenth century, which we recognize today as the autoimmune disorder multiple sclerosis. In short, if you're convinced that your problems have a physical basis that outweighs any psychological component, avoid those who attempt to label you as emotionally ill and seek help elsewhere.

For colorectal cancer survivors who have an ostomy, resuming sexual activity may be a significant hurdle for either the survivor or a loved one. See "Sexuality and ostomy," later in this chapter.

General points

Although full coverage of sexuality after cancer is not possible in this brief chapter, a few of the points made by Dr. Schover and others are worth mentioning specifically:

- Communicate about sex. Communicate not just during or after attempting sex, at which times emotions are too highly charged, but always. In particular, tell your partner if you're experiencing pain.

- Cuddle, touch, and be affectionate, even if you're temporarily not up to sex as you used to know it. A sexual relationship based on love can be described as one of continual foreplay. Just walking side by side touching can be an act of lovemaking.

- If you're a female who has had pelvic irradiation for rectal cancer, the scarring of radiation fibrosis can develop in the vagina over several years. It's important to use the vaginal dilator the doctor recommended, or to have frequent sexual intercourse to prevent this scarring. Use these techniques three times a week, or as your doctor recommends. Not only will sex be less painful, but the gynecologic exams that you must have as a follow-up for cancer care will not become excruciatingly painful over time.

- If you're male, bear in mind that male orgasm without erection and without ejaculating is possible. Moreover, many partners consistently report sexual pleasure that does not require penetration by an erect penis. Good options for achieving an erection exist, such as medication or hydraulic implants, if failure to obtain or maintain an erection continues to be a concern.

- Be patient, expect new sensations, and keep an open mind about new experiences. Sex may be very good after cancer, but it might not be exactly the same as it was before cancer. Some colorectal cancer survivors report that sex after cancer—after symptoms are diminished by surgery or other treatment—is better than before.

- Ask your oncologist if the partner being treated with chemotherapy should protect the other partner from drugs that may persist in sperm or vaginal secretions. The amount of chemotherapeutic agents present in body fluids is likely very low, but it may be best to be careful (radiotherapy poses no similar risk). Wearing a condom or a vulvar shield might be recommended, for example.

- Cancer cannot be "caught" during sex, although some viruses that may cause certain cancers can. In addition to HIV, human T-cell lymphotropic virus I (HTLV-I) is transmitted by sexual contact, as is the papillomavirus thought to be linked to most cases of cervical cancer.

- The endorphins released during sexual pleasure reduce pain elsewhere in the body.

Sexuality and treatment

Psychological perceptions and misconceptions regarding sexual drive and satisfaction may be compounded by frank physical damage from treatment. Many colorectal survivors report a variety of problems with sexuality following surgery, chemotherapy, or radiotherapy. Dry ejaculation, impaired valve function that causes painful ejaculation of semen backward into the bladder, difficulty gaining or maintaining an erection, vaginal and vulvar pain during intercourse, loss of sensation in the genitals, and surgical sites that ache or are numb for up to a year after surgery are not uncommon among colorectal cancer survivors.

> I have vaginal dryness, and it makes having intercourse painful at times. This has decreased my desire. I have not ever heard of a stretcher. I

do think that, due to my surgery, I have been changed internally. I certainly feel pressure in different places, but my husband doesn't feel them.

Many medical and surgical remedies exist for these problems. Consulting a reproductive endocrinologist, a gynecologist, or a urologist for advice would be wise. Ask for details regarding these solutions:

- Devices or medications to gain or maintain erection

- Vaginal dilators to offset the formation of scar tissue following surgery or radiotherapy

- Lubricating or hormone creams to ease vaginal or vulvar pain during intercourse

- Microsurgery to correct damaged valves that cause ejaculation of sperm backward into the bladder

- Stretching the male urethra to ease pain during ejaculation caused by strictures

For sexuality affected by early treatment-induced menopause, see "Menopause," later in this chapter.

Sexuality and ostomy

Those living with an ostomy may have unique aspects of sexuality to address. These concerns can be very distressing for colorectal cancer survivors, even if they would assess their pre-surgical sexual relationship as good, because the survivor or the partner may be struggling against taboos about bodily waste that they've addressed in the bathroom, but not the bedroom.

If either the colon cancer survivor or the survivor's partner is bashful, frightened, or repelled by the thought of resuming sexual activity, one or more discussions about this with each other, with an ET (enterostomal therapist) nurse, and with ostomy support group members are highly recommended.

In general, though, sexual activity may simply require more planning and less spontaneity. Considering the following points may help:

- With today's ostomy appliances, virtually no odor exists, although trial and error may be necessary to find well-fitting appliances.

- Consider avoiding foods that produce gas, such as the broccoli and cabbage family of vegetables.

- Empty the pouch before lovemaking to reduce the chance that an embarrassing accident may occur. If it does, you might consider making light of it by resuming sexual activity in the shower.

- Pouch covers are available to hide the ostomy bag during lovemaking. Specialty stores carry lingerie designed with the female ostomate in mind, such as crotchless panties that cover the pouch but leave the genitals free for activity.

- Some survivors might not need an ostomy bag while making love. Those who have had a colostomy rather than an ileostomy produce more solid waste, and only periodically. A colostomate might be able to forego wearing a bag for a time (ileostomates, on the other hand, produce liquid waste more or less continuously). Ostomy plugs and covers are available to accommodate activities such as lovemaking, sports, swimming, and so on. Ask an ET nurse about the usefulness of irrigation prior to using a plug for these occasions.

- Once the stoma has healed—several weeks is typical—you can't hurt it if you bump it or press against it during lovemaking.

- During the few weeks that the stoma is healing following surgery, you can engage in sexual activity or cuddling that avoids the area.

- Nothing should be inserted into the stoma as part of sexual activity: the risk of tissue tearing or infection is too high.

- For the squeamish, lovemaking with the lights off might be useful.

- After some time living with an ostomy, you may become aware when it's least active, and can plan lovemaking sessions accordingly.

- Keep a supply of smaller pouches on hand, or pouches that fasten to the side instead of downward, if you find that the pouch itself gets in the way when you're in your favorite positions for lovemaking.

- Find a practical, factual sex manual to discover new positions and techniques for lovemaking.

- You may have concerns about body image after ostomy surgery that go beyond having a stoma and a pouch to cover it. For excellent and detailed discussions about these issues, see the books about ostomy that are listed in the bibliography.

- If you're an ostomate without a sexual partner but are seeking one, consider discussing your ostomy before engaging in sex. This topic is a hefty one that, owing to differences in personalities and situations, might best be addressed within an ostomy support group. In general, though, allowing a potential partner to discover by touch or by sight that you're an ostomate, with no preparation, is probably not the best approach.

- Keep in mind that your partner sees parts of your body that you never see, and that some of these "vantage viewpoints" are not always flattering. It's likely that your partner, already acquainted with your good and bad features, will be much less concerned about your ostomy appliance than you think he or she will be.

- Your partner is likely to view the ostomy as the means by which your life was saved rather than a negative feature.

Fertility

If you've been treated for colorectal cancer with surgery, chemotherapy, or radiotherapy and are still in your reproductive years, you may experience temporary or permanent fertility problems, such as an inability to conceive, cessation of menstruation, blocked sperm ducts, or sperm of poor quality or quantity. When the choice is saving the patient's life versus saving his fertility, the surgeon must opt for full excision of all cancerous tissue, even if damage to healthy reproductive tissue results. You should discuss with your oncologist the potential risk to fertility that your specific treatment may entail, and what solutions are available.

See also "Menopause," later in this chapter.

Fertility and surgery

Various surgical procedures can cause subsequent problems with fertility in both female and male colorectal cancer survivors. Surgical removal of ovaries, uterus, testes, or other structures of the reproductive system as part of en bloc surgeries to remove tumors entangled with reproductive organs may result in reduced fertility or sterility. Most patients do not require such extensive surgery. Scar tissue (adhesions) can immobilize and constrict the reproductive organs and limit the blood supply to the sexual organs, a blood supply necessary for erection in males and for nurturing the growing fetus in females.

For females, the path from the ovary through the fallopian tube to the uterus must remain open for a successful conception and implantation, and the end of the fallopian tube nearest the ovary must be free to move in order to channel the fertilized egg into place. If this path has been blocked by scar tissue, a second surgery later in life may be necessary to remove adhesions and straighten or reopen these pathways, or, more commonly, in vitro fertilization will be recommended.

For males, certain surgeries or the adhesions of the healing process can bind or damage the vas deferens, part of the network of sperm production and transport. In addition, males needing to have lymph nodes within the pelvis biopsied are at risk for neurologic damage that may make erection or ejaculation incomplete or impossible. Nerve-sparing surgery might be used to avoid this problem. For those suffering this damage who wish to father a child, techniques such as stimulation of ejaculation with electricity or micro-surgery to retrieve sperm from within the testes are possible.

Discuss nerve-sparing surgical technique with the surgeon you've chosen for your surgery. If you are dissatisfied with his responses or have reservations after your discussion, consider getting second and third opinions from other surgeons before proceeding with surgery.

Fertility and chemotherapy

Although some reports exist regarding temporary suppression of sperm counts among men who receive fluorouracil for colorectal cancer, no such reports exist regarding suppression of ovulation or menses among females who receive the commonest adjuvant chemotherapies, such as fluorouracil for colorectal cancer. Reports that do exist for drugs used against colorectal cancer in females assess these drugs in combination with other agents, such as cyclophosphamide used with fluorouracil against breast cancer. In this context, few conclusions can be drawn about the permanent effects of fluorouracil on female fertility.

Owing to the scarcity of information regarding fertility directly related to adjuvant chemotherapy and to the ongoing development of new treatments for colorectal cancer, it's critical for you to discuss these issues with your medical oncologist and a reproductive endocrinologist.

Men might be advised to have sperm harvested and frozen before treatment. Women still interested in childbearing might be advised to use oral contraceptive pills during chemotherapy in order to suppress ovarian activity, sparing more follicles for the future, or to have embryos or ovarian tissue harvested and frozen, although the freezing of ovarian tissue still is experimental.

For those able to conceive after treatment ends, carrying a baby for the full term and giving birth to a healthy baby who develops normally appears likely for couples of which one has been treated with chemotherapy. There appears to be no increase in cancer or other health problems, nor in cognitive problems, among the children of those treated for colorectal cancer with chemotherapy, except among children born to families with one of the cancer family syndromes that increase the risk of colon cancer and certain other cancers (see Chapter 3, *What Is Colorectal Cancer?*).

Fertility and radiotherapy

Radiation therapy places future fertility at high risk if the brain, pelvis, abdomen, or testes are irradiated.

Radiotherapy is clearly harmful to the ovaries, testes, and associated reproductive structures, with demonstrated dose effects such that low doses cause subtle damage and increasingly higher doses eventually cause outright sterility.

If an ovary or testis is the site of the colorectal cancer tumor or the site of likely spread, treatment with radiation therapy may be essential for survival, and fertility may have to be sacrificed. In this instance, harvesting and storing sperm or ova in advance of treatment is clearly the best and perhaps the only option for preserving fertility.

Following radiotherapy to the ovaries, older females are more likely to experience loss of fertility than younger females, owing to the decreasing number of viable ova within the ovary as females age. Some studies have found that the fertility of young males is affected more strongly by radiotherapy than that of older males; other studies have not.

In addition to outright sterility following radiation therapy, subtle damage among ovulating, menstruating women who appear to be capable of conceiving a child may include compromise of the blood supply to the uterus and changes in uterine size. Structural and functional changes such as these may make conception and implantation more difficult, and miscarriage more likely.

Subtle damage in the male may include ducts within the pelvic reproductive array that are constricted or totally blocked, cells in the testes that can no longer produce sperm, sperm that are decreased in number, are misshapen, or have impaired motility. The blood supply to the penis that is responsible for erection may be compromised if the veins are constricted from the scarring (fibrosis) that can follow radiotherapy.

Ovarian or testicular function that has not been totally destroyed by radiotherapy may return to normal levels in the years following treatment. This can be tracked indirectly by following blood levels of pituitary follicle-stimulating hormone and luteinizing hormone (FSH, LH) in females and FSH in males. FSH and LH are hormones that act as messengers from the pituitary to the ovary and testis to stimulate egg growth and sperm production. In some instances, even seemingly inadequate ovulation or sperm production, as indicated by abnormally high values of FSH or LH, nevertheless may result in a pregnancy

Cranial irradiation for brain metastases can interrupt the function of the pituitary and hypothalamus. Because these two organs within the brain control the function of ovaries and testes, there can be a corresponding disruption of the production of reproductive hormones when the pituitary and hypothalamus are affected. This may result in failure to ovulate or menstruate in females or impaired production of sperm in males.

Methods to protect the ovaries and testes from radiation, such as surgery to temporarily or permanently move them out of the radiation field (oophoropexy and orchidopexy, respectively), are available to preserve fertility and are generally successful, although temporary or permanent infertility may result in spite of these precautions. In some instances, a second surgery to restore the ovaries to a position realigned with uncontorted fallopian tubes is necessary. Lead shields can be constructed to protect ovaries and testes from almost all of the radiation administered, but internal scatter—an echoing of x-rays among internal organs—still may affect them adversely.

Menopause

Colorectal cancer survivors who are treated with pelvic irradiation or surgical removal of the ovaries may experience early permanent menopause.

A survivor who was treated with surgery, chemotherapy, and radiotherapy discusses her early menopause:

> I began with hot flashes both during the day and at nighttime. I would awaken from a sound sleep with them. As one who had always been a cold person, this was quite a change for me. I was throwing the covers off many times a night, quite to my husband's surprise. Then I'd be cold again—on they went, only to shortly be thrown off again.

> I have night sweats also, and an aching in my hips so bad it wakes me. My joints have all begun aching, some days worse than others. I can be sitting, and then when I try to get up, I can hardly walk for a few minutes. I was on an over-the-counter pill called "Hot Flash" for a few months, but have stopped taking it. I thought it was helping, but then decided it really wasn't, so I quit. I cannot take hormone replacements as I have had a blood clot, but the gynecologist wants me to get some soy and see how I do with that.

Menopause and sexuality

Female colorectal cancer survivors are sometimes surprised by permanent cessation of menstruation (menopause) that may be associated with pelvic irradiation or surgery to remove the ovaries (oophorectomy). The biologically compelling event heralded by menopause is cessation of ovulation, but to the female experiencing it, the systemic symptoms—hot flashes, vaginal dryness, insomnia, loss of libido, hair thinning, and so on—are often much more disturbing than the inability to conceive. Symptoms associated with abrupt menopause may be more severe than the symptoms occurring with natural menopause. The complaint voiced most often by female colorectal survivors in early menopause is pain during and after intercourse, usually owing to vaginal dryness, but also attributable to radiation fibrosis.

In some cases, hormone replacement therapy (estrogen, estrogen and progesterone, or any of these with testosterone) might be appropriate to reduce or eliminate the overall symptoms of early menopause.

When hormone replacement therapy is not appropriate, local estrogen-containing creams, estrogen rings, or water-based lubricants that are used in the vagina and on the vulva can provide relief from vaginal dryness and pain during intercourse. Moreover, local estrogen-containing creams and estrogen rings are to some degree absorbed by the body and may provide relief from other symptoms as well.

Frequent intercourse or a vaginal stretcher should be used by all women who have had pelvic irradiation in order to keep vaginal tissue flexible. Radiation therapy can cause scar tissue (fibrosis) to develop in the vagina during the years following therapy.

Menopause and infertility

If you have time before treatment that places fertility at risk, you might want to consider banking ova or embryos for future pregnancies.

Infertility associated with pelvic irradiation can best be addressed by a reproductive endocrinologist. Ask your oncologist for a referral to one or more of these gynecologic subspecialists. You can also get a referral from the ABMS Public Education Program in Atlanta, Georgia ((800) 733-2267 or *http://www.certifieddoctor.org*).

See also the sections on "Fertility" and "Fertility treatments," which appear elsewhere in this chapter.

Fertility treatments

A full discussion of techniques to enhance fertility is beyond the scope of this book, but several general methods are discussed. For greater detail, see Leslie Schover's 1997 book, *Sexuality and Fertility After Cancer*.

Infertility that occurs after chemotherapy or radiotherapy may be treatable by fertility specialists, called reproductive endocrinologists, using techniques such as:

- Stimulation of ovulation (ovulation induction)
- Concentration of sperm
- Selection of healthy, motile sperm
- Assisted penetration of the ovum by sperm
- In vitro fertilization/embryo transfer and micromanipulation techniques
- Insemination

- Sperm retrieval techniques
- Egg or sperm donation

Pregnancy during colorectal cancer

Perhaps one of nature's cruelest tricks is the development of cancer during a pregnancy. For the mother diagnosed with cancer, grave concern for the well-being of the unborn child exists amidst terror for herself. For the father diagnosed with cancer, concern about the heritability of cancer may exist along with fear that the unborn child soon may be fatherless.

It is rare for any cancer to arise in the mother during pregnancy, and rarer still for colorectal cancer to develop during pregnancy. Unfortunately, colorectal cancers that arise simultaneously with pregnancy usually are diagnosed at a late stage because symptoms such as nausea are mistaken for those of pregnancy.

There is no evidence that the hormones of pregnancy can cause a colorectal cancer to develop when no underlying disease exists before pregnancy, and colorectal cancer cannot be "caught" by an unborn child.

You should discuss with your oncologist how your illness and treatment might affect your unborn child, and what options are available to you. When a cancer does arise, the mother might opt to defer treatment until after the child is born. Accordingly, an early induced delivery might be planned, allowing treatment to begin more quickly. Some studies have shown that cancer itself may interfere with the healthy growth of the fetus. It might be wise to prepare for the fact that some oncologists suggest termination of pregnancy to save the mother's life.

Pregnancy and chemotherapy

Owing to the scarcity of information directly related to colorectal cancer and pregnancy and to the ongoing development of new treatments for colorectal cancer, you should discuss with your oncologist the potential for damage to the fetus that your specific treatment may entail. The drug most commonly used today as adjuvant therapy against colorectal cancer, 5-fluorouracil, is known to cause damage to unborn laboratory animals, and avoiding this drug during pregnancy usually is recommended, especially during the first trimester.

If adjuvant treatment commences after the birth of the child, breastfeeding may be dangerous to the newborn child owing to chemotherapy drugs in breast milk. Verify this possibility with your oncologist.

Pregnancy and radiotherapy

Irradiation of the abdomen or pelvis for either diagnostic testing or treatment must be avoided to protect the fetus. Irradiation of other organs may be possible if the developing fetus can be properly shielded.

Pregnancy after colorectal cancer

If you are a colorectal cancer survivor who becomes pregnant, your chances of carrying a baby to full term and giving birth to a healthy child who remains healthy are very good, except in cases of familial colon cancer, in which the offspring are at increased risk of developing cancer later in life.

You can have a successful pregnancy and a healthy baby in spite of having an ostomy.

If you had surgery for rectal cancer that required low rectal anastomosis, you might require a delivery by cesarean section in order to protect the anastomosis.

You should be evaluated as a possible high-risk pregnancy. Ask your oncologist for a referral to an obstetrician who is experienced in treating cancer survivors and has a subspecialty in fertility techniques and high-risk pregnancies.

An interval of at least one year after treatment is recommended before conception, in order to insure that there is no recurrence of cancer.

Summary

Issues of sexuality and fertility surrounding treatment for colorectal cancer are common and treatable. Take advantage of the resources available by finding a gynecologist, urologist, or andrologist who specializes in post-cancer care, and consider consulting a sex therapist if needed.

Temporary or permanent fertility problems may arise if you were treated for colorectal cancer while still in your reproductive years. Very effective treatments to boost fertility and aid in conception are available.

Adjusting to an ostomy may impede full enjoyment of sex for some colorectal cancer survivors. Your doctor, an enterostomal therapist, or a support group for ostomates can help you.

If you are pregnant, you should discuss with your oncologist how your treatment might affect your unborn child, and what options are available to you, such as delaying treatment, early induced delivery, and avoidance of chemotherapy and radiotherapy.

CHAPTER 19

Recurrence of Disease

We do not know what we mean by cure
because there is a great difference
between cure and long-term survival.

—Arthur Holleb

AFTER EXPERIENCING CANCER AND ITS TREATMENT, at times it is almost impossible for one to think of anything except the possibility that disease will return. This fear might be fleeting; or it could be trenchant, obsessive, and compelling, occupying both waking and sleeping thought processes.

Depending on the stage at which your colorectal cancer was diagnosed, and what you've learned about it, you may be somewhat prepared intellectually and emotionally for recurrence, perhaps with a new treatment plan already selected. Others among us may be utterly broadsided by the news.

This chapter will begin with a definition of recurrence of disease, and then will describe who is likely to experience a recurrence, how recurrence is detected, in what areas of the body it may emerge, when it's most likely, and why it occurs. There are indeed instances of test results mistakenly being interpreted as recurrence of disease—and we'll discuss what findings may constitute equivocal results—but chiefly this chapter will focus on true recurrence. A discussion of the difficult emotional issues that arise at this time, which often are different from those we encounter at first diagnosis, will follow.

Treatment of recurrence is discussed in Chapter 6, *Modes of Treatment* and Chapter 20, *Clinical Trials*.

It's possible to mistake some aftereffects of treatment for symptoms of recurrence. It may relieve you of some anxiety if you review Chapter 17, *Late Effects, Late Complications*, which describes most of these physical changes.

The definition of recurrence

As defined by Altman and Sarg in *The Cancer Dictionary*, relapse or recurrence is the return of disease in a patient who, by the best measures available, appeared to be disease-free for longer than 30 days after treatment ended. The patient who experiences a return of disease within 30 days of treatment, or who had quantifiable evidence of tumors remaining after treatment, is said to experience a progression of disease rather than recurrence. Some colorectal cancer survivors have tumors that remain the same size for some period of time, a condition called stable disease that is almost always a precursor of recurrent disease.

True absence of disease after treatment of any kind is very hard to determine with complete certainty. The surgeon's eyes and the specific imaging tools and blood tests used today to detect remaining or recurring disease unfortunately are not foolproof.

How recurrence is detected

Some colorectal cancer survivors experience old, familiar feelings of malaise in the abdomen or pelvis, or notice other alarming symptoms, which trigger a visit to their oncologist. Other survivors note entirely new symptoms that they might not think of as related to colorectal cancer, but somehow they know that things just aren't right. Still others may be feeling fine, yet a routine imaging study, blood test, or colonoscopy indicates a possible return of disease.

If you have worrisome symptoms, contact your doctor immediately. Do not allow concerns about being thought a hypochondriac interfere with getting timely medical care that may save your life.

It's likely that your oncologist will order one or more tests if either you or she notice anything that hints at a return of disease. Many of these tests, such as imaging scans, colonoscopy, barium enema, or blood testing, will be familiar from your experiences during your initial diagnosis and follow-up care.

Clinical recurrence

When symptoms or signs of returned disease are noticed by the survivor, a loved one, or a medical professional, and the return of disease becomes likely during a subsequent physical examination or imaging study, it's called a clinical recurrence. Chest x-rays may show suspicious lesions in the lung, for instance, or computed tomography (CT) may show lesions in the liver.

Pathologic recurrence

Pathologic recurrence is recurrence detected by one or more tests on suspected cancerous tissue at the cellular level. Biopsy specimens of lung or liver tissue, or of colonic tissue retrieved via colonoscope, might upon examination confirm the return of disease.

Rebiopsy

If suspicious lesions reappear in the vacated tumor bed or in the abdominal cavity, liver, lungs, or brain where masses known to be malignant were found previously, treatment might proceed with no rebiopsy. If no lesions ever appeared in these organs before, however, or if imaging studies show that original lesions are gone, but lesions in new areas exist, your doctor might wish to confirm the re-emergence of disease with a second biopsy or second-look surgery before proceeding with treatment.

Often these decisions depend on the stage of the original disease: a person originally diagnosed at stage IV is considered more likely to experience metastases to other organs eventually, whereas a person diagnosed at stage I has a lower chance of recurrence. Thus liver lesions appearing on an imaging scan for a stage I survivor might be questioned as benign scarring or fatty lesions, but for a stage IV survivor, they might be interpreted as very likely representing a spread of disease.

Why disease recurs

The most widely accepted theory for recurrence is that not all colorectal cancer cells were removed or killed by the original treatment. In the strictest sense, progression of disease is probably a better description of these events than recurrence of disease.

Recent research has shown that remaining cancer cells can acquire resistance to chemotherapeutic drugs by turning on genes that block the cellular intake of certain drugs and others related to them, a phenomenon called multiple drug resistance (MDR). Other theories hold that genetic predisposition or continued or repeated exposure to environmental or bacterial toxins might be responsible for the return of disease, but it can be argued that these latter instances are independent (metachronous) cancers, and not recurrence, progression, or spread of the first cancer.

Who experiences recurrence

Very broadly, and only in the context of today's treatments, one can say that those who were diagnosed in advanced stages of illness and those diagnosed with aggressive tumors are more likely to relapse than those diagnosed in early stages or with tumors of low malignant potential.

With many new treatments being developed for colorectal cancer, however, it's not wise, correct, or ethical to adhere to generalities without continually revisiting the progress of research, and without noting exceptions. Solitary liver metastases, for instance, often can be surgically removed, restoring very good odds for long survival. Chapter 4, *Prognosis*, discusses these exceptions in detail.

Where disease recurs

The return of disease can be classified as local, regional, or distant.

Local recurrence

The most common sites of recurrence for most colorectal cancers are at or very near the site of original tumors, called the tumor bed (which includes incision lines from bowel resection), and the abdominal and pelvic organs closest to the original tumor.

If the primary tumor occurs in a portion of bowel held in place by other body structures (several such places exist), it may be difficult for even the best surgeon to be certain that all disease was surgically removed, particularly for later-stage disease that has breached the bowel wall. If the primary tumor occurs in portions of bowel that are free-moving (labile), the odds are somewhat lower that disease will recur in adjacent structures.

The medical community continues to debate the meaning of colorectal cancer metastasis along surgical incision lines. Some argue that, ironically, surgery with curative intent can cause cancerous tissue to rupture, spread, and implant along incision lines and the lining of the abdomen, whence chemicals released during the healing process stimulate subsequent growth. Others argue that incision-line metastasis represents the incomplete removal of disease without clear margins—that is, that microscopic disease already existed in this nearby tissue even as the surgeon was removing more visible disease from adjacent tissue.

Regional and distant recurrence

For those diagnosed at an advanced stage of disease or with aggressive tumor types, sites of possible recurrence include the liver (which, unlike many other organs, has a direct blood supply from the intestines, facilitating spread of disease), abdominal lymph nodes, or the lining of the peritoneal cavity. Lung and brain metastases, and other distant metastases—some in very unusual places such as the foot—are possible as well.

Metastasis

When cancer recurs in sites not initially involved with the first tumor, the disease is said to have spread, or metastasized.

Grey areas and delays

In the last ten or fifteen years, we have benefited by the tremendous progress made in medical science's ability to detect cancers at much earlier stages. Nevertheless, we forget at times that our sophisticated imaging tools still provide just a glimpse into the body's complex workings. Consequently, blood tests and imaging studies sometimes yield equivocal results that must be qualified with additional testing or with a second biopsy.

Following some types of chemotherapy, for example, fatty lesions can form in the liver. Following liver (hepatic) surgery or chemotherapy channeled directly to the liver, scarring (sclerosis) may occur. These benign lesions may appear upon CT scanning as liver metastases. Positron emission tomography (PET) is better able than other imaging tools to distinguish benign lesions from colorectal cancer that has spread to the liver.

Carcinoembryonic antigen (CEA), a blood test that is widely used to track possible re-emergence of disease, is not always a reliable indicator of recurrence in the absence of other findings. CEA can become elevated as a result of other bodily or disease processes, or as a result of changes in smoking or alcohol consumption habits. Tumors that are either highly differentiated or poorly differentiated are less likely than moderately well-differentiated tumors to produce abnormally high levels of CEA; mucinous tumors or tumors that are localized are less likely to elevate blood levels of CEA. One study has shown that liver metastases are more likely to elevate CEA than tumors in other locations.[1] Some clinicians say that CEA might not become elevated upon recurrence, even when gross metastatic disease is present, and that changes from initial test values often are meaningful even if the patient's level remains within laboratory normal ranges. Different laboratories sometimes use different manufacturers' assays to measure CEA level, and their results cannot always be compared with accuracy. Thus, some clinicians say that at least two consecutive increases in CEA must be found before recurrence is likely.

Shelly illustrates his sound understanding of the necessity of an upward trend in CEA, that conclusions cannot be drawn from a single value:

> I only had one upward CEA two weeks ago, from 4.4 to 10. For some reason the oncologist wanted to put me on CPT11 at the first sign of an upward movement. Now that it is going down again maybe he will opt to keep me on 5-FU. I'm going to suggest, no, demand that I stay on 5-FU until there is a more defined trend upward. No need to go to a more aggressive and debilitating chemotherapy if I don't have to. I am on 5-FU/leucovorin once a week, six weeks on, one week off. Hopefully it will stay that way. CEAs can rise and fall, sometimes for unknown reasons. I guess we just have to go with the flow.

Nonetheless, an increase in one's CEA value almost always causes great fear among colorectal cancer survivors. Additional testing becomes necessary, often after an agonizing watch-and-wait period of several weeks is endured, to determine either an upward trend or a false positive.

Other blood-borne tumor markers that are more specific than CEA in predicting recurrence of disease are being assessed, including CA19-9, but at this time no other blood test is as widely used as CEA.

Shelly Weiler describes his fears about a continued rise in his CEA levels:

> Yesterday I got news from my oncologist that my CEA is up. This is very alarming to all of us, my wife, me, and my doctor. He will retake the CEA this Wednesday when we meet for my regular chemo session. Hopefully it will show a lower number. If it's higher he will switch my chemotherapy to CPT11.

If I go on CPT11 how much worse will the aftereffects get? I know everyone is different, but I had all the side effects from 5-FU but the mouth sores. Food now tastes like crap and my appetite has greatly declined.

So far I've not lost too much weight, maybe five pounds in the last month and a half. I really don't know what lies ahead for me, just know that I'm still here fighting the fight, but getting ready to concede round one to the disease.

When does risk abate?

In general, the longer you remain disease-free, the less likely you are to experience a recurrence of disease. You might be considered by insurance companies, for example, to be cured of the primary tumor once you have been in remission for five years. Indeed, guidelines for follow-up testing relax around the fourth year.

It is known, though, that those who have had colorectal cancer face a very high risk for a second colorectal cancer if any colonic or rectal tissue remains. It's thought that the same environmental or genetic aberrations that triggered the first tumor remain to cause a second tumor—that is, a tumor whose development is distinct from a recurrence or metastasis of the first tumor. This means that, for some people, the quest for cure of the original tumor might be only half the battle.

If the survivor has hereditary nonpolyposis colon cancer (HNPCC), Lynch syndromes, ulcerative colitis, or multiple primary malignant neoplasia (MPMN), he should never relax the vigilance of follow-up testing to detect second cancers or recurrence. These genetic disorders predispose one to multiple cancers of the colon and, in some cases, of other organs.

All colorectal cancer survivors, with and without hereditary gastrointestinal disorders, should continue to have periodic colonoscopy and other tests at intervals determined by your oncologist.

Treatment options

How recurrence will be treated depends on how your first appearance of disease was treated.

- If you were treated with surgery alone, a second surgery followed by chemotherapy or radiotherapy might be used.

- If a second surgery is deemed too risky because disease appears too widespread, because your stage at initial diagnosis was advanced, because surgery would endanger a vital organ, or because your general health is too frail, chemotherapy or radiotherapy, alone or in combination, might be planned without a second surgery to obtain material for rebiopsy.

- If only one organ such as the liver is affected, therapies that target only the liver, such as surgical removal, radiofrequency ablation, or hepatic artery infusion might be used. Single lesions in the lung might be surgically removed; brain lesions might be reduced with radiotherapy.

If chemotherapy is planned and you have received chemotherapy previously, your oncologist might assume that the drugs you were given at first, at least at their initial doses, would not be the best choice for treating recurrence. The thinking is threefold:

- If these drugs were very effective, your disease would not have recurred.

- Colorectal cancer cells can become resistant to drugs, making them ineffective.

- Some drugs are toxic to various organs, and their lifetime dose must be limited.

This means that, for subsequent chemotherapies, it's usually the case that a second drug or series of drugs will be attempted. Because colorectal cancer treatments are evolving continually, any attempt to describe herein the specific treatments your doctor might suggest would be quickly outdated. See Chapter 6, Chapter 20, and Chapter 23, *The Future of Therapy*, for specific information on treatment of recurrence.

If you didn't familiarize yourself with clinical trials during your first experience with colorectal cancer, now is a good time to do so. Clinical trials are a good way to gain access to newer, possibly more effective treatments before they are made available to the general public. Having some familiarity with what agents and surgical techniques are being tested in clinical trials will position you well to make decisions about subsequent treatment.

Emotional issues

Clearly, recurrence is an emotional lowland for almost anyone affected by colorectal cancer, including the survivor, the family, friends, and the oncologist.

The emotional issues faced at recurrence are different in quality and scope from those encountered at first diagnosis and endured during treatment. What follows are some of the reactions that many colorectal cancer survivors describe having.

Fear and terror

Feelings of fear or raw terror may overcome you, even if the odds remain in your favor. A sense that your options are narrowing may grow stronger, even if you are aware that, by medicine's best assessment, they are not. Thoughts of death that you may have been able to put aside during and after treatment crowd back in, even if you know that there are still treatment options open to you. Fear of different, stronger, more damaging treatments may emerge.

> *I'm scared, afraid of the outcome inevitably. My emotional outlook is not good. I keep focusing on the inevitable.*

Abandonment

There may be a sense that you fought the good fight, and now you deserve peace, contentment, and normalcy. Not only are you not getting these just rewards, you're getting something that could hardly be worse. You may wonder why unethical, unkind humans go about happy and healthy. You may find yourself wishing that certain particularly unpleasant people would get cancer, too.

Anger

Anger over life's unfairness, perhaps kept in check or rationalized during surgery and the first rounds of treatment, may now emerge and may cause you, and those around you, much discomfort. What psychological adjustments you may have made to your illness may go out the window, seeming to be a waste of time. Anger may manifest as rage, irritation, cynicism, or depression.

Shelly says:

> *I'm trying to refocus on the battle and stop feeling sorry for myself.*
> *Also trying to get rid of the underlying anger I have for my ex-primary*
> *doctor. This will take time. All I have is time.*

Grief

Many people grieve from the moment of diagnosis. They grieve for lost health, energy, and diminished opportunities of many kinds, from career opportunities they had to forego to have treatment, to loss of sexuality, loss of bodily integrity, or ruptured relationships.

Not surprisingly, an expanded sense of grief may emerge upon recurrence. Some people can't help but remember having heard that, for many cancers, failure of first-line treatment entails a poor prognosis. Although you may know that this generality does not apply to all colorectal cancer survivors, it's still a frightening thought that makes some people grieve for the life they may lose.

Despair

The initial diagnosis of colorectal cancer and first-line treatment often are addressed with a can-do attitude that may be difficult to sustain at recurrence, even if your chances of long-term survival are just as good after an additional therapeutic regimen that achieves a solid remission. There's something about facing the battle all over again that might make you weary at the very thought of it. You may feel that the difficult treatment you've already endured was a waste of time. You may question the quality of your life. You may contemplate suicide.

Shelly continues:

> *How do I now keep focused on the battle and don't start feeling sorry*
> *for myself and just giving up? That's what I've wanted to do this week,*
> *give up. With the diarrhea, fatigue, and nausea from chemotherapy, and*
> *the pain in my shoulders, life doesn't seem worth living, frankly.*

Loss of trust

You may lose trust in the medical system in general or in your oncologist in particular. If a strong faith sustained you during diagnosis and first-line treatment, you might find yourself questioning this faith now. You might lose confidence in your own ability to meet physical and emotional challenges.

Acceptance

Many colorectal cancer survivors marshal their emotional resources to start additional treatment. Shelly concludes:

> *I've now come to grips with my situation and will continue the fight. I've not struck out yet. Still have my sense of humor even though I might be typing a little slower due to the pains in my shoulders.*

> *We changed our oncologist appointment to tomorrow to speed things up a bit and also hope he will give me the chemotherapy tomorrow so that I can possibly enjoy Thanksgiving this week. I know I have to be thankful for each day and I want to make the best of the time I have left. My only wish is that it be discomfort-free. I may be asking too much, but it doesn't hurt to ask.*

Family and friends

The reactions of friends and family may be completely supportive, positive, and loving, or particularly inept. Unless they're kept well informed about your illness and its likely patterns, they may give up on being sustaining, instead treating you as if you have one foot in the grave. They may mourn prematurely; they may practice living without you emotionally. One way to forestall these negative reactions is to inform them from the beginning that, often, colorectal cancer can be retreated at recurrence.

Employers may begin to lose patience with you at the prospect of yet more absenteeism. Your children or grandchildren may once again exhibit earlier, less adaptive behaviors that they had outgrown, such as clinging, aggression, bedwetting, or temper tantrums.

Getting help

Cancer counselors have a considerable amount of exposure to and experience with those who are dealing with cancer as a chronic, recurrent illness, and sometimes are cancer survivors themselves. You can locate a cancer counselor by contacting your hospital's social worker for referrals, the local Wellness Community, or the local office of the American Cancer Society.

Support groups are an inestimable resource for regaining emotional footing and a balanced outlook. If you didn't examine options for finding support during your first experience with colorectal cancer, it would be wise to do so now. It's not an overstatement to say that you'll be overwhelmed by feelings of hope and energy when you discover how many other people have gone through what you're experiencing, and came through it in good shape.

Many forms of support are available for cancer survivors in general and colorectal cancer survivors in particular. Chapter 14, *Getting Support*, details these options.

Summary

Recurrence of colorectal cancer is an extremely difficult time for most people. Fear, hopelessness, anger, and overwhelming sadness are common feelings.

Recurrence is not a death sentence. There are good options available for retreatment, and many people report feeling very much better after they familiarize themselves with the options available.

Key points to remember:

- Any suspicious or worrisome symptoms you experience should be reported to your doctor immediately. Do not concern yourself with fears that others will think you're a hypochondriac.

- A rise in blood levels of carcinoembryonic antigen (CEA) is not an indisputable sign that disease has returned. Other factors, such as changes in smoking or alcohol habits or the presence of noncancerous liver disease can cause CEA to rise.

- The most likely places for disease to recur are in organs near the site of the original tumor, in lymph nodes near the tumor, in the lining of the abdomen, in the liver, or in the lungs.

- Re-emergence of disease is not an automatic death sentence. Certain tumors that recur or spread can be treated in some instances.

- Clinical trials of new treatments can be found at the National Cancer Institute's web site (*http://cnetdb.nci.nih.gov/trialsrch.shtml*) or by calling the NCI at (800) 4-CANCER.

CHAPTER 20

Clinical Trials

"Come to the edge," he said. They said:
"We are afraid." "Come to the edge," he said.
They came. He pushed them ... and they flew.

—Guillaume Apollinaire

WHY WOULD ANYONE CHOOSE AN EXPERIMENTAL THERAPY over standard colorectal cancer treatments that have well-known risks? Aren't clinical trials of new treatments dangerous? Aren't these experimental treatments just for people who have no other choices left? And why are they called clinical trials?

Colorectal cancer is the subject of a great deal of very promising research. These new and possibly better treatments are available to colorectal cancer survivors in carefully controlled settings called clinical trials.

Many of the treatments now in the pipeline are of very low toxicity, unlike some traditional, standard chemotherapeutic agents. Many experimental treatments, such as monoclonal antibodies, use natural cancer-fighting body products that are amplified outside the body and then reinserted. Others, such as idiotype vaccines, use our own white blood cells that are retrained to attack tumors. Other treatments aim for and destroy the parts of the cancer cell's chromosomes that make cancer cells immortal.

Critical information on clinical trials will be shared in this chapter. We'll discuss the structure of clinical trials, and how they're run. Their advantages and disadvantages, safeguards for the patient, and the patient's rights are outlined. We will show you why it's often to your advantage to do your own searching instead of relying on trials your doctor may recommend, and how to evaluate different trials. What to expect and what to do when you're finally enrolled are explained.

This chapter focuses on finding and evaluating clinical trials for treatment, not on trials for support, prevention, or detection. For the sake of readability, we will use the word "substance" throughout this chapter, with the understanding that either new substances or new methodologies can be the objects of testing.

Who should examine clinical trials?

The National Cancer Institute recommends that if you have stage II or higher colorectal cancer, or colorectal cancer that has not responded to standard treatment or that has relapsed, examination of clinical trials may be very much worth your while. The factors that contribute to this statement are discussed at length in Chapter 4, *Prognosis*.

Nonetheless, *all colorectal cancer survivors should become familiar with methods for finding trials, and with the general structure and function of trials.* If you wait until you need a trial to attempt to learn these things, you may run out of time.

What are clinical trials?

Clinical trials are the tests by which new treatments are evaluated to see if they offer more benefit than existing treatments. Success of a new treatment in the highly structured, controlled environment of a clinical trial is required by the US Food and Drug Administration (FDA) before treatment can be approved for wider use by doctors and patients in less controlled settings. When clinical trials show that a new treatment is better than older standard care, and these results are verified by objective third parties, the treatment that was used in the clinical trial becomes the new standard for care.

Clinical trials are tests run in the clinic, or—more clearly stated—on humans. The word "clinical" distinguishes these trials from tests done on tumor samples or on animals. Clinical trials are not started on humans until a substance has shown promise when tested first on human tumor samples, and then on animals, usually mice.

There are many kinds of clinical trials. The ones that usually interest most colorectal cancer survivors are the ones that focus on treatment, but trials also exist to improve cancer support, detection, and prevention. A clinical trial can test either a new substance, a new combination of substances, a new surgical technique, or a new method for administering treatment.

Clinical trials are designed and structured such that the results can withstand the minute and critical scientific scrutiny necessary to determine if a new treatment is effective. Three study designs that aid in ensuring that the results of treatment are attributable to the new agent and not to chance or confounding factors are randomization, blinding, and double-blinding. Blinded and double-blinded trials are rare in the testing of new cancer therapies, but an explanation of these concepts is included here so that you will be well informed should you be asked to participate in a blinded trial.

- A randomized trial is one in which a large number of patients with the same disease are assigned via computer to receive either the new treatment or existing, standard treatment. This means that you might not receive the new substance at all. Randomization is used to demonstrate as clearly as possible that a group of similar patients did either better or worse, and that *only* the treatment given explains the difference in outcome. The ideal randomized clinical trial would treat only patients who are alike in every respect except for the treatment given. This would ensure that the *only* difference that accounted for success or failure is the treatment used. In reality, this regimentation is not possible because each individual is unique.

- In a blinded trial, not only are patients randomized, they also are unaware of which treatment they're being given. This is considered necessary to rule out the *placebo effect*, defined as the ability of the human body to respond differently to treatment in measurable, physical ways, based on complex psychological and motivational factors experienced by the patient. Some patients might respond better to a treatment, for example, simply if they know they're getting a new treatment as opposed to an older one. Passive, compliant patients might report responses that they think will please the doctor and staff. The placebo effect is the subject of some controversy, with some researchers maintaining it's truly measurable, while others believe its supposed effects can be attributed to other phenomena, such as inaccurate metrics or patient subjectivity.

- A double-blinded trial is one in which the patients and some of the medical staff are unaware which substance is being given to whom. For example, the patient, the nurse who measures vital signs, and the pathologist who examines tissue samples might be unaware of which substance is being given. The doctor writing orders as outlined by the trial's protocol is aware, though, as he or she must be prepared to deal with side effects that arise. Double-blinding is used to eliminate the possibility that subtle factors, such as motivation and mood on the part of the nursing staff, might be sensed by the patient. These could account for differences seen in the progress of the group receiving the new treatment compared to those receiving the old—see the placebo effect, described in the previous paragraph.

- A case-control study is one in which patients are matched on as many characteristics as possible, then one group is given a particular treatment and the other group is not. For cancer clinical trials, the characteristics on which patients are matched are disease characteristics. Very few case-control studies are designed for cancer treatment, although they are for cancer prevention.

Here are examples of trials both randomized and double-blinded currently in NCI's clinical trials database:

- Phase II randomized, double-blind, placebo-controlled study of high-dose folic acid for the prevention of colorectal cancer in patients with resected adenomatous polyps

- Phase III randomized, double-blind study of Warfarin versus placebo for chemoprevention of thrombosis in central venous access catheters in cancer patients

- Phase III randomized, double-blind study of Megestrol versus Dronavinol versus both in patients with cancer-related anorexia and cachexia

- Phase III randomized double-blind study of intratumoral CDDP/Epinephrine injectable gel for recurrent or refractory squamous cell carcinoma of the head and neck

In these respects, clinical trials differ from less rigorous tests designed and administered by doctors and researchers working independently on new substances in for-profit clinics. These researchers, some of whom are well respected by the broader medical community, some of whom are not, often lack complete records and consistent evidence that can be verified by impartial observers. Often their patients are not subjected to the necessary long-term evaluation—five years or more—that determines whether the new treatment truly made a sustained difference in patient survival.

In general, if trials are run by a university, an NCI-designated regional cancer center, or a pharmaceutical company adhering to NCI and FDA guidelines, the chances are very good that safeguards for the patient are part of the design, and that the substance being tested has been reviewed and approved for use by a committee of responsible and knowledgeable researchers. Therapies offered by independent researchers in their own for-profit clinics, especially those that involve ingesting or injecting an untested substance, should be avoided or, at the very least, approached with extreme caution.

Why use clinical trials?

Aside from the altruistic aspect of participating in a trial in order to benefit others—an aspect that may or may not motivate you—clinical trials offer you a good chance to receive more effective treatment, and perhaps a cure, years before it's available to the general public. For example, a monoclonal antibody treatment for colorectal cancer, Panorex, has been available for several years to those with colorectal cancer who were willing to enroll in clinical trials testing this substance. Intron-A, a manmade version of interferon-alfa, a human body product that fights infection and cancer, was approved by the FDA in December 1997, but was used by patients in clinical trials for years beforehand.

Steve Dunn is a nine-year survivor of metastasized kidney cancer. In Cancer-Guide, he tells of his difficult experience with this cancer, which, prior to the availability of interleukin-2 therapy developed at NCI, had five-year survival statistics in the 2 to 3 percent range. Like most of us, Steve started at ground zero with no medical background or insider information to assist his search.

Steve's story is available at the CancerGuide web site at *http://www.cancer-guide.org*, one of the best cancer sites on the Internet. His personal story alone is probably enough to convince most people of the benefits of finding the best clinical trial for their circumstances. Moreover, his advice to patients on locating, examining, and choosing a clinical trial is unparalleled in the scientific and lay literature.

Won't I be just a guinea pig?

In the US, the long and not altogether honorable history of the clinical trial process has resulted in laws, procedures, and methods that safeguard the patient. For example, each clinical trial has a lengthy plan, called a protocol, that will be given to you *if you ask for it*. The protocol describes what will be done when, and what action will be taken if certain undesirable effects occur. You should always ask for a copy of the full protocol, and read it thoroughly.

Informing the prospective patient and obtaining consent from the patient are time-consuming and repetitive processes done to ensure that all risks and benefits are made clear. For example, the patient should be made aware that she can drop out of the study at any time, and that care cannot be denied her if she does so.

Unfortunately there still remain cases of patients being pressured to sign clinical trial consent forms without full information, or at the last minute, without time to consider other options. Remember that very few colorectal cancers progress fast enough to require a same-day, or even a same-week, decision.

- Always ask that the consent forms and the protocol be sent to you well in advance of your scheduled visits.

- Do not sign a consent form until you have received and read a copy of the full protocol, and have considered all other clinical trials for which you might be eligible.

Only institutions funded by the federal government, or governed by pertinent local laws, are required to abide by consent guidelines. If you're being treated in a for-profit hospital that receives no government support, it's possible for you to be treated in a study without your knowledge or consent, thinking that you're getting standard treatment. Ask your doctor if your treatment represents state-of-the-art treatment as defined by NCI, or if you're being treated in a study. In addition, phone your state health department to determine if your state has its own laws regarding consent issues.

Placebos

For cancer clinical trials, true placebos are almost never used. A true placebo is a drug or treatment that has been made to look exactly like the active substance or the effective procedure, but it has no effect. In clinical trials of antihistamines, for instance, the placebo used most often is a sugar pill.

For randomized cancer treatment trials—usually phase III trials, of which more is said later—the new treatment is compared to existing, accepted treatment, not to a placebo. Exceptions to this ethical policy are new treatments for which no corresponding previous treatment exists, such as trials of the earliest efforts to purge bone marrow of cancerous cells prior to bone marrow transplantation. In that instance, standard care was represented by reinfusion of unpurged marrow, and the test treatment involved reinfusion of marrow purged using an experimental technique.

How are clinical trials run?

Clinical trials are organized into three stages: phase I, phase II, and phase III. Each phase attempts to address different and increasingly complex issues concerning the success of the new treatment. Some drugs are tested in trials that are a combination of two phases, such as phase I/II or phase II/III. Usually this is done if some knowledge of the new treatment's effect in humans is already known so that its development and testing can be expedited.

There may be clinical trials in which you can participate locally on an outpatient basis, but many require travel and in-patient stays.

Phase I clinical trials

The primary purpose of a phase I clinical trial is to measure the safety and toxicity of different doses of a new substance in the human body. Some phase I studies may also assess tumor response, therapeutic effectiveness, the amount of drug that accumulates in the body, and a substance's general behavior (pharmacokinetics) in the body.[1]

Phase I trials are preceded by animal studies that measure toxicity, so an estimated safe human dose is already known. Rigorous controls are enforced to be sure that no patient suffers adverse effects. For example, blood or urine values of certain body substances may be measured several times a day to ensure that the liver and kidneys are not compromised. Doses that are found to be unacceptably toxic are lowered.

Phase I trials usually enroll just a few patients, perhaps ten to thirty. Often these patients have a variety of different cancers. Sometimes one cohort of patients will receive only a low dose of the drug, and a different group will receive higher doses, but in other studies, the same patients who initially receive a low dose may be given a higher dose later if toxicity is not too profound.

The advantages of a phase I trial are:

- You may receive a treatment that may be better than anything else currently approved by the FDA years before it becomes available to the general public.

- If this drug is already in use for other illnesses, its toxic effects might not be completely unknown.

- Candidate substances for cancer treatment are not approved for phase I trials unless the substance has shown reasonably acceptable toxicity, and activity against cancer, in cultured tumor cell lines and in animal studies. Of every 5,000 substances tested in animals, only 5 enter phase I trials.

- Doses found to cause unacceptable toxicity are lowered.

The disadvantages of a phase I trial are:

- For every 100 drugs tested in phase I trials, only 70 will prove successful or safe enough to carry forward into phase II trials.

- Because phase I trials are chiefly concerned with discovering dose-limiting toxicity, they are brief compared to phase II and III trials. You may receive too few doses of the test substance to destroy all of your cancerous cells.

- Phase I trials usually test one substance alone, yet experience has shown that, at least for the chemotherapeutic agents commonly used today, combined drug regimens are more effective against most cancers than single-drug regimens.

- The substance, although it may be an approved drug for other illnesses or even for other cancers, most likely has never before been used in humans for your illness. Although it has been tested in cultured tumor cell lines, and in animals implanted with tumors, it may not be effective against your tumor, or it may be no better than existing treatments.

- The substance, although it may be an approved drug for other illnesses or even for other cancers, may be administered to you at a much higher, more toxic dose.

- The dosage will be varied among those enrolled, thus its effects on your tumor may not be directly comparable to the effects on the tumors of others enrolled in the trial ... and patients do talk among themselves.

- The use of patients with different tumor types makes it difficult for you to compare your progress to that of other patients.

- Toxicity may cause substantial discomfort, illness, or permanent damage, in spite of the safeguards designed to prevent damage.

- Often phase I trials are run by one principal investigator at one institution. You may have to travel to participate in a phase I trial.

Here are the titles of a few phase I trials for colorectal cancer selected from the NCI clinical trials database. Note that the titles state the phase number, and at this phase make no reference to randomization or blinding. Don't be distracted by the overly technical verbiage in these titles. You'll become more familiar with the terminology as you read more about your illness:

- Phase I Pilot Study of Flt3 Ligand Prior to Resection of Hepatic Metastases of Colon Cancer

- Phase I/II Study of Irinotecan and Radiotherapy in Patients with Unresectable or Locally Recurrent Large Bowel Cancer

- Phase I Study of Iodine I 131 Humanized Monoclonal Antibody A33 in Patients with Advanced Colorectal Carcinoma

- Phase I Study of Sequential ICI D1694 and Fluorouracil in Advanced Colorectal Carcinoma

- Phase I Study of Oral Capecitabine as a Radiation Enhancer in Patients with Locally Unresectable, Residual, or Recurrent Colorectal Cancer Localized in the Pelvis

Phase II clinical trials

Phase II trials measure the effectiveness of new treatments against cancer after phase I trials have demonstrated the maximum safe dose. Some phase II trials also attempt to measure how best to deliver the drug to the tumor— orally, by infusion, and so on—and how often the dose should be given.

Phase II trials enroll many more patients than phase I trials, perhaps 15 to 80, so that the substance will receive a more thorough test and the statistics collected will be more meaningful.

Sometimes, but not always, phase II clinical trials are divided into arms, with one arm getting one version of the experimental treatment and a second arm getting another—perhaps the same experimental agent combined with an established, FDA-approved cancer-killing drug, or delivered by another route, or on a different dose schedule.

Because some phase I trials seek preliminary evidence of efficacy against disease, a clearer idea might exist regarding what cancers will benefit most from this treatment when it's used in a phase II trial.[2] Nonetheless, the types of cancers that will be addressed in a phase II trial usually are determined by the researchers designing the trial. Sometimes parallel phase II trials for different cancers will be designed and funded.

Phase II trials take more time than phase I trials because, unlike phase I trials, more of the new agent is administered for a longer time in an attempt to cause tumor regression.

The advantages of a phase II trial are:

• Candidate substances for cancer treatment are not approved for phase II trials unless phase I trials have shown that the substance is safe at a given dose and, in some trials, that the substance has some activity against cancer in humans.

• You'll be receiving a treatment that may be better than anything else currently approved by the FDA several years before it becomes available to the general public.

• Only doses of acceptable toxicity, determined during phase I testing, are utilized.

• Randomizing and blinding usually are not used in phase II trials. Therefore, you are assured of receiving the experimental treatment.

The disadvantages of a phase II trial are:

• More than half of the drugs used in phase II trials will be found ineffective against cancer or too problematic for use. Of the original 100 drugs that entered phase I trials, of which 70 survived to pass to phase II, only 33 will survive phase II testing.

• The substance, although it may be an approved drug for other illnesses or even for other cancers, may not prove to be better than existing treatments for your illness.

• Although its toxicity was determined in the phase I trial of this substance, the substance is still an evolving treatment with the potential for unexpected side effects.

- More of your time will be needed for a phase II trial than for a phase I trial.

- You may have to travel to participate in a phase II trial.

Here are a few examples of phase II trials for colorectal cancer selected from the NCI clinical trial database. Note the occasional use of randomization, and the trend toward fewer cancer types being eligible, as opposed to phase I trials:

- Phase II Study of Flavopiridol in Patients with Metastatic or Recurrent Colorectal Cancer

- Phase I/II Study of Amifostine as a Protective Agent for Irinotecan Toxicities in Patients with Metastatic Colorectal Cancer

- Phase II Study of MOAB 17-1A/GM-CSF for 5-FU-Resistant Metastatic Colorectal Cancer

- Phase I/II Study of Active Immunotherapy with Carcinoembryonic Antigen RNA Pulsed Dendritic Cells in Patients with Resected Hepatic Metastases from Adenocarcinoma of the Colon

Phase III clinical trials

Phase III clinical trials test a new substance's efficacy compared to existing standard treatments.

Phase III trials are much larger than phase II trials, and are almost always multi-center trials—that is, trials run in many sites simultaneously. They run for years, including perpetual follow-up of the patient's cancer status and overall health.

The large number of patients in a phase III trial tends to flatten any aberrant statistics that result from patient differences that lessen the usefulness of statistical data collected in a smaller trial. For this reason, patients in a phase III randomized trial can be of various ages and both sexes, for example, as long as they're all colorectal cancer patients, or all lymphoma patients, and so on.

Phase III trials are almost always randomized (case-control studies are not), but are rarely blinded or double-blinded.[3] When blinding is used, patients might discover which treatment they're receiving based on side effects, comparison in conversations with other patients, or other overt or subtle phenomena.

The advantages of a phase III trial are:

- A substance that has survived the scrutiny of phases I and II is very likely to be better than current treatments: either more efficacious, or equally effective but less toxic.

- You'll be receiving a treatment that may be better than anything else currently approved by the FDA a year or two before it becomes available to the general public.

- If, during the trial, a new treatment shows itself to be profoundly superior to existing treatment, those receiving the existing treatment are switched to the arm of the study utilizing the new substance.

- If a new treatment shows itself to be clearly or dangerously inferior to existing treatment, those receiving the new treatment are switched to the standard treatment regimen.

The disadvantages of a phase III trial are:

- Of the 33 drugs that survived phase II testing, only about 25 will be found effective in phase III trials.

- Randomizing and blinding may not appeal to those who are determined to receive only the new treatment, not the contrasting current treatment.

- The new substance may prove to be just as effective as, but no better than, the existing treatment.

Here are a few examples of phase III trials for colorectal cancer selected from the NCI clinical trials database:

- Phase III Postsurgical Maintenance Immunotherapy with Corynebacterium granulosum P40 for Patients with Colon and Breast Cancer and Melanoma Residual Following Surgery

- Phase III Randomized Study Comparing Two Adjuvant Chemotherapy Regimens with Fluorouracil and Leucovorin Calcium in Patients with Stage II or III Colon Cancer

- Phase III Randomized Study of Conventional Versus Laparoscopic-Assisted Surgery for Colorectal Cancer

- Phase III Randomized Study of Leucovorin Calcium Plus Fluorouracil with Either Irinotecan or Oxaliplatin in Patients with Recurrent Metastatic Colorectal Cancer

- Phase III Postsurgical Maintenance Immunotherapy with Corynebacterium granulosum P40 for Patients with Colon and Breast Cancer and Melanoma Residual Following Surgery

Which phase is best?

This chapter cannot offer you absolute advice about which type of clinical trial is best for you. This decision should be made only by you and your treatment team. Several aspects can be considered, though:

- A phase III trial that offers randomization to either standard therapy or a new therapy might be the choice that's right for you. The relative safety of receiving a known regimen might be reassuring to those who discover that they have not been randomized to the new treatment arm.

- A phase III trial in which all patients receive the new drug and only an ancillary feature of treatment (such as one antibiotic against another to control infection) is randomized might be as good a choice as a phase II trial of a less well-known substance.

- A phase II trial of a very promising substance might appeal to patients who find phase I trials too risky and phase III trials too controlled.

- A phase I trial of a drug with a long, safe history of use for another illness might be a reasonable choice for you if animal studies have shown that the agent is active against colorectal cancer and if you have tried several other treatments without success.

Where are clinical trials run?

Clinical trials are found most often at the NCI-designated Comprehensive Cancer Centers and Clinical Cancer Centers, and at other university medical hospitals that receive federal funding and cooperate with NCI on clinical trials. Your community oncologist may participate through association with NCI's community clinical oncology programs. See Chapter 2, *Finding the Right Treatment Team,* for more information on NCI-designated cancer care centers.

How can I find trials for colorectal cancer?

If you're an adult with colorectal cancer, you must take an active role in finding the best care for your disease. Adults with cancer are seldom asked to join a trial unless they are being treated in a regional cancer care center. The approach is different from that used for children with cancer, whose families are commonly approached regarding enrollment in clinical trials, and 75 percent of whom eventually are enrolled in clinical trials. The NCI estimates that less than 5 percent of adults eligible for clinical trials enroll, and that minorities are underrepresented in the clinical trial process.

You can use several methods to find clinical trials:

- You can ask your oncologist which trials would suit your medical circumstances. This has its advantages and disadvantages, one advantage being that you need do very little except trust. The disadvantages are described later in the section called "Why research trials on your own?"

- You can call the National Cancer Institute at (800) 4-CANCER and ask about trials for your subtype of colorectal cancer, being sure to specify whether you're willing to travel—otherwise they'll send you local trials only. Be sure to ask for the full document, not the summary. Be warned that if you call often with this request, which is not an unreasonable thing to do, because new trials are added every month, eventually they may decline to send you any more listings. This has been the experience of some cancer survivors who've used this service, which is provided by various regional cancer care centers under the auspices of NCI.

- You can research US and international clinical trials on your own at the NCI's web site. This, in conjunction with learning to use Medline, is by far the most comprehensive way to check on new treatments being tested. This service alone may be worth the cost of a personal computer and the time spent learning to use it. Once available only to those who subscribed to the NCI's Information Associates' program for $100 per year, now the NCI provides this tool free of charge on the Internet.

We strongly suggest that you examine all trials available for colorectal cancer, not just those in your area. At the time of this writing, the URL for the protocol search geared to physicians (another, less edifying tool is available for patients) is: *http://cnetdb.nci.nih.gov/trialsrch.shtml.*

- You can use CenterWatch on the Internet to track new cancer treatment trials. CenterWatch has improved their service greatly in the last few months, adding new information showing what agent is being tested and at what center the trial is being held, instead of only a general trial title and city. (This additional information is imperative if you're searching for trials at a top-notch cancer center in a large urban area.) The listings are still by state, however, forcing you to review some of the same information over and over for each state if you're willing to travel and want to be familiar with all trials available. The web address for Center-Watch is: *http://www.centerwatch.com.*

- You can use the services of commercial Internet service providers such as America Online (AOL) to receive email press releases from pharmaceutical companies concerning new products in development. Be aware, though, that press releases often will simply echo in less detail the medical information you may already have found elsewhere. Furthermore, press releases typically are written to attract or reassure investors, rather than impart information to cancer survivors.

- To find trials specifically for children, you can search the National Childhood Cancer Foundation site at *http://www.nccf.org* in addition to the NCI site listed earlier.

Why research trials on your own?

Some people who have depended only on their oncologists for comprehensive and up-to-date information on clinical trials have been disappointed. In many cases, oncologists in clinical practice—and that means most oncologists—are aware only of the high-priority trials that receive emphasis in publications such as *Oncology Times*, or those that are offered nearby. Some still do not use a computer to search the NCI's database for *all* applicable trials. Perhaps they haven't the time to do so: remember that most oncologists in the trenches must track information on every cancer known, whereas you have the opportunity to focus intensely on your own cancer, subtype, and stage.

At the other end of the colorectal cancer oncologist spectrum is the oncologist associated with a university medical school or cancer research center. You can usually expect very good to excellent treatment from such a specialist, but often when consideration of clinical trials is appropriate, they may be biased toward their own research, or toward trials run by colleagues at their own institution.

The following story is an all-too-common example of our need to educate ourselves about clinical trials:

> Several months ago I had a phone call from a friend who now has a second cancer, a lymphoma, following treatment as a child for bone cancer. She thanked me for sending her information on the FDA's approval of a new monoclonal antibody treatment for lymphoma.
>
> She was originally enrolled in an antiviral trial at a prestigious East Coast cancer center, but the trial was halted following concerns about safety. When she showed her doctors the information on the new monoclonal antibody, they immediately put her on it. "They had never heard of it," she said. Today, ten months later, she continues in remission.

The ideal oncologist is one somewhere in the middle: educated about all trials and aware of what's a good fit for you, but not biased toward her own work or that of colleagues.

Life doesn't often approach the ideal, so it's a good idea to learn to search for clinical trials on your own, and to repeat your search every month, because new trials are constantly opening. Once you have found a trial for which you believe you qualify, you should bring it to your doctor's attention. Suppose you find several trials that seem to admit patients with your profile? How can you tell which trial would be best for you? Clearly this is one of the most important questions that will arise in your experience with colorectal cancer.

At this point, you need to acquire skills for searching Medline and reading the studies that result from your searches. The substances used in each clinical trial may have results published regarding their previous use in animals or in humans. These studies should be found, evaluated, and compared, by you and your doctor, to single out the substance most likely to benefit you. Detailed techniques for searching Medline are discussed in Chapter 24, *Researching Your Illness*.

If your oncologist is unwilling to help you, is negative, or is at best ho-hum about your proactive attitude toward searching for trials, find a new doctor, because you'll need a doctor's recommendation to get admitted to a trial.

Getting admitted to a trial

Once you have found one or more clinical trials that you think you're eligible for, you must ask your oncologist to consult with and refer you to the treatment center running the trial for an evaluation to be admitted. If your doctor is unwilling to do so, seek a second opinion. You might try phoning the principal investigator listed in the trial description. Often they'll speak directly with patients about what's involved, but a few may insist on speaking first with your doctor.

You and your medical records will be scrutinized closely by your doctor, the doctors at the institution offering the trial, and perhaps your insurance company, to see if you're truly a candidate. Various physical parameters such as the condition of your lungs and liver may be factors. The kind of tumor you have, how large it is, or whether your disease is progressing must be considered.

One of the chief considerations in evaluating patients for most clinical trials is how much previous treatment they've had, and what kind. Some trials want only those who have been heavily pretreated; others require patients who have not had any treatment resembling that proposed for the trial. Still others seek patients who have had no treatment at all.

You should read all of the entry criteria listed for the clinical trial and should become very familiar with the results of your various tests so that you'll have a good idea whether you're eligible before you approach your doctor for a referral. Questions that many other cancer survivors feel overwhelmed by—questions such as how long the trial will run, where is it located, and what are the side effects—will not be a problem for you, because the description of the study will have answered many of these questions for you.

In order to be accepted, there may need to be a great deal of rapid cross-communication among you, your medical care providers, your insurance company (which will almost certainly insist on pre-approval), the oncology nurse in charge of administering the trial at the center you've targeted, the social worker, the housing assistant (if you must travel for this care), and the principal investigator, an MD, running the trial. You may need to make one or more trips to the cancer center for an evaluation. You may be pleasantly surprised by how kindly you're treated—some doctors phone personally, for instance—or you may be dismayed by lost records, lack of communication, and red tape. Other patients experience heartache and anger when, after passing all the benchmarks, a reviewing MD employed by their insurance company denies payment for the treatment after finding some discrepancy. More on this topic is discussed later, in the section called "About payment."

The evaluation process is the time to ask for your own copy of the full protocol. The protocol is the document that describes what will be done when, and what action will be taken if certain undesirable effects occur. You should always ask for a copy of the full protocol and read it thoroughly.

Do not sign a consent form until you have received and read a copy of the full protocol, and have considered all other clinical trials for which you might be eligible.

Many principal investigators are willing to speak directly with prospective patients about the details of the trial and the patient's medical history. The names and phone numbers of the principal investigator and participating doctors can be found at the end of the document that describes the clinical trial.

You can expect to feel conflicting emotions at this time. The excitement of finding a treatment that may be more effective than current treatments, the fear that the treatment might have unknown effects, concerns about being away from home, nagging worries about financial considerations, and the thrill of empowerment on finding the best care may suddenly emerge as overwhelming feelings after months or even years of relatively calm feelings about coping with your illness.

Questions to ask

No doubt the very detailed information that is part of the full protocol will answer many of your questions, and will trigger many others. In addition, consider these less-than-obvious questions, which are adapted from Nancy Keene's book *Working with Your Doctor*:

- Who reviews this study, and how often?
- Who monitors patient safety?
- Why do the principal investigators believe that this treatment is better than standard treatment?
- What are all of the potential physical side effects of this treatment, both short- and long-term?

- Will participation in the study mean that I have to change oncologists?

- Must I be hospitalized to participate?

- What will be my costs, and what will my health insurance pay?

- Does the study follow patients for the long term?

- Who pays for any care I'll need if the treatment has unexpected negative effects?

Once you're in

Detailing exactly what to expect after you're enrolled in a clinical trial is not possible in this or any book, because each trial is quite different, but in general, most people find they feel well cared for in a trial setting. It might be wise, however, to expect the unexpected. One cancer survivor, for example, traveled a great distance to take part in a clinical trial, only to be told upon arrival that the trial had been closed owing to safety concerns. Others meet delays because the paperwork necessary was never forwarded by those who promised to do so, especially insurance company pre-approvals for payment.

Once treatment is underway, some people are surprised that the extensive and detailed protocol outlining the treatment really is just a guideline. Although a great deal of homage is paid to adhering to the protocol for the sake of science, the truth is that the protocol can be changed if you're suffering adverse effects. Often a change in protocol will not adversely affect your chances of succeeding on the treatment. This is particularly true in a phase I trial that's measuring toxicity.

If at all possible, have a friend or relative with you during treatment to verify what medications are given, to provide emotional support, and to be an advocate if you need one. This is especially important if you have traveled some distance for care, or are using morphine, for example, to control side effects.

Remember that you have the right to withdraw at any time from a clinical trial, to read your medical records, and to ask that deviations from the protocol be made if you're experiencing very bad side effects.

Experimental drugs outside clinical trials

There are several ways, other than clinical trials, to obtain drugs that are still in testing phases.

Investigational new drugs (IND)

Thanks to activism by AIDS patients, gaining early access to drugs still being tested is possible under the FDA's Treatment Investigational New Drug (IND) program, sometimes called the compassionate use program. This access is reserved for those with life-threatening diseases that have no other satisfactory treatment. According to FDA statistics, more than 20,000 patients with cancer have received treatment under a treatment IND since 1987. For more information, contact your doctor, the drug manufacturer, and the FDA at (800) 532-4440.

Paralleling a trial

Once the FDA approves a drug for a given condition (commonly referred to as its indication) a doctor is free to prescribe this drug for *any* illness. This is called off-label use, and demonstrates the FDA's faith in the medical community's integrity and knowledge.

If a clinical trial is testing drugs that are already approved by the FDA, but in new combinations or at new dose levels, your doctor might be willing to administer these drugs to you as they would have been given within the trial. Contact your doctor for more information.

Importation of a foreign drug

If an illness has no cure using drugs currently approved by the FDA, drugs made in foreign countries might be imported. Only those drugs meeting strict FDA regulations, though, are permitted. Among other requirements, the manufacturer must file an investigational new drug application with the FDA, and a letter justifying importation must accompany the request. For more information, contact your doctor, and contact the FDA (CDER Executive Secretariat (HFD-8), Center for Drug Evaluation and Research, Rockville, Maryland, (800) 532-4440).

About payment

Many people have found that they have difficulty getting their insurance companies to approve payment for care administered under the auspices of a clinical trial or for an investigational new drug.

One might surmise that, because cancer is a very expensive chronic disease, it would be to the financial benefit of insurance companies if better treatments were found. Nevertheless, individual companies often are unwilling to assume the costs of these studies.

The trend, however, is that more companies are paying for trials than in the past, or can be convinced to make exceptions for those who need treatment in trials. The federal government has set a good example by ruling that federally insured employees will be covered for their treatment within NCI-sponsored clinical trials. Rhode Island has passed a law requiring insurance companies to pay for cancer clinical trials. The state of Maryland has passed similar legislation that will require payment of fees for treatment given as part of a clinical trial for any illness, as long as the trial is NIH-approved.

Some cancer survivors have had success getting insurance payment approval by having their doctors supply evidence that previous tests of the new treatment showed some superiority over existing treatments, or by writing "letters of necessity" demonstrating that this experimental treatment is the only good choice available. Others have luck when their employers intervene. Still others use the news media to generate publicity that is embarrassing for the insurance company. Some cancer facilities offering clinical trials make provisions for those who want to participate but cannot pay.

Investigational new drug (IND) programs may offer drugs at a reduced price.

Importation of foreign drugs for single-patient use under the FDA's strict guidelines will almost certainly be an expense you'll have to bear on your own, but do check with your health insurance company, as policies vary widely.

An excellent source of additional information on negotiating for payment of treatment is Nancy Keene's book *Working with Your Doctor: Getting the Health-care You Deserve.*

Free treatment

In the following list are several institutions that charge little or nothing for participating in clinical trials:

The National Cancer Institute in Bethesda, Maryland, offers free treatment for those who qualify for their trials. This is a top-notch scientific institution run by the federal government, having some of the best cancer researchers in the country. Those who have used their services sometimes say, though, that they were very aware that they were in a research setting, as opposed to a setting oriented toward patient care and comfort. Call (800) 4-CANCER.

Non-US citizens are also admitted to trials at NCI at the discretion of the principal investigator. Criteria that are weighed in making this decision include whether a US citizen would be denied treatment if a non-US citizen were enrolled, and whether treating this particular individual's illness would benefit medical progress.

For children being treated at NCI, the Children's Inn at NCI provides free room and board for the children and their families. The Children's Inn accommodates both US and non-US citizens.

Shriners' Hospitals, 22 free children's hospitals across North America, are supported by the Shrine of North America, an international fraternity. These hospitals specialize in orthopedic and burn care. Children under age 18 who suffer spinal cord injury from radiotherapy might benefit from clinical trials offered at the Shriners' Hospitals. In the United States, call (800) 237-5055. In Canada, call (800) 361-7256.

The St. Jude Children's Research Hospital in Memphis, Tennessee, offers free treatment for children, and is on the forefront of developing successful treatments for children's cancers. Highly successful treatment for childhood leukemia was developed at St. Jude's in conjunction with other pediatric cancer groups. Call (901) 495-3300.

Summary

The National Cancer Institute recommends that clinical trials, a means of testing new therapies in order to improve cancer treatment, can be a good choice for those with stage II or greater colorectal cancer, colorectal cancer that has failed to respond to first-line therapy, or colorectal cancer that has relapsed.

Clinical trials are organized into three phases that evaluate increasingly complex aspects of treatment success. Each phase has its advantages and disadvantages. A careful assessment of all clinical trials is necessary to choose the one that's best for your circumstances.

Patient rights and safeguards are carefully observed in the clinical trial setting. You are free to withdraw at any time, and you cannot be denied care if you do so.

You can find information on clinical trials by asking your doctor, calling the National Cancer Institute at (800) 4-CANCER, or searching for trials on your own. See Chapter 24 for more information on searching for trials.

Being admitted to a trial may be preceded by a flurry of administrivia surrounding your evaluation that may thrill you with its cut-to-the-chase aspect, or may disappoint you with delays and miscommunications. The administrative offices of certain cancer care centers can be quite disorganized in spite of the institution's fine reputation for practicing excellent medicine.

Plan to have a friend or loved one act as an advocate for you during your treatment. It can be difficult to resolve certain problems, especially if you're far from home or using morphine, for example, to control side effects. Your emotional reactions might be surprising and conflicting, but overall you can probably expect to be confident that you've made a good choice.

CHAPTER 21

Traveling for Care

I traveled among unknown men,
in lands beyond the sea...

—Wordsworth

ROBUST RESEARCH IS UNDERWAY ON COLORECTAL CANCER at many prestigious national cancer centers. This means that there might be times when, after you have researched progress in treating your illness, you realize that the best care for your type or stage of colorectal cancer is provided at a major treatment center away from home—perhaps very far from home.

This, of course, adds several layers of complexity to your treatment plans, not the least of which are financial considerations. Some health insurance policies cover airfare but not lodging; some pay a per diem to apply to food and lodging, but do not cover airfare; still others pay only so much per travel mile. Some policies pay nothing for travel and lodging.

This chapter doesn't have answers to all of these questions, but it will help you with the financial aspects of traveling for care. It is organized to address monetary needs, and focuses on free services. Resources for children being treated for colon cancer are included as well as resources for children who will accompany parents who are ill. Canadian resources are reiterated in a separate section.

Assess needs and benefits

Your first step should be to verify what travel expenses your health policy will cover, because this coverage varies greatly.

Next, do some planning. If airfare isn't reimbursed by your health policy, driving might be an option. Driving may be out of the question, though, if the distance is great, if your car isn't in such good shape, or if you feel just plain awful. Lodging for family members who go with you is yet another expense. And who will remain behind, if young children need care in your absence?

Air travel

In many instances, the only practical way to travel to the treatment center of your choice is by air. There are charitable groups that exist to fly you, free of charge, to distant treatment centers.

Some of these groups have requirements, for example, that the patient be able to embark and disembark the plane without airline assistance, or that support equipment, if needed, be manageable without airline intervention.

Each service is described below, but the best starting point if you're pressed for time is Mercy Medical Airlift's National Patient Air Transport Helpline (NPATH), the only national toll-free number that can direct patients to the nearest and best air travel resource for their travel needs: (800) 296-1217.

Mercy Medical Airlift

Mercy Medical Airlift is the coordinating organization for three sectors of charitable air services in the US. They utilize fixed-wing (not helicopter) aircraft to help financially needy patients go to and from care centers for previously scheduled evaluation, diagnosis, treatment, and rehabilitation appointments. They do not provide emergency transport. Mercy Medical Airlift can be contacted at (800) 296-1191.

The three sectors of aviation involved in MMA are:

- The corporate aviation sector, consisting of 750 corporations that allow cancer and multiple sclerosis patients to use empty seats on regularly scheduled flights. The Corporate Angel Network (CAN) is the focal point for this program. In 1997, 900 patients were transported. You do not need to demonstrate financial hardship to use CAN; there is no limit on the number of trips you can make. Cancer patients, their companions, or bone marrow donors are eligible. Children may be accompanied by two parents. Patients must be able walk up stairs to board the plane without assistance, and must be able to fly without any form of life support or medical assistance. Call (914) 328-1313 for other requirements.

- The private aviation sector, consisting of 4,500 pilots within 32 volunteer pilot organizations across the US who use their own time and aircraft to fly patients free of charge to care centers. Organizationally, these groups cluster under Air Care Alliance. In 1997, more than 8,000 patients were transported. You may call ACA at (888) 662-6794 in the US; elsewhere call (757) 318-9145.

- The commercial airline sector. Several commercial airlines offer, at times, special ticket prices or free tickets to those who need to travel for medical care, but cannot afford full ticket prices. These special offers vary by airline, and are not necessarily ongoing offers.

In addition, Mercy Medical Airlift operates the Patient Assistance Center (PAC: (888) 675-1405), whose programs are:

- The National Patient Air Transport Helpline (NPATH) is, as mentioned earlier, the only national toll-free number that can direct patients to the nearest and best air travel resource for their travel needs. (800) 296-1217.

- Special-Lift and Child-Lift Programs to assist with transport of those needing care for pediatric or rare diseases at medical research centers.

- Programs to develop the charitable services of the private air sector, under the auspices of the Air Care Alliance.

- Programs to encourage and unify charitable ticket use programs among the commercial airlines.

The Red Cross

For military personnel only, the Red Cross can assist with emergency travel and communication. Call (202) 728-6400, or their 24-hour line at (202) 728-6401, to find the chapter nearest you or your destination.

Mission Air Transportation Network

This Canadian group uses corporate, government, or commercial aircraft to fly Canadians who need medical care but cannot afford air transport. Call (416) 222-6335.

Mission Aviation Fellowship

MAF supports air ambulance services and medical assistance in 57 countries. Call (909) 794-1151.

Land travel

Fewer organizations exist to help with land travel than for air travel.

American Cancer Society

The ACS regional offices in many cities have networks of volunteers who can provide transport by car to and from your treatment center. Call your local office or (800) ACS-2345.

Traveler's Aid Society

Traveler's Aid provides emergency travel and lodging for those in dire financial need. Check local phone books for contact information. For the Traveler's Aid phone number at your destination, check your public library for phone books for other major cities.

Lodging

Having the means to pay for travel for care is part of the solution; however, finding affordable housing remains a barrier to travel for some colorectal cancer survivors. Several groups offer lodging for free or for a nominal fee.

Note that the cost of meals usually will be your responsibility. Facilities such as Hope Lodge, however, have kitchens that you can use to reduce your expenses by avoiding the higher cost of restaurant meals.

American Cancer Society's Hope Lodge

The American Cancer Society sponsors free lodging in various cities for cancer patients being treated at nearby hospitals and their families. Their service is also offered to non-US citizens traveling within the US for medical care. Lodging is free and is provided on a first-come, first-served basis, so contact the ACS for the phone number of the Hope Lodge nearest the hospital you'll be using to verify that space is available. Each Hope Lodge has kitchen and laundry facilities. Call (800) ACS-2345.

National Association of Hospital Hospitality Houses

NAHHH offers a list of member hotels who provide reduced rates and special services to patients at nearby hospitals. Call (301) 961-3094, (317) 883-2226, or (800) 542-9730.

Ronald McDonald Houses

Ronald McDonald Houses, sponsored by the McDonald's Corporation, offer free lodging to children who must travel for medical care and their families. Pregnant women considered high-risk pregnancies also are eligible. Financial need may be a prerequisite for entry at some sites. A nominal fee of ten dollars a night may also be charged, but this may be waived if financial hardship is demonstrated. Call (312) 836-7100.

Adult care at the National Cancer Institute

Adult patients who have been treated at NCI report that their spouses were allowed to stay overnight in the patient's room. You should verify this with NCI and with the nurses on the floor.

Hospital-hotel agreements

Many hospitals have agreements with nearby hotels for reduced rates for patients and families. Contact the hospital's social worker or the admitting desk in advance of traveling for such information.

Hospital Outpatient Facilities

Some major cancer centers, such as Johns Hopkins in Baltimore, have outpatient lodging run by the institution for those requiring long-term follow-up care. Discuss these resources with the hospital admitting staff before you travel. The cost of you and your family staying in such hospital-run facilities may be covered by your insurance policy.

Children's Inn at the National Cancer Institute

The National Cancer Institute offers free meals and housing for children under age 18 who are being treated at NCI. Lodging might also be available for family members on a case-by-case basis. Both US and non-US citizens are accommodated. Call (800) 4-CANCER for more information.

For family members who cannot be lodged at NCI in Bethesda, Maryland, the American Cancer Society's Hope Lodge in nearby Baltimore is an alternative, as are nearby hotels who have agreements with NCI to offer reduced rates to the families of cancer patients treated at NCI.

St. Jude Children's Research Hospital

The St. Jude Children's Research Hospital in Memphis, Tennessee, offers free treatment for children, and is on the forefront of developing successful treatments for children's cancers. Call (901) 495-3300.

Travel insurance with medical features

Your health insurance might not cover out-of-state emergency medical care, so before you travel for pleasure, you should verify your health policy's coverage. If it's restrictive, consider getting travel insurance that covers emergency medical care. This ensures that if you take a vacation out of state, and need, for instance, to get a transfusion or other emergency care while you're away, you'll have coverage to do so.

Here's a partial list of companies that offer such coverage, although this list does not imply recommendation or endorsement:

- Travel Assistance International: (800) 821-2828
- Medex: (888) MEDEX-00
- Travel Emergency Assistance (TEA): (281) 364-7726

Schooling

Some treatment centers, such as the Fred Hutchinson Cancer Center in Seattle, offer on-site schooling for sick children and their siblings. Contact the cancer center you're planning to use to see if they accommodate children who travel for care or who accompany others.

Your child's school, of course, might be willing to design a lesson plan that you can oversee to continue schooling your children who must travel.

Canadian assistance

This section describes Canadian services, some of which also are discussed elsewhere in this chapter.

- The British Columbia Medical Services Plan coordinates sharing travel expenses with commercial transportation firms such as airlines and ferries. Your doctor must fill out a Travel Assistance form. Call (800) 661-2668 toll-free or (250) 387-8277.

- The Mission Air Transportation Network uses corporate, government, or commercial aircraft to fly those who need medical care but cannot afford air transport. Call (416) 222-6335.

- The Canadian Cancer Society offers various forms of assistance. Call (604) 872-4400 or (416) 961-7223.

- Canadian Cancer Society resource numbers by province:
    - Alberta, (403) 228-4487
    - Manitoba, (204) 774-7483
    - New Brunswick, (506) 634-6272
    - Newfoundland & Labrador, (709) 753-6520
    - Nova Scotia, (902) 423-6183
    - Ontario, (416) 488-5400
    - Prince Edward Island, (902) 566-4007
    - Quebec, (514) 255-5151
    - Saskatchewan, (306) 757-4260

Summary

The search for excellent care sometimes leads us far from home. The emotional issues regarding care away from home, and the logistics of accommodating family members who must remain behind are difficult. Adding the expense of travel to these often seems overwhelming. This chapter offers ways to make traveling for care financially easier.

Key points to remember:

- Free air travel for cancer patients is available. Call the National Patient Air Transport Helpline at (800) 296-1217.

- Cancer care at the National Cancer Institute is free if you agree to enroll in an NCI clinical trial. Call (800) 4-CANCER.

- Free lodging for patients receiving outpatient care, and for their families, is available in many cities at the American Cancer Society's Hope Lodge. Call (800) ACS-2345.

CHAPTER 22

If All Treatments Have Failed

Death, the refuge, the solace, the best
and kindliest and most prized friend ...

—Mark Twain
Adam

NOT SURPRISINGLY, THE PERSON WHO HAS HAD COLORECTAL CANCER, or indeed any cancer, sometimes feels compelled to consider what experiences he faces if his treatments do not succeed, and likely will do so with more clarity, urgency, and fear than the person who perceives himself to be reasonably healthy.

This chapter will discuss what dying appears to be like. Before reading further, please consider carefully whether reading this chapter will be bad for you emotionally, if you still have options remaining, as this chapter assumes that one's treatment options have been exhausted, or are potentially too uncomfortable or damaging to continue.

Speaking to and for the patient is our chief goal, not for family and friends, as this chapter must attempt to communicate a great deal in limited space, and many books already exist for those who will grieve. We will offer information about dying as an incipient event rather than addressing the problems of living well with colorectal cancer. The physical and emotional aspects, but not the philosophical, religious, or financial aspects of approaching death will be discussed.

In the last twenty years, and especially in the last few years, many good books have become available on the topics of dying and dying well. Some, such as several by Elisabeth Kubler-Ross, tend to address those nearest the dying rather than speaking directly to the dying person. Others by Kubler-Ross, and such books as *How We Die*, by Sherwin Nuland, *The Art of Dying*, by Patricia Weenolsen, *The Dying Time*, by Furman and McNabb, and *A*

Graceful Exit, by Lofty Basta, speak directly to the dying person. Please see the bibliography for these and other books.

Preparing emotionally for death

There are probably as many emotions about dying as there are human beings, and there is no one correct way to die. If death is somewhat expected and not too rapid, the emotions of loss that we experience are likely to mirror those felt at first diagnosis of colorectal cancer. In fact, the evolving feelings associated with loss that were described in Chapter 1, *Symptoms, Diagnosis, and Staging*, were first described by Elisabeth Kubler-Ross following her observations of the dying. They are common to many people in the time approaching death:

- Initially, *denial* that death is approaching

- *Anger* that you're being taken too soon, or unfairly

- *Bargaining* with God, or with others, for more time, less pain, or comfort for your loved ones

- When bargaining fails, *depression* and *sadness* that death is inevitable

- Finally, *acceptance* that death will occur

Not everyone goes through all of these stages, nor do all people evolve through them in the same order, nor does one linger in these stages for the same amount of time. The person experiencing great pain, for instance, is likely to long for and accept death's approach quickly rather than be angry.

These stages are not necessarily sequential and discrete: you don't necessarily feel anger until it's spent, and only then move on to bargaining, for instance. The stages often are overlapping or concurrent.

A wife discusses her husband's acceptance of his approaching death:

> We are facing the details of J's death head on. When we first discovered his illness, we prepared living wills and medical power of attorney documents. We're now working on his obituary and a letter to be sent to business clients and friends. He's also taken on a new project and in the time remaining will be recording his story of the re-development of the historic heart of the city. He's always felt that the story of saving the inner city should be told by the people who did it, and he's one of them. I'm tell-

ing you this tale because I know that many of you have stories to tell—about your lives, your towns, your loves. DO IT NOW! Share your memories, tell the tales that no one else knows. Leave your footprints in the sands of time.

Asking for honesty

You might not be able to prepare to die as you would like if those around you are not willing to admit it's imminent. At the very least, one can expect and ask for honesty from doctors, even if family members continue to deny your approaching death in order to protect themselves a little longer.

If you have trouble getting honest answers from those around you, you might try pointing out how much it means to you to make sense of this final experience, to be ready for it, to be as comfortable as possible. You might also attempt to tell those you love if you are convinced that death will occur soon, as often the patient is more aware than others—sometimes even more aware than medical personnel—that the end is quite near.

Difficult family issues

Unfortunately, at this very difficult time one often needs to deal not only with one's own feelings, but with those of loved ones. This may be made even more difficult if their experiences with loss and grief are out of phase with your own. Your relatives' denial that you are dying is not the only issue that may sadden your final days. They may grieve earlier than you do, anticipating your death before you yourself have accepted it—or indeed, perhaps before you're dying at all. They may lag behind you in the stages of acceptance, continuing to bargain with medical personnel for life-support measures when you're ready to let go. Or perhaps your family will express anger toward you for asking questions about dying, railing against any sign that you've given up.

You might be able to ease your family's acceptance of your death by reassuring them that they will be taken care of, by telling them that you love them, that you're weary of the battle and you welcome death, and by saying goodbye in loving ways, both overtly and symbolically.

What to say to children

Dependent children and grandchildren need unique reassurances that they will be loved and well cared for after you're no longer available to love and help them. Of course, if you have dependent children, by now you've most likely done your best to arrange loving care for them, and they probably know of these arrangements.

Fortunately, there are many good books you can use to help your child or grandchild understand death in general: see Appendix A, *Resources*, and the bibliography, and in particular *I'm with You Now*, by M. Catherine Ray. In general, it's considered wise to give children as much honest and pointed information as possible, in terms that are appropriate for their age. For instance, it may be upsetting for your child to hear you say that you're in pain and are taking medicine for pain, but it's likely to be much more damaging if she sees you suffering and wasn't prepared to see this, and thinks your suffering cannot be mediated.

Make it clear to your children or grandchildren that your circumstances were not caused by anything they did. Children are egocentric, and must be reassured repeatedly that their thoughts and actions did not cause this illness.

Make it clear as well that your spouse and the child's siblings and parents are not to blame. Expect that young children will be openly or secretly angry with you for leaving them: spurts of this anger are natural and inevitable. At the same time, they may understand that it's not acceptable to blame you for dying. This doesn't leave the anger anywhere to go. Thus, the path that the young psyche may take—if they cannot blame you, and the burden of anger and self-blame is too great to carry alone—is to blame the surviving grandparent, parent, or a sibling. Make it as clear as possible that nobody is to blame, and that everybody is feeling sad and sorry about your dying.

Tell them over and over that you love them, and that you would not leave them if you had a choice.

There are specific points to be avoided, though, when talking to a child about dying. In her book *The Art of Dying*, Patricia Weenolsen suggests you avoid saying the following:

- Do not say you're simply going to sleep for a long time. Children may develop a fear of falling asleep if it's compared to dying, this phenomenon which is making all the grown-ups act so sad. They may even fear that they will never wake. If your faith includes a belief in an afterlife during which one awakes and is reunited with loved ones, try to explain using an analogy that does not parallel the child's normal daily actions.

- Likewise, don't tell them you're going on a long trip. They may never accept that you've died, and they may never again trust others to return. Your death may raise enough issues with trust as it is; don't add to these issues by using allegorical detail with children who are too young to do other than take what you say literally.

- Be cautious about suggesting that your spiritual presence will remain nearby if your children believe in, and act fearful of, ghosts. They may become fearful of haunting after you've died.

Forgiveness and other emotional closures

Some religions emphasize that, before one dies, certain spiritual life tasks must be completed, such as forgiving those who have harmed you, forgiving yourself, and admitting your wrongdoings.

Only you need to be satisfied with the state of your inner being as you prepare to die. You may choose to adhere closely to religious beliefs, or you may decide they're bunkum, that you wish to die peacefully without trying to contact everyone you've wronged, for example.

Detachment

Just as one may have withdrawn quite naturally from healthy, unaware friends after diagnosis, cleaving instead to other cancer survivors, as death approaches, you may find yourself wanting and needing to withdraw from the living. This is a natural process, partly physical as you weaken and perhaps suffer physical pain, but it might also be a shift in the spiritual or emotional needs of the non-physical self.

You may sense that people who have died are trying to communicate with you; you may dream about those who have died, or of places distinctly not of Earth's confining dimensions. While it's beyond the scope of this book to speculate on the meaning or veracity of such events, others who are dying have reported such happenings and appear to be much comforted by them. Often these dreams and perceptions occur in the last week or so of life.

The outside observer sometimes is appalled by the sight of the family sitting in the dying person's room, talking among themselves as if the patient had already died. While ignoring the dying person's need to communicate does sometimes happen, at other times it's a reflection of the family's tacit understanding that the dying person is withdrawing from the living.

Permission to die: the last gift of love

Many reports of the experiences of the dying tell us that some people need permission from their loved ones to let go. If you are blessed with time, you might discuss this in advance with your family. Particularly if you are in pain, try to make it clear to them that they give you a great gift when they give you permission to die.

At times, even among those who have had this discussion, a final gesture of letting go by the family, verbal or tactile, appears to be necessary in one's final moments to allow death to occur.

One colon cancer survivor who has faced her death writes:

> I am 63 years old, have had three surgeries for colon cancer, have had a colostomy, and still have unremovable cancer in my body. I began this adventure in November 1996. My husband and I have five grown children (ages 26 through 42) and two grandchildren (17 months and 2 months). We are due another grandchild in September.
>
> Dealing with my children is mostly okay. My oldest daughter was the first to look up colon cancer on the Net and knows just about as much as I do about the subject. She is also the one, along with my husband, who talks to the surgeon and oncologist after each surgery. We know there is no cure and only time to fight.
>
> I am very lucky as I am still using the original chemotherapy (5-FU with leucovorin) and it still seems to be working. My last surgery was in April of this year, when I received my colostomy after finding the tumor had affixed to the abdominal wall in the rear.
>
> Only my daughter is willing to talk in reality, with my sons only questioning how I feel. Good is good and bad is not so good. I think all of them know that this disease is only going to allow me so much time and I certainly plan on making the best of it.
>
> I have spent a good deal of time weaving my kids and their families into a large mosaic to continue loving and working together after I am

gone. I watched my husband's mother, who was the one who kept every-one together for outings and such, die and the rest of the family go their own way, not really being close to each other. It pains me to think that could happen to mine even though they are close now.

My God has given me the gift of not being afraid of death (not now, anyway). But I certainly plan on living up until I can't, and I make no secret of my feelings when talking to my children. Being prepared is some-thing I truly believe in, and am truly grateful for the time that has been allowed me to do the preparation. I sometimes think of the people who leave for work one day and never come home. I have had at least time to do and say the things that are very important for my family and myself.

Physical aspects of dying

Many colorectal cancer survivors and their families ask what dying will be like.

How will we die?

Dying from colorectal cancer can occur in several ways depending on which organs are most affected by disease. Life-threatening symptoms usually will be related to the failure of organs invaded by or near a tumor mass. Colorectal cancer metastasized to the brain may suppress the brain center that controls breathing or may cause seizures. Colorectal cancer spread to the liver or kidney may cause toxins to accumulate in the bloodstream, which in turn causes coma. A large lung or liver tumor may cause the lungs or heart to fail; a blocked intestine might cause death from lack of nourishment. Because colorectal cancer can manifest in several ways, your oncologist is the best person to prepare you for the physical symptoms you are most likely to face, and what level of pain, if any, you may need to counter with medication.

Even a death preceded by great pain and discomfort sometimes is, in its very last stage, peaceful and illuminated by a brief cognizance.

When will it occur?

No human knows the answer to this question: not for colorectal cancer or for any other form death may take. There are well-known physical signs associated with the very last stage of life, yet some people have revived after all signs of life are extinguished. Many people have rallied for months or years after feeling so ill they wished for and surrendered to death, or after their doctors had given up all hope for survival. We can know only that our death will occur in our lifetime.

The final moments of life

Most people at this stage of death seem not to be aware of what is happening to their body, or they seem to drift in and out of awareness. The perception of family members looking on at this stage is that the patient is in great discomfort, but those who have had near-death experiences do not report remembering great distress at this stage. The truth is unknown.

The visible physical signs seen most often just before death comprise the *agonal* stage, and might include muscle spasm, one or more large gasps for breath, breathing that starts and stops, heaving of chest or shoulders, a single deep exhalation, clear or unclear vocalizations, or noisy breathing. All muscles relax, including bowel and bladder sphincter muscles. This might release no body waste, though, if no food was taken recently.

These signs may be visible for just an instant, or may last for several minutes.

How medical staff define death

Currently, brain death is the criterion used to ascertain that death is irrefutable, because other classic signs of death such as cessation of heartbeat or breathing can be misleading, or can be reversed using twentieth-century medical technology.

Signs of brain death include loss of all reflexes such as the blink reflex or the pupil's response to light, failure to respond physically or verbally to urgent or painful stimuli, and the absence of electrical activity within the brain as measured by an electroencephalogram (EEG).

If a colorectal cancer patient dies in a hospital or under hospice care, though, and death has been expected, medical workers are very likely to simply check for pulse and breath as death approaches. Under these circumstances, an EEG would most likely be unwarranted.

Can we make dying easier?

Easing death can take several forms: receiving physical and emotional comfort, finalizing affairs, or perhaps forgiving one's self and others for old grudges and sins. Some of these topics are addressed in other chapters; spiritual comfort and philosophical adaptation are addressed in many fine books.

Pain control

The most pressing concern for many people with terminal colorectal cancer is the control of pain. In the past, several studies have shown that dying cancer patients did not receive adequate medication to control pain owing to misconceptions on the part of medical doctors about addiction or accidental overdose. In the time since these studies have been published, however, many physicians have become better informed about pain control for the dying cancer patient. They're doing a better job of providing palliative care, but patients and especially caregivers must remain vigilant about insisting on adequate pain medication.

It's wise to plan in advance on having a say in the comfort of your death. If you have the luxury of choices and the time to make them, draft a living will or advance directives, or both, and plan to die at home or in hospice care instead of within the hospital. Studies of care administered in hospitals show that advance directives expressing wishes against extraordinary life support measures often are ignored by doctors when care is administered in the hospital. Hospice care or care by loved ones is more likely to assure your comfort than life-saving hospital measures are.

> The best thing both my parents did was to have a living will, a power of attorney for health, and general power of attorney assigned to me years before they got sick. We never needed it for my dad, but for my mom I did. After my parents' death my aunt did the same thing, and I used the power of attorney (especially the health one) many times for her at the end. I was faxing that precious document everywhere so they had to deal with me instead of bothering her. She was so grateful, and the caretakers knew they'd better ask me first if they wanted to do anything to her.

Hospice and hospice home care

One of the most useful resources for the comfort of the dying person and his family is hospice care, a comfort-centered concept that emerged in Europe and migrated to the US following many years' failure of medical technology to provide comfort for the dying. Hospice care is devoted only to making one comfortable and loved in her dying days, not to prolonging life. A peaceful and less expensive variation of hospice care is hospice home care, now quite common in the US.

Hospice nurses are on call for you 24 hours a day. They might visit one or more times daily if needed, or perhaps once a week or less if your needs are minimal. They are able to administer pain medication, provide skilled nursing care such as monitoring vital signs, are trained to recognize the signs of impending death, and can help the family with the arrangements that are necessary just after a death in the home has occurred. Their focus includes the physical and emotional comfort of the patient, and the well-being of the surviving family members after death.

Under many hospice programs, home health aides also are available to help caregivers with some household chores and certain kinds of patient care such as bathing.

Some hospice services charge little or nothing for those who cannot afford the service; others provide free hospice care regardless of one's financial status.

To qualify for hospice Medicare benefits and for many private insurance companies' benefits, a doctor's statement is necessary stating that the patient has less than six months to live.

Our journey ended last Friday afternoon. My husband died, at home, quietly. He had been able to visit with friends and to listen to the basketball game yet on Thursday night. But in the night, things changed, he began vomiting blood.

The nurse was here most of the morning. She helped me to plan for his care for the next few weeks, but by the time she left at 12:30 she told me to call his family and let them know they should be making plans to come if they wanted to speak to him before he died. Our older son came home from school at lunchtime, just feeling the need to check on how things were going and decided to stay. My husband's partner from the firm came to visit in the afternoon, and while my husband couldn't speak, he did respond. Our younger son arrived home from school about 3:30.

My husband took his last breath at 4:37. He very much wanted to be at home and not to have this phase of the journey drag on. That wish was granted.

Euthanasia

Unfortunately, there can be painful preludes to death for which no amount of medication is adequate. In some cases, the dying and their loved ones are willing, indeed almost compelled by horrific suffering, to end life earlier than the disease would end it.

Euthanasia, the hastening of the end of life by active intervention, has been much discussed in the US recently. Groups such as the Hemlock Society and the American Medical Association have expressed divergent points of view. The American Medical Association states that doctor-assisted suicide violates their standards. The Hemlock Society publishes literature on dying and the right to die, including the book *Final Exit*.

In his book, *How We Die*, Dr. Sherwin Nuland, a surgeon, says:

> *In my medical practice, I have always assured my dying patients that I would do everything possible to give them an easy death, but I have too often seen even that hope dashed in spite of everything I try. At a hospice too, where the only goal is tranquil comfort, there are failures.*

Some doctors will privately state that they have broken the law to ease a patient's going. A geriatric neurologist I know stated that among her fellow medical doctors, about half will help a patient of their own to die when medicine and technology cannot relieve suffering.

Planning your own memorial ceremony

It's an odd fact that many people who cannot bear to think of the dying process, who cannot even conceive of their mortality, are quite happy to plan their own memorial ceremony and burial. As death becomes a certainty, many people find comfort in planning how others will remember them and celebrate their life.

Some of the things you might want to consider are:

- Whether you would like to be buried or cremated, where and how you would like your remains to be preserved or honored

- What memories of your life you'd like retold at your funeral or memorial service

- If there are special songs or poems you want sung or read
- Whether the ceremony will be a religious one
- If your interment or the scattering of your ashes will be private

Summary

Dying cannot be described accurately by the living, much less by the well. Nonetheless, we have tried to listen to those preparing for death, to learn from what they say, from those nearest them, and to share these insights with you.

We are blessed to be living during a renaissance of interest in society about dying and death, and to benefit from cultural considerations of how to die well. You will find many books available to make the journey called dying as peaceful as possible.

Key points to remember:

- Adequate control of pain is possible and should be discussed in advance with your doctor.
- Hospice care is an excellent choice for those facing death, as they provide extraordinary physical and emotional support for the dying person and her family.
- If you have time, prepare wills, living wills, and advance directives so that your wishes about dying will be known and honored.
- Communicate with your loved ones about dying. The last days or weeks of life can be beautiful and peaceful if you have the support, acceptance, and love of those around you

CHAPTER 23

The Future of Therapy

*Every great advance in science has issued
from a new audacity of imagination.*

—John Dewey

THE SPIRIT OF COOPERATIVE ACADEMIC ENDEAVOR, a coalescence of insights from multiple medical disciplines, governmental prioritization, a highly developed research infrastructure, and the uninterrupted scientific focus of nations at peace have positioned us well for the development of promising new cancer therapies in the years ahead.

This chapter will discuss peer-reviewed mainstream medical therapies for colorectal cancer. The first section is a brief overview of what causes cancer, followed by a section discussing broad trends in research. Next is an encyclopedic reference list of treatments now in trials, organized by mode of action, then trials for prevention of colorectal cancer. Finally, we discuss therapies we're likely to see in the more distant future, consisting of substances and approaches, such as tissue regeneration, that are not being tested against colorectal cancer at this time.

The purpose of the chapter is to give you an idea of the kind of research that is currently underway. None of the descriptions that follow should be construed as a recommendation for treatment. Any treatment that you find here or elsewhere should be carefully evaluated by oncology experts before your treatment decisions are made. You can gain access to new treatments that are still in clinical trials if you and your doctor decide it would be advantageous to do so. See Chapter 20, *Clinical Trials*, for more information.

Although the timing for testing and approving a typical cancer treatment is measured in years, cancer treatments are being improved constantly. This chapter represents merely a snapshot of new therapies at the time this book was written. Information presented here concerning how various anticancer substances work, for instance, reflects the knowledge currently available in the medical literature, and is subject to change as research progresses.

The sources of information for this chapter are the National Cancer Institute's clinical trials database and research papers accessible through the National Library of Medicine's Medline, a collection of more than 9 million published medical papers.

What causes cancer?

Many of the descriptions of newer treatments being developed today will be easier to understand if the known causes of cancer are understood. This topic is covered in detail in Chapter 3, *What Is Colorectal Cancer?*, but certain key points are reiterated here.

Cancer is an illness resulting from damaged genes. Many if not all instances of cancer are accompanied by changes in the tumor cell's DNA. At times, a gene is entirely missing, or has been half-spliced with another gene after DNA strands from two entirely different chromosomes accidentally overlap, break apart, and rejoin. In other cases, one chromosome will break, flip, and rejoin at the wrong ends. A third kind of damage involves deletion of one base pair of nucleic acids from an amino acid encoding sequence in a gene. All of the body's work is accomplished using proteins built from genes. If the gene is damaged by chromosome breakage, for example, a protein built from it may be partly or completely nonfunctional, toxic, or even tumor-promoting.

A tumor may arise because such genes are:

- Incorrectly transcribed into aberrant proteins
- Not transcribed at all or are overexpressed
- Expressed at the wrong time
- Two erroneously spliced genes are being transcribed into a hybrid protein that is impotent or oncogenic
- A combination of any of these

When these aberrant genetic changes occur in, or very near, genes that regulate cell growth, trigger orderly cell death (apoptosis), or regulate maturation or cell division and reproduction, cancer may result. For almost all cancers, an accumulation of genetic damage is needed before a cell becomes cancerous—that is, capable of uncontrolled growth and able to invade other tissue.

An overview of research trends

Over the last five to twenty years, broad trends in cancer research in general and in colorectal cancer research in particular have taken several concurrent paths:

- A much more targeted approach to identifying and testing potentially useful anticancer substances, enabled by our much improved understanding of the genetic origin, development, and metabolic milieu of tumors within the body.

- An altered (and, to date, not entirely successful) effort in fighting cancer with substances our own bodies make, instead of using external plant-based or manmade substances.

- Interdisciplinary cooperation that yields coordinated treatments with better results.

- An emphasis, at the request of many patients, to design drugs and procedures for supportive care—drugs that do not destroy cancer, but instead contribute significantly to survival by eliminating the secondary effects and illnesses related to treatment. The drugs that control nausea or stimulate growth of new blood cells after chemotherapy, for example, fall into this category.

- An interest in preventing cancer and examining its causes.

- Development of exquisite imaging tools that reveal the smallest of tumors and metastases.

- Refinements in surgical technique that permit sparing of healthy tissue and more thorough removal of tumors.

Substance identification and testing

For many years, anticancer drugs were discovered by testing many natural and manmade substances wholesale—often in excess of 5,000 per year—against tumor samples that were kept alive in laboratories. Substances that worked in this setting were then tested in mice; those that worked in mice were tested in humans. Those that worked better in humans than existing drugs became part of standard treatment—all without understanding the drug's mode of action until afterward, if ever.

While this approach is still often used, a trend toward understanding a drug's mode of action before its use has emerged, owing to great advances in biochemistry, genetics, molecular biology, and many related fields of science such as engineering and computer science. You'll see this trend reflected in almost every drug category discussed later in this chapter—indeed, that they can be categorized at all reflects this new understanding.

For instance, a problem that often emerges in cancer therapy is the inability to deliver a high dose of toxin directly to the tumor, either because it's encapsulated within or entwined with healthy tissue, is many cell layers thick, or has high internal pressure that makes penetration difficult. Many of the newer approaches to cancer therapy target specific barriers such as these, rather than just a wholesale killing of the tumor by unknown mechanisms.

This refined testing relies on our much improved understanding of the genetic causes and biologic pathways of cancer. Using this understanding, a researcher might be able to identify the portion of a molecule that's responsible for the specific anticancer activity the researcher is hoping to accomplish. Often this design and simulation is computerized, atom by atom, including animation showing how the molecule will interact with the binding site of the tumor or other bodily substance that aids cancer growth. This isolation of design is followed by a computerized search of a database of millions of substances, retrieving all that match this characteristic. Sometimes among the substances that match will be a tried and true drug for another illness; sometimes it will be a drug tried for other purposes, but abandoned, such as thalidomide. Sometimes it will be a new plant-based biological compound found during a pharmaceutical company's last foray into the rainforest or ocean to collect samples of all flora.

Some researchers take this understanding several steps farther and attempt to build from scratch custom-made drugs that have a lock-and-key fit to the tumor cell type, or to some biological mechanism that supports tumor growth. This approach is called rational drug design.

Biological anticancer substances

Almost any anticancer substance could by definition be called biological in that it has an effect on the body, but in this book the term includes only those substances made by the body to fight enemy substances. These substances have accumulated a tremendous following among many patients and some researchers as potential cures for cancer. As a distinct class of drugs, they are appealing for many reasons. One fairly overt reason is the popular contemporary cachet of "natural substances" and their alleged low toxicity. Another less obvious reason is the sense of balance provided by the theory that cancer is an internal process run amok, and that a corresponding internal substance may correct it. The third and best reason is that they may work, as interleukin-2 and interferon-alfa-2B have against some kidney cancers and melanomas.

Four biological anticancer substance types are in clinical trials for use against colorectal cancer at the time of this writing. Each of these is discussed in detail in the following sections:

- Monoclonal antibodies

- Tumor vaccines

- Leukocyte therapy

- Cytokines

Much work remains to be done in the area of biological substances, because the concept is very promising and has hardly been tapped. Combining monoclonal antibodies with toxic substances that permit targeting only of the tumor instead of healthy tissue is being pursued hotly. Combining the interferons with some of the interleukins, notably interleukin-2, may yield better results than interferons alone have yielded. Combining these natural substances with traditional chemotherapies is the target of many clinical trials now being run. Creating a version of one or more of these molecules that's slightly different from those found in nature may make them more potent than those produced by our bodies.

It's useful to keep in mind, though, that some substances that have long been used against cancer also are "natural." Mitomycin C, for example, is derived from a fungus. In other words, natural substances are not always harmless and magically effective, just as steroids—including such substances as estrogen, vitamin D, and cholesterol—are not necessarily rage-producing, dangerous, and illegal.

A subcategory of drugs that are considered biological therapy are the biological response modifiers, another somewhat ambiguous name, as any substance that modifies a bodily response might in theory fit this category. In this instance, though, we include only substances made by the body and replicated in the lab, such as:

- Cytokines, including the interleukins and interferons

- Tumor necrosis factor
- Colony stimulating factors for red and white blood cells and platelets, discussed later under "Supportive care"

Interdisciplinary cooperation

Cancer survivors sometimes report that a medical oncologist's assessment of their condition includes a recommendation for chemotherapy, while a radiation oncologist's assessment suggests that radiotherapy is the best choice.

While this unenviable dilemma still arises for some cancer survivors, now more than ever, the surgeon, medical oncologist, and radiation oncologist work as a team.

For colorectal cancer, this is demonstrated in the use of presurgical chemotherapy or radiotherapy to debulk tumors, facilitating more complete surgical removal; intraoperative radiotherapy to target precisely and only diseased tissue; or radioactive implants inserted during surgery.

Supportive care

Although this chapter does not discuss many investigative drugs used for supportive care simply because space is limited, they should not be underestimated. Many of the gains made in lengthening life or curing cancer have come about because of drugs for supportive care, such as:

- Zofran for controlling nausea and permitting the individual to retain nutrients more successfully
- G-CSF and GM-CSF for reestablishing adequate levels of infection-fighting white blood cells
- Epoetin (Epogen, Procrit) for reestablishing adequate levels of red blood cells
- Amphotericin for overcoming previously fatal fungal infections

Progress in supportive care is responsible for the success of certain cancer therapies that depend more on ancillary care for success than on the procedure itself. Marrow ablation followed by stem cell reinfusion, for instance, a process just beginning to be tested against colorectal cancer, is in itself a straightforward procedure, but exacting and copious supportive care is required to avoid and control infection until marrow is reestablished.

Cancer prevention

Years ago, cancer epidemiology consisted of asking those already diagnosed with cancer to recall incidents and lifestyle habits from many years ago. Their answers were examined for patterns that might correlate to the incidence of cancer in a population.

Today, we're seeing different kinds of detection and prevention trials, such as those designed to examine lifestyles, diet, and environmental factors as they're occurring, and to tally and track all cases of cancer in these groups as they develop. This is a more accurate way of assessing risk and correlation than asking patients in a highly stressful setting to recall, for example, dietary habits from 30 years ago.

Other trials include asking participants to adhere to a specific diet for a number of years, and then recording the incidence of cancers in this group as opposed to the incidence among those who had no dietary restrictions.

Still others may involve participants who are taking vitamin supplements, exercising to a schedule, using estrogen supplements, or losing weight. These groups are followed for many years, and any cases of cancer that occur are recorded and followed.

Imaging tools

The ability to visualize body organs and to delineate the status of disease without invasive procedures truly is one of the great gifts of twentieth-century medicine. X radiation, computed tomography (CT), magnetic resonance imaging (MRI), positron emission tomography (PET), scintigraphy, and ultrasound (US) give us better information than ever before regarding the health and disease status of individual organs.

The use of such tools has shown us, though, that even better tools are needed. Computed tomography, for instance, does not clearly display soft tissue, while MRI does; and while one or the other may delineate an unusual internal mass, they may be unable to determine if it's a cancerous or harmless lesion. Positron emission tomography, on the other hand, can distinguish the metabolic rate of glucose in tissue, and by this measure may identify a mass as cancerous or benign.

Surgical technique

The surgeon operating today has many new advantages to offer you. Some are aimed at improving the removal of all tumors; other aid healing; others extend the surgeon's ability to perform less invasive surgery:

- Bloodless surgery
- Camera-guided microsurgery
- Computer-enhanced imaging tools
- Nerve-sparing surgery
- Radioimmunoisotopes to highlight hidden cancerous cells for removal
- Imaging dyes to track cancer's spread to specific lymph nodes
- Gamma-knife radiologic surgical tools
- Skinlike suturing and bandaging materials to reduce postsurgical complications
- Materials to layer between organs to prevent formation of adhesions
- Tools that access and repair areas not reachable with human hands
- Manmade materials to replace diseased organs
- Laparoscope-assisted surgery

Current trials of drugs, techniques, and devices

Currently, there are 93 clinical trials of treatment for colon cancer and 75 trials of treatment for rectal cancer. Some are trials of treatments already approved by the FDA, but with restructured timing or dosage for better results; some are of entirely new substances, techniques, or devices.

Note that the substances and techniques listed here were in trials at the time this book was being written. For the most current information on substances in clinical trials, use the National Cancer Institute's clinical trials search engine at *http://cnetdb.nci.nih.gov/trialsrch.shtml*.

Novel substances by mode of action

Novel substances being used in trials for colorectal cancer are listed below, grouped alphabetically by modes of action. You'll note that some substances, such as phenylbutyrate, fit more than one category.

Alkylating agents

DNA strands are held together by a variety of forces, one being electrical bonds. Alkylating agents form new electrochemical bonds within the DNA strand. This disrupts many normal functions of DNA, including its ability to divide. Alkylating agents are able to affect a cancer cell's DNA even when the DNA is not uncoiled and separated—in other words, they are not cell-cycle specific—which may explain their relatively high activity against many cancers.

New alkylating agents being tested for colorectal cancer are carmustine, cisplatin, carboplatin, Melphalan (L-PAM), and 6-hydroxymethylacylfulvene (HMAF or MGI-114), an extract of a mushroom toxin.

Antiangiogenesis therapy

Most tumors trigger growth of many new blood vessels to support the increased metabolic needs of the tumor. This growth of new blood vessels is called angiogenesis. Antiangiogenic agents interrupt the ability of the body to grow new blood vessels, causing tumors to shrink.

Some of the substances being studied now to reduce the blood supply to starve tumors, an approach called antiangiogenesis, cause concern because they also are likely to reduce the blood supply to normal tissues. The normal tissues of concern are found near the healing wound and, for example, in the uterus of a menstruating woman. Refined methods of curtailing a tumor's blood supply are being examined, such as triggering clots only in tumor blood vessels by preferentially binding clotting substances to proteins found only on tumor cells.

Antiangiogenesis drugs now in clinical trials for colorectal cancer are thalidomide, heparin, and BAY 12-9566.

Antibody therapy

Antibodies are substances, proteins, secreted by white blood cells called B-cells. They attach to foreign material and pathogens so that the invaders can be destroyed by other white blood cells called T-cells and macrophages.

Antibodies engineered in the lab to attach to only one cell surface receptor—monoclonal antibodies—have long been used in research and cancer diagnosis to tag cancer cells for visibility and quantification. Now they're beginning to be used to treat cancers.

Monoclonal antibodies (moabs) being tested for colorectal cancer include:

- A33, attached either to iodine I-131 or to cisplatin-epinephrine (intradose MPI-5010)

- LMB-9 for tumors that express the Lewis Y Antigen (B3 antigen)

- Moab 17-1A

- The bispecific antibody 520C9xH22 (MDX-H210) for HER2/neu-positive (p185) tumors, in combination with interferon gamma

- The monoclonal antibody F19 (BIBH-1), an antibody expressed on fibroblasts, in those with fibroblast activation protein-positive tumors

Anti-cytokine therapy

This is a broad category of anticancer drugs that contains some agents also in other categories.

By definition, cytokines are proteins our bodies manufacture to trigger activity in other cells, "cyto" meaning cell, and "kine" meaning activity. Using this definition, almost any protein or enzyme is a cytokine, but for cancer and inflammatory processes, special cytokines are in play. All of the interleukins and interferons are cytokines, as is tumor necrosis factor and the colony stimulating factors.

Some cytokines appear to cause cancer growth under certain circumstances, such as interleukin-6 (IL-6) in myeloma studies. Some cytokines work in opposition to each other, such as interleukin-10 and interleukin-12.

The substances being tested as anti-cytokines for colorectal cancer are interleukin-12 and low molecular weight heparin (Dalteparin).

Antimetabolite therapy

As the word antimetabolite implies, these substances in some way impede the cell's metabolism, its building up and breaking down of cell parts. Each of the antimetabolites used for colorectal cancer works a bit differently from the others, and some may fit into other categories described in this chapter, such as the antifolates.

- Gemcitabine (difluorodeoxycytidine) is an antimetabolite that substitutes for an enzyme in the process that constructs DNA from RNA, causing the process to fail.

- Hydroxyurea, a cell cycle-phase specific antimetabolite, blocks the enzyme ribonucleotide reductase. This enzyme is responsible for converting ribonucleotides to deoxyribonucleotides. DNA, but not RNA, synthesis is impaired.

Antisense molecules (antisense oligonucleotides)

DNA wants to exist in paired strands, except when a cell is dividing. Because cancer cells are known to have one or more faulty genes somewhere along the length of their DNA, some researchers are experimenting with delivering to the tumor short pieces of DNA or RNA that will match the faulty genes and couple with single strands of the cancer cell's DNA. In theory, these short pieces of DNA or RNA might interfere with a cancer cell's division and replication in a variety of ways.

Antisense substances being tested against colorectal cancer are ISIS 3521 and ISIS 5132.

Chemoprotectants

These agents are used to offset dangerous effects of chemotherapy by shielding healthy cells from damage, or by promoting their regrowth.

A substance being tested for this purpose among those being treated for colorectal cancer is Amifostine (Ethyol), which protects bone marrow, the central nervous system, and kidneys.

Chemosensitization/potentiation

Research has shown that some drugs, while having no direct ability to kill cancer cells, appear to heighten the cancer cell's vulnerability to other drugs. Other studies have shown that some drugs can both kill cancer cells and improve the ability of other drugs to do so.

Substances being tested for these purposes are ethynyluracil, hydroxyurea, and O6-benzylguanine.

See also Drug modulation and Radiosensitization.

Colloidal drug delivery

Certain drugs are not absorbed well by the body because they are not readily soluble in blood, or cannot survive the acid of the gastrointestinal tract.

Attempts to overcome these drawbacks include creation of these drugs in soluble forms, or attached to vehicles that traverse inhospitable biological environments.

A form of 9-aminocamptothecin (9-AC) has been created in a colloidal dispersion that is injected directly into the abdominal cavity in an effort to improve its concentrations within cancerous tissue.

Colony-stimulating factor therapy

Some treatments, particularly those that target the immune system, may work better if red or white blood cells or platelets are abundant when the substance is administered.

Trials for colorectal cancer exploiting this theory include:

- Phase I Study of Mutant MGMT Gene Transfer into Human Hematopoietic Progenitors to Protect Hematopoiesis During O6-Benzyguanine and Carmustine Therapy of Advanced Solid Tumors and Non-Hodgkin's Lymphoma
- Phase II Study of Vaccine Therapy with Tumor Specific Mutated Ras Peptides in Combination with Interleukin-2 or Granulocyte-Macrophage Colony-Stimulating Factor for Adults with Metastatic Solid Tumors

- Phase II Randomized Study of Autologous Tumor Cell Vaccine in Patients with Advanced Cancer

- Phase I/II Study of ALVAC-CEA-B7.1 Vaccine Alone or in Combination with Sargramostim (GM-CSF) in Patients with Recurrent or Refractory CEA-Expressing Adenocarcinoma

- Phase II Study of MOAB 17-1A/GM-CSF for 5-FU-Resistant Metastatic Colorectal Cancer

Cyclin-dependent kinase inhibitor therapy

Cyclins are proteins that govern the progression of the cell from one stage of cell division to the next. The cyclin-dependent kinases are enzymes that join with cyclins, forming several unique cyclin/cdk complexes, to mediate this progression. Substances that can inhibit these enzymes inhibit tumor growth.

Flavopiridol is being tested for this purpose.

Cytokine therapy

Cytokines, as discussed earlier under Anti-cytokine therapy, are proteins our bodies manufacture to trigger activity in other cells, such as the release of prostaglandins at the site of injury or the growth of new white blood cells. All of the interleukins and interferons are cytokines, as is tumor necrosis factor and the colony stimulating factors. Cytokines such as G-CSF are used in clinical trials in conjunction with other substances to boost an immune response or to support patient recovery.

Manmade cytokines being tested for use against colorectal cancer include:

- Interferon-alfa

- Interleukin-2

- Intraperitoneally administered interleukin-12 (IL-12)

Dendritic cell vaccines

Dendritic cells are accessory cells of the immune system. They can be educated to stimulate other white blood cells to kill tumors.

Current clinical trials for dendritic cell vaccines include:

- Phase I/II Study of Active Immunotherapy with Carcinoembryonic Antigen RNA Pulsed Dendritic Cells in Patients with Resected Hepatic Metastases from Adenocarcinoma of the Colon

- Phase I Study of a CEA Peptide-Pulsed Dendritic Cell Vaccine for Metastatic Breast or Gastrointestinal Cancer

- Phase I Pilot Study of Active Immunotherapy with Carcinoembryonic Antigen (CEA) Peptide-Pulsed Autologous Dendritic Cells in Metastatic Adenocarcinomas that Express CEA

Differentiation therapy

Cell differentation into distinct functional types is part of the normal cell's maturation process. When cancer cells are continually dividing, however, they might not mature and differentiate into the adult, functioning form of the tissue in which they arose. The result is a large group of cells that not only fail to carry out the function the organ was designed to do, but that also crowd out other cells, and commandeer a disproportionate share of the body's resources. Some cancer cells are so poorly differentiated that it's not possible to tell what organ gave rise to the tumor, and the diagnosis is by default carcinoma of unknown primary origin (CUP).

Some substances can force cancer cells to mature as normal cells do, stopping the cycle of uncontrollable cell division that characterizes cancer cells.

Bryostatin 1 and phenylbutyrate are possible differentiators being tested for colorectal cancer.

DNA adduct formation

Drugs that form DNA adducts interfere with the cancer cell's ability to copy its DNA for cell division. Adducts confuse and derail the enzymes responsible for cell division and replication.

Oxaliplatin, a platinum-based substance, is a DNA adduct forming drug being tested against colorectal cancer.

Drug modulation

Certain anticancer drugs seem to make other drugs more effective in killing cancer cells for reasons that vary. Fluorouracil (5-FU), for example, works more effectively in the presence of methotrexate, trimetrexate, interferon-alpha, leucovorin, or N-(phosphonacetyl)-L-asparte acid (PALA).

Being tested with 5-fluorouracil and leucovorin for use against colorectal cancer are:

- Trimetrexate glucuronate

- N-(phosphonacetyl)-L-asparte acid (PALA)

See also Chemosensitization.

Farnesyl transferase (FTPase) inhibitors

In several cancers, including colorectal cancers, a gene called ras, which, along with other genes, is responsible for orderly cell division, is mutated. Certain substances can inhibit the growth of cancerous cells that contain a mutated copy of ras, while leaving normal cells unaffected.

L-778,123 is a substance being tested for this purpose.

Folate antagonist therapy

Folate is needed to make the building blocks of DNA, purines and thymidy-lates. Without these, new copies of DNA cannot be made. Because cancer cells divide more rapidly than most normal cells, and because they commandeer major supplies of the body's nutrients, treatments such as folate antagonists are expected to affect cancer cells more strongly than most healthy cells.

Phenylbutyrate and Tomudex (also called raltitrexed, ICI D1694, or ZD1694) are classified as antifolates. See also Thymidylate synthase inhibitors.

Gene therapy

In its broadest sense, gene therapy is a name applied to several kinds of cancer treatment that involve modifying genes, such as triggering the body's white cells to attack tumors. Conforming to the strictest definition of gene therapy are experiments to reinsert genes into cancer cells lacking properly functioning copies of these genes, or inserting a manmade suicide gene into the tumor cell that will make the cell more susceptible to the toxic effects of certain drugs.

Modification of white blood cells to attack a tumor can occur, for example, if a weakened virus, modified genetically to contain a piece of the tumor's DNA, is inserted into the white blood cell. When this weakened virus is unleashed in the body, our white blood cells recognize it as an enemy, and destroy it. Because the virus also is expressing part of the tumor's DNA, white blood cells become sensitized to this tumor protein as well, and attack it wherever they find it, that is, either on the virus coat or on the tumor.

Currently, these gene therapy trials are underway:

- Inserting a working copy of the p53 tumor suppressor and apoptosis (cell death) gene into liver tumors, using one of the common cold viruses as a carrier. This therapy is infused directly into the liver by way of the hepatic artery.

- Inserting a copy of the cytosine deaminase gene into colon cancer tumors using one of the common cold viruses. The cytosine deaminase gene will cause the otherwise impervious cell to react to the harmless prodrug Flucytosine (5-fluorocytosine) and convert it to 5-fluorouracil, a drug that can kill colorectal cancer cells. Cytosine deanimase in cells makes nearby cells more likely to be killed by 5-FU.

- Transfer of a mutant copy of the alkyltransferase gene, MGMT, into young blood cells to protect them from chemotherapies such as O6-benzylguanine and carmustine (BCNU). These chemotherapies target the enzyme alkyltransferase, which results in cell death, a desirable outcome for colon cancer cells but not blood cells.

- Gene therapy using SCH-58500, a recombinant adenovirus with a modified p53 cell death gene, via hepatic artery infusion in those with liver tumors.

Growth factor antagonist therapy

This approach is similar to antiangiogenesis therapy, which aims to stop growth of blood vessels supplying tumors with nutrients. Growth factor inhibition aims at depriving the tumor of other substances and structures needed for growth.

A substance being tested for this purpose is suramin.

Idiotype vaccines.

See Tumor-cell derivative vaccines.

Leukocyte therapy

This approach uses white blood cells to challenge a tumor. The patient's blood cells are extracted from a vein, resensitized to the tumor, and reinserted.

The following trials using leukocyte therapy are underway:

- Dendritic cells, which are accessory immune system cells that can be pretreated to recognize carcinoembryonic antigen (CEA). They are reinserted into the body to attack tumor cells that express CEA.

- Injection of a tumor-specific vaccine containing either the cell-death p53 gene, or ras, a growth signaling gene, with or without cellular immunotherapy with peptide-activated lymphocytes plus interleukin-2.

Liposomal encapsulation

Some drugs appear to work better, to be less toxic to liver or kidney, and to be effective when taken orally if they are first encased in a layer of lipids.

A drug being used in this way is doxorubicin.

See also Colloidal drug delivery.

Monoclonal antibodies

See Antibody therapy.

Non-specific immune-modulator therapy

Nonspecific immune modulators are substances that aid in redirecting, suppressing, or boosting the immune system in ways that are either somewhat general or perhaps poorly understood.

Vaccine adjuvants may contain aluminum or small pieces of protein, for instance, that are not related to the vaccine material, but are known to elicit a stronger immune response.

The vaccine adjuvant QS-21, like vaccine adjuvants in general, has been shown to heighten the immune response, and thus the effectiveness of a vaccine created from tumor cells. (See Tumor-cell derivative vaccines.)

The following substances are being tested as nonspecific immune stimulants against colorectal cancer, in combination with vaccines or traditional chemotherapy:

- Corynebacterium granulosum P40

- Alum precipitate

- QS-21 adjuvant

- Flt3 ligand, which appears to boost the antitumor activity of NK (natural killer) white blood cells

Prodrugs

Prodrugs are substances that have no activity against cancer until some biological event converts them to another drug that is tumoricidal.

Uracil-tegafur (UFT, Orzel), currently being tested against colorectal cancer, is a prodrug of 5-fluorouracil (5-FU), and is slowly metabolized to 5-FU in the cancer cell and by the liver.

Peripheral blood lymphocyte therapy

See Leukocyte therapy.

Radioimmunotherapy

These substances are compounds usually consisting of manmade monoclonal antibodies (see Antibody therapy) and a radioactive isotope. The antibody attaches preferentially to tumor cells; the isotope decays within, upon, or very near the tumor, damaging or killing the cell, and in some cases, other nearby tumor cells, with radiation.

Monoclonal antibodies conjugated to radioisotopes for colorectal cancer include yttrium-90 joined to Biotin.

Radiosensitization

Certain drugs can make tumors more sensitive to damage by radiotherapy.

5-FU prior to or during radiotherapy appears to make colorectal cancer cells more sensitive to radiotherapy.

Recombinant viral vaccines

Viruses engineered to target only cancer cells are being considered as one way to damage tumors and spare healthy tissue. The virus itself could attack and kill the tumor, or it could insert its DNA or RNA into the tumor—DNA that has been modified in the lab to contain a killer sequence or to weaken the tumor's defenses or ability to replicate.

A vaccine made of combined carcinoembryonic antigen (CEA) and Vaccinia virus, with postvaccination CEA protein injections as a booster, is currently being tested against colorectal cancer.

Stereotactic radiotherapy

Stereotactic surgery is surgery guided by a three-dimensional image of the tumor and by multiple targeting criteria that allow precisely aimed microsurgeries. Stereotactic radiosurgery is the aiming of one or more small, precise beams of radiation at cancerous tissue using these stereotactic guiding systems.

A clinical trial of fractionated stereotactic radiotherapy following surgical removal of brain metastases is being conducted to determine the efficacy of this method as follow-up treatment for brain metastases.

Thymidylate synthase inhibitors

Certain anticancer drugs such as 5-FU inhibit the enzyme thymidylate synthase, which in turn affects DNA synthesis. Certain newer drugs in this class are capable of avoiding degradation inside the tumor cell, thus increasing its presence in the cell.

Two drugs that behave as thymidylate synthase inhibitors and are being tested for colorectal cancer are:

- Tomudex (also called raltitrexed, ICI D1694, or ZD 1694)

- Uracil-tegafur (UFT, Orzel)

Topoisomerase inhibitor therapy

Topoisomerases are enzymes that our cells use to untwist DNA before copying, and to repair breaks in DNA after copying. Topoisomerase inhibitors interfere with DNA repair, causing the cancer cell to die because damaged DNA cannot be translated into proteins, such as transport and digestive proteins, that each cell needs to breathe or eat.

Topoisomerase inhibitors being tested against colorectal cancer include aminocamptothecin, doxorubicin, and oxaliplatin. Oxaliplatin appears to be the most promising of the three at this time and might be approved by the FDA soon.

Tubulin inhibitor therapy

When a cell has made a copy of all of its chromosomes and is ready to divide, spindles made of tubulin form to pull the two copies of each chromosome apart into two identical clusters of 46 chromosomes apiece. Tubulin inhibitors stop spindles from forming, thus stopping the tumor cell from dividing.

A novel tubulin inhibitor being tested is dolastatin 10, a substance found in a marine animal.

Tumor-cell derivative vaccines

Vaccines made from tumor cells that have been removed from the body and cultured in the lab can cause our bodies to become resensitized to tumors, resulting in renewed attacks against the tumor by our immune systems.

The trials currently underway that exploit this technique are:

- Vaccine therapy with tumor-specific mutated ras peptides, aimed at causing an attack against tumor cells expressing this mutated protein (peptide) in the cell's membrane. Ras proteins, a product of the ras gene, frequently are mutated in human cancers, where they are known to be involved in the development of tumors by incorrectly signaling for ongoing growth and cell division.

- Intralymphatic immunotherapy with interferon-alfa-treated tumor cells. Tumor cells are incubated with interferon-alfa, then the tumor cells are reinjected directly into lymphatic ducts. Some patients show an antibody response to tumor cells after this treatment.

- Tumor-specific vaccines made with either the cell-death gene p53, or the ras oncogene; with or without cellular immunotherapy consisting of peptide-activated white blood cells and the cytokine interleukin-2.

Vaccines

Vaccines against cancer also can be made without using tumor cells as a basis, using instead synthetically engineered molecules thought to stimulate an immune response in any one of a variety of ways.

The following vaccines are being tested against colorectal cancer:

- ALVAC-CEA-B7.1 vaccine, which targets two cell surface antigens, CEA and B7-1.

- A vaccine made of Carcinoembryonic Antigen Peptide-1 (CAP), a protein expressed by colorectal cancer cells.

Novel techniques and devices

Not only new substances are tested for efficacy against colorectal cancer, but new techniques and devices as well. Listed below are novel methods and devices currently being funded by NCI.

Bone marrow ablation with stem cell support

See High-dose therapy with stem cell support.

Chronomodulated therapy

Several clinical trials have shown that some drugs are more effective against cancer if administered at certain times of the day, week, or month. One trial for colorectal cancer, using fluorouracil, leucovorin calcium, and oxaliplatin, attempts to exploit this theory.

Continuous infusion therapy

Several trials are underway to exploit the observation that fluorouracil may be more effective against colorectal tumors and appears to operate biochemically in different ways if it is administered slowly over long periods, instead of injected all at once during a brief office visit. As with other cell-cycle-specific anticancer drugs, 5-FU will kill cancer cells only if it is present as they divide. Continuous infusion allows 5-FU to be present continuously as cancer cells enter the process of cell division across several days or weeks.

Cryosurgery

Freezing of colorectal cancer cells that have lodged in the liver is being examined as a possible alternative for those whose tumors are not removable using standard surgeries:

- Phase II Study of Cryoablation for Treatment of Unresectable Colorectal Hepatic Metastases

- Phase II Study of Multiple Metastasectomy Combined with Systemic 5-FU/CF and Hepatic Artery Infusion of FUDR in Patients with Colorectal Carcinoma Metastatic to the Liver

Embolization

Some trials are designed to eliminate the blood supply to the tumor or to halt the flow of chemotherapy out of an organ (during isolated perfusion) by causing a blood clot in the tumor or in one or more blood vessels exiting an organ. This technique is known as tumor embolization or simply embolization.

Hepatic arterial infusion (HAI)

Also see Isolated perfusion. Isolated perfusion in the purest sense targets a single organ with chemotherapy. Hepatic arterial infusion targets the liver, but some of the drug administered also travels to other organs. Nonetheless, the National Cancer Institute currently classifies HAI as isolated perfusion, for which see their web site at *http://cnetdb.nci.nih.gov/trialsrch.shtml*.

High-dose therapy with stem cell support

Very high doses of chemotherapy and radiation therapy may kill all tumor cells, but they also quickly kill bone marrow, which causes death when new blood cells cannot be created. Marrow can be harvested and frozen, however, and reinserted after chemotherapy has ended. This technique has been used with success against the lymphomas and leukemias.

Trials using doses of drugs that do not kill all marrow, but are followed by infusions of one's marrow, stem cells, or white blood cells also are underway.

Two trials are underway to gauge the success of this approach for colorectal cancer:

- Phase II Study of Nonmyeloblative Allogeneic Peripheral Blood Stem Cell and Donor Lymphocyte Infusions in Patients with Refractory Metastatic Solid Tumors

- Phase I Pilot Study of Sequential High-Dose Cisplatin, Cyclophosphamide, Etoposide and Ifosfamide, Carboplatin, Paclitaxel with Autologous Stem Cell Support for Advanced Carcinomas

Interstitial laser photocoagulation

This technique, typically used for liver metastases, causes tumor cells to die by generating heat within the tumor, coagulating its blood supply. Optic fibers that conduct laser light are inserted through the skin and into the tumor while the tumor is being visualized with ultrasonography.

Intraoperative radiotherapy

Irradiating the tumor bed during surgery after tumor removal is considered by some researchers to be a good means of destroying any remaining cancerous tissue, while sparing a large amount of nearby healthy tissue from unnecessary radiation exposure. Moreover, the single large dose delivered in this setting is thought to be more effective than the fractionated doses usually administered over many days or weeks.

Intraperitoneal chemotherapy

Chemotherapy administered directly to the abdominal cavity may be more effective against tumors than is intravenous chemotherapy. Several trials are testing this theory:

- Phase I Study of Intraperitoneal Interleukin-12 for Mullerian and Gastrointestinal Carcinomas with Abdominal Carcinomatosis

- Phase I Study of Recombinant Human Interleukin-12 in Refractory Advanced Stage Ovarian Cancer and Other Abdominal Carcinomatosis

- Phase I Study of Intraperitoneal Aminocamptothecin Colloidal Dispersion in Patients with Cancer Predominantly Confined to the Peritoneal Cavity

- Phase III Adjuvant Study of Levamisole versus Alfa Interferon 2a Plus Fluorouracil and Leucovorin Calcium for Intraperitoneal Colorectal Cancer

Isolated perfusion

Targeting only a specific organ with chemotherapy is an attractive goal, as it may allow much higher doses of cancer-killing drugs to be delivered to the tumor while sparing healthy tissue. Isolated perfusion in the purest sense targets a single organ with chemotherapy. The National Cancer Institute currently classifies these trials as isolated perfusion therapy, however, although some of the drug administered during hepatic arterial infusion also travels to other organs. Trials include:

- Gene therapy with SCH-58500 (rAd/p53) via hepatic artery infusion

- Intravenous versus intrahepatic arterial infusion of 5-fluorouracil and leucovorin

- Hepatic perfusion with escalating dose Melphalan followed by postoperative hepatic arterial floxuridine (FUDR) and leucovorin calcium

- Hepatic artery floxuridine, leucovorin calcium, and dexamethasone versus systemic 5-fluorouracil and leucovorin

Portal vein infusion

This technique is similar to hepatic arterial perfusion, but uses the portal vein:

- Phase II Study of Hepatic Resection Followed by Adjuvant Portal Vein Infusion of Floxuridine plus Systemic Fluorouracil/Leucovorin Calcium in Metastatic Colorectal Carcinoma

See Isolated perfusion.

Radiofrequency ablation

This technique, like interstitial laser coagulation, is typically used for liver metastases, and causes tumor cells to die by generating heat within the tumor, coagulating its blood supply. Insulated electrode needles are inserted through the skin and into the tumor while the tumor is being visualized with ultrasonography.

Prevention trials

Trials of substances such as tamoxifen, vitamin E, and beta-carotene have shown some success in preventing cancers in certain groups of people. High levels of calcium and vitamin D, for example, have been linked to decreased rates of colorectal cancer.

More such trials are likely to be held, perhaps testing substances found in vegetables, such as limonene from orange peel, lycopene from tomatoes, and resveratrol from grapes, dietary fiber, exercise, or perhaps testing manmade substances that mimic products found in nature.

The following trials currently are underway to assess prevention of colorectal cancer:

- Celecoxib, a COX-2 and prostaglandin modifier, for hereditary nonpolyposis colorectal cancer patients and gene carriers
- Two-part trial of rutin, quercetin, and curcumin versus sulindac, or of curcumin only
- High-dose folic acid for the prevention of colorectal cancer in patients who have had adenomatous polyps removed

- Aspirin in patients with curatively treated Dukes stage A/B1/B2/C colorectal cancer

Future trials

The strategies detailed below are being discussed with vigor among scientists, and some are being tested against other cancers, but they are not yet ready for human trials against colorectal cancer. Some may prove suitable for treating colorectal cancer; others may not.

Cellular matrix exploitation

The cellular matrix is a medium somewhat like cement along which cells propel themselves, and in which cells eventually become anchored in order to thrive.

For either normal or cancerous cell growth to occur, the cellular matrix has to provide a foothold for new cells migrating to their home. Studies of the behavior of cellular matrix proteins such as laminin and some collagens, and the enzymes that interact with them such as the matrix metalloproteases, may shed light on cancer pathways that are amenable to normalization.

Some molecules involved with growth of new blood vessels—angiogenesis—appear also to be involved with activities of the cellular matrix.

Death receptors

Normal cells, cells being transformed into cancerous cells, and fully cancerous cells have on their surface certain proteins that act as binding regions for a protein, TRAIL (also called Apo2L), that triggers orderly cell death. Cells being transformed into cancerous cells can be destroyed by TRAIL, but normal cells protect themselves from this destruction by using "decoy" receptors: they bind TRAIL, but do not transport it inside the cell, thus seeming to render it ineffective. Cancerous cells also appear to have many ways to avoid cell death. Future cancer therapies will examine these differences in behavior among normal, cancerous, and soon-to-be-cancerous cells.

In vitro sensitivity-directed chemotherapy

This approach requires a sample of one's tumor, against which a variety of anticancer compounds are tested to see which works best. In practice, there are problems with this approach, because tumor cells that respond well in a test tube may be inaccessible to the apparently useful drug when the same scenario is attempted within the body, and because substances that appear to be inactive in the test tube may become active in the body after biochemical interaction with various substances.

In other words, this technique cannot yet be used with accuracy to determine agents to which the tumor will respond.

Some clinicians offer this service now, but its use is not widespread.

Mitochondrial DNA

Science and medicine have focused primarily on the activity of genes within the cell's nucleus, but DNA also exists within the mitochondria of each cell.

Mitochondria are small organs (organelles) within each cell that burn oxygen to accomplish cellular tasks. It's theorized that mitochondria are bacteria that were enslaved by the cells of larger species many millions of years ago, because each mitochondrium contains its own DNA, and resembles a bacterium in certain other ways. All of the cells of all higher species contain mitochondria; cells requiring higher levels of oxygen consumption, such as muscle cells, contain more mitochondria than do others.

Mitochondrial DNA can only be inherited from the female. Ova—being fully functioning cells—contain mitochondria, but spermatozoa do not.

These facts are meaningful for cancer research for at least three reasons:

* For diseases that are linked to colorectal cancer and found in both males and females, but found consistently only on the mother's side of the family, mitochondrial DNA may play a role.

* Mitochondrial DNA sometimes exhibits damage that is known to cause cancer, as does the much more closely studied nuclear DNA.

* Mitochondria appear to respond to chemotherapy and radiation therapy, and mitochondrial DNA can be modified to improve cancer treatment.

Molecular oncology

A tumor may arise because a gene is being incorrectly transcribed into an aberrant protein, is not transcribed at all, is overexpressed, or expressed at the wrong time; because two erroneously spliced genes are being transcribed into a hybrid protein that is impotent or oncogenic; or owing to a combination of any of these.

Molecular oncology attempts to substitute the correct or missing gene product for a faulty or missing gene. For example, the protein normally produced by the DCC (deleted in colon cancer) gene missing in some familial forms of colon cancer might be a target for molecular oncologists.

Proto-oncogenes, oncogenes, and tumor suppressor genes

As with many areas of cancer research, this is a well-studied but not yet fully understood area of genetics.

DNA in normal cells contains oncogenes and precursor genes called proto-oncogenes. Both can trigger growth, but these genes normally are tightly regulated, sometimes kept quite literally under wraps with methylation, so that they cannot be transcribed into proteins that would trigger growth until it's time for the cell to divide.

In contrast, and for biological balance, there are about nine known tumor-suppressor genes (of which p53 is the best known) sensitive to the activity of the dividing cell, that signal when to demethylate and transcribe growth genes, when to arrest growth, and when to initiate cell death if irreparable errors are found in the cell's DNA.

Errors in or near any of these genes can cause a cell to become cancerous.

Some studies are examining ways to regain control of oncogenes that have run amok, or to substitute for the products of tumor suppressor genes that have been damaged.

Telomerase inhibitors

At the end of each chromosome is a long string of repeating, non-translated genetic material called a telomere. Not too long ago, it was discovered that, as a normal cell ages, the telomere, or tail, shortens. When it is entirely gone, the cell dies in an orderly, shrinking, dissolving way (apoptosis).

The telomeres of many cancer cells, however, never shorten.

Some researchers believe that an enzyme called telomerase is faulty in certain cancer cells, and that by manipulating this enzyme, the cancer cell might be forced to age normally and eventually die.

Tissue engineering

Currently, tissue engineering is in limited use to regrow skin damaged by burns and to repair damaged cartilage within joints. Artificial kidneys that are half human tissue, half mechanical device are being tested in animals. Although tissue engineering is not used yet following cancer therapy, it's conceivable that someday new vocal chords, breast, or colon tissue might be regrown in the laboratory and implanted into a cancer survivor weeks or months after laryngectomy, mastectomy, or colectomy.

The obstacles to this approach are several, the first being that usually a small piece of the patient's own tissue is required to grow the much larger quantity on a base consisting of anchor material and nutrients. For cancer survivors, the risk exists that microscopic cancer growths that might be included in this sample would survive, thrive, and subsequently be reimplanted. The second problem is that even seemingly simple tissues can be quite complex. Cartilage, for instance, is composed of several layers, each having a separate function. Results of cartilage implantation are too new to be certain that the tissue functions as it should for many years after. Although multilayered skin has been regrown and used successfully in burn therapy and is FDA-approved, it's not known at this time whether all tissues, in all their complexities, can be regrown. A third obstacle is expense. One square inch of nutrient matrix for regrowing skin costs several thousand dollars. Tissue engineering for a very complex organ might be beyond reach, simply owing to expense.

Triplex molecules

In some cases, the antisense molecules (described in an earlier section) which bind to single strands of dividing DNA or RNA also can bind with double-strand DNA that is not in the process of dividing. When antisense molecules do bind to double strands, they form a triplex molecule. Some researchers are pursuing this strategy as a means of cross-binding DNA so that it cannot even begin replication, thus causing the cancer cell to become static or to die.

Summary

Many new concepts and treatments are evolving for cancer in general, and colorectal cancer in particular. This chapter has addressed some of the treatments now in clinical trials and those still in the planning stages.

It's wise to keep in touch with new treatments being developed for colorectal cancer by consulting your doctor, by browsing the NCI clinical trials database, or by calling NCI and asking for a list of trials for colorectal cancer. Chapter 20, *Clinical Trials*, and Chapter 24, *Researching Your Illness*, contain information regarding evaluating clinical trials.

Key points to remember:

- The National Cancer Institute web site for searching for clinical trials is *http://cnetdb.nci.nih.gov/trialsrch.shtml*.

- The National Cancer Institute telephone number for getting help finding clinical trials is (800) 4-CANCER.

Researching Your Illness

Chance favors the prepared mind.

—Louis Pasteur

THIS CHAPTER WILL OFFER YOU BASIC WAYS TO FIND information about your illness, outside of simply relying on your doctor. First a few generalities about approaches to learning are covered, then we discuss using medical libraries and research journals; the National Cancer Institute's Internet, phone, fax, and clinical trials services; and hiring a search firm to do the legwork for you. Methods for checking drug side effects, verifying your chemotherapy dosage, finding support groups, interpreting test results, and evaluating unproven remedies are offered.

For each type of information, ways to access the source with and without a computer are outlined when it is possible to do so. For instance, the Merck Manual section on laboratory results is available both on paper and on the Internet. Certain unique resources, however, are found only on the Internet.

Reasons to research

Colorectal cancer survivors and their loved ones choose to search for information for many reasons. Many feel a compelling need to learn all they can as quickly as possible about what they'll be facing, or they feel that they must do something to contribute to their recovery. Some just like to verify that the doctor is relaying accurate and up-to-date information, even when the care they've received has been very good. Others are faced with having to assume a greater responsibility for their healthcare, owing to living in areas with few doctors, or perhaps owing to having had a bad experience with a doctor's lack of knowledge. HMO policies that are based on cost control and that may deny the best care in order to keep expenses down are a driving force for many. Loved ones of cancer survivors sometimes need to feel they're doing something to help, and finding information may satisfy that need.

The decision to research your illness is the beginning of an empowerment that will do more than just serve you in good stead for making decisions. Research on stress and cancer hints that a proactive attitude may contribute to long survival. The more you learn, the more control you have over how events unfold, not only because you'll be making better health and treatment choices, but because you can take back some of the control that is lost in the clutter of automation that now accompanies cancer diagnosis and treatment.

Prerequisites and perspectives

Before you start, you need to know a few specific facts about your diagnosis to make searching more fruitful. You also will benefit by knowing what to avoid, and what to insulate yourself against.

Prerequisites

You'll need three things before you start: the exact name of your colorectal cancer subtype, its stage, and a medical dictionary.

If you don't know your precise diagnosis, you'll waste a lot of time and precious energy reading the wrong material. You may even frighten yourself unnecessarily by finding distressing but wrong information, not realizing that it doesn't pertain to you.

Your doctor's staff can read you the exact name of your colorectal cancer subtype from your pathology report. Better yet, ask them to send you a photocopy of this, and of all your medical records. Crosscheck this information against Appendix D, *Staging System Equivalents*, to see how your stage is identified in other systems. This way, if you find your stage of colorectal cancer referred to in research papers by an unfamiliar term, you'll be better equipped to assess what you're reading.

Purchase a medical dictionary for between five and twenty dollars to help you with the terminology you will encounter, which becomes increasingly easy to understand with greater exposure. Several reasonably priced medical dictionaries are listed in the bibliography. One of the most useful is *The Cancer Dictionary*, by Altman and Sarg.

Perspectives

The following perspectives are helpful to keep in mind while researching your condition.

Persistence

Please don't feel intimidated by the volume of information on colorectal cancer or its seeming complexity. As with any other task of assimilation, small steps ultimately will yield great gains. If you're wary of trying to search for information because medicine seems like an alien frontier to you, it might be helpful to know a few interesting facts:

- Academic success does not account for all that much of success in life. Success also is a result of being flexible, adaptable, developing social skills, having luck, being persistent, patient, and so forth.

- If one person can understand something, generally so can another person, and if the second person doesn't understand, it might be because the first person isn't explaining it very well.

- Contrary to popular mythology about kids being computer whizzes and older people not, the fastest growing group of Internet users is the group consisting of those over age 65.

In short, if you're persistent in asking about, searching for, and trying to absorb medical information—and in turning away from doctors who are condescending, seeking instead those who respect you—you'll succeed. You won't need a degree in medicine or an abnormally high IQ to understand what you find, just a medical dictionary and the motivation to acquire new skills. It might take you 20 minutes longer to understand a certain medical concept than it takes an MD, but it's worthwhile if that 20 minutes makes the difference of a lifetime.

Clarity

When asking for help, be specific about what you need. If you ask friends for help, or hire a search firm to do a medical search, the same considerations about clarity and intent apply.

Educate yourself first as to what options are available. We suggest you ask for full information, rather than edited versions that may exist. For example, when communicating with the National Cancer Institute (NCI), consider requesting the information for physicians, not for patients, if you already are somewhat familiar with colorectal cancer. (The patient information statement is quite basic, and, while it may be useful to you initially, soon it will seem less than edifying. If you find that this is the case, it's time to request the physicians' version of PDQ information.) Likewise, ask for the full information on clinical trials, not the summaries. Specify a national search, unless you want to limit yourself to only those trials in your area.

Humility

Don't forget that you should always verify what you find with your oncologist. It's imperative that you focus on correct, current information, and that you understand what it means regarding your specific circumstances. At times people simply are not equipped to evaluate what they've found, but it's almost a certainty that your doctor has a good frame of reference for doing this evaluation.

Courtesy

Good manners dictate that you make an appointment to discuss lengthy topics with your doctor or other health professional, or that you offer to pay for a telephone consultation. See Nancy Keene's book *Working with Your Doctor* for a good discussion of improving patient/doctor relationships.

Diplomacy

Some doctors react badly to the idea that their patients find information on the Internet, because the information available on the Net ranges from abysmal to superb. If you use the Internet to research your illness, avoid using the word "Internet" when discussing your findings with your oncologist. Instead, use terminology that credits the original sources on which your Internet findings are based: Medline, the PDQ database of the National Cancer Institute, CancerLit, certain reputable medical journals, and so on.

Self-respect

If your doctor is not interested in what you find, or seems threatened by your efforts, consider discussing this attitude with him, or consider changing doctors.

Serenity

When you have started researching your illness, you may find some information that's upsetting, such as survival statistics. Keep in mind that statistics always describe composite results of studies involving numbers of people, and cannot be applied to the progress and circumstances of a single individual. For example, when a researcher averages the survival times of 80 patients treated with drug XYZ whose survival ranges from 2 months to 212 months, he may calculate that the average survival following treatment is 13 months. Nobody has an idea where to place himself on this continuum, however, unless he knows intimately the health factors of all 80 people and can match himself to at least one of them. For the researcher, the average will tell her whether the treatment is worth further development, but for the individual, statistical averages are just data, not information.

Ways to find information

Here's a summary of ways that you can obtain information about colorectal cancer. The sections that follow describe these methods in detail.

- If you have a computer, you can find an almost limitless amount written about colorectal cancer on the Internet, some of which is highly accurate, some of which is of lesser quality. The highly reliable information at the National Cancer Institute's site should be your starting point, and the latest medical research papers are an ongoing source of information.

- If you have siblings, children, or grandchildren with a computer, and you don't feel like starting from scratch using a computer amidst your worries about cancer—and who would blame you?—ask them to do Internet searches for you. Make sure you tell them the specifics of your diagnosis, and what you're looking for: treatment options, complementary therapies, stories of other patients, clinical trials, and so on.

- If you're friends with a doctor, nurse, or librarian, ask them to do searches of various resources, such as the National Library of Medicine's Medline database and NCI's Physician's Data Query (PDQ).

- Pay a commercial firm that specializes in this activity to do a search for you.

- Visit an academic or medical library to research the medical journals in the periodicals section and their medical texts.

- Ask your doctor for help getting copies of research papers from medical journals, but offer to pay for any photocopying that's needed.

- Contact the American Cancer Society, and ask for information that can be mailed to you.

- Call the National Cancer Institute at (800) 4-CANCER and ask for information, or ask for help using their CancerFax service.

How to obtain NCI's information

The information on cancer amassed and maintained by the National Cancer Institute, a division of NIH, is the granddaddy of all cancer databases, and should be your starting point for learning the basics about colorectal cancer. It's accurate and current. You can access this information in several ways.

By phone

You can call NCI at (800) 4-CANCER and request that information on colorectal cancer be sent to you by mail free of charge. Remember that the information geared to physicians is much more useful and detailed than that written for patients. If you feel uncomfortable asking for physician information, you can give some justification or even make something up. For example, you could say that your doctor asked you to request this information. One patient said that he was writing a newspaper article that required indepth material. You might want to ask as well for literature that describes all of the NCI publications that one might order, such as tracts that describe dealing with fatigue or depression.

By fax

The information available by phone request is also available by fax. Call (800) 4-CANCER and ask for instructions for faxing.

By personal computer

If you have a computer, you can read the National Cancer Institute's state-of-the-art colon or rectal cancer treatment statements for physicians, as well as an immense collection of other literature, at their CancerNet web site (*http:// wwwicic.nci.nih.gov*). Follow the path for *health professionals*, to PDQ information and the word *treatment*.

You may retrieve the NCI physician's statements on colon cancer via email by keying *help* into the message area, with no other information, such as your signature, included in the message area. Send this email to *cnet@icicc. nci.nih.gov*.

How to obtain medical research papers

Reviewing the research papers published in medical journals is the best way for a colorectal cancer survivor to get the most current information. Textbooks are out of date almost as soon as they're printed owing to the time delays of production. NCI PDQ information is a good foundation, but doesn't reflect every emerging trend still in the test phase—just state-of-the-art standards for care.

If you'd like to read about basic cancer research that's years away from becoming treatment, the journals *Science*, *Cell*, and *Nature Biotechnology* are good choices.

Many medical journals are now on the Web, including *Science*, *The Journal of the American Medical Association*, and *The Journal of the National Cancer Institute*. Some of these cannot be viewed online unless you're a subscriber to the standard paper edition.

Reading medical research papers is arguably the most difficult part of learning about progress against colorectal cancer, as well as the best way to keep abreast of progress. A medical dictionary will serve you well in this effort, and you should ask your doctor about parts that are not clear. Usually the abstract (summary) of a paper will suffice, as abstracts of cancer research studies normally contain conclusions, but at times obtaining the full text of the paper will be necessary.

If you use the full text of a paper, don't try to understand the whole thing at first. Just read the introduction, the conclusions, and the discussion. The middle sections deal with scientific methodology that's important in verifying that the research was performed to strict scientific standards, but this part has been peer-reviewed by other scientists and the editors of the journal. This material is usually, but not always, less important to a patient trying to find good prospects for care. As you become better acquainted with research papers and their terminology, occasionally you may want to read the remaining sections as well.

By subscription

Subscription costs for journals such as these usually start at about one hundred dollars per year, and can go much higher. The disadvantage of subscribing to individual journals, besides the accumulation of hard-to-index paper copy, is that good research articles on colorectal cancer will be spread among all of these, and subscribing to several becomes prohibitively expensive.

By using Medline

Medline, a database maintained by the US National Library of Medicine (NLM), is an indispensable resource—some say the most important resource for library research on medical issues. Various Medline search engines, such as NLM's, which at the time of this writing is free, are available on the Internet, giving you access to the 9 million medical research papers in the National Library of Medicine.

If you don't have a computer, ask a friend or relative to do a search for you. Alternately, a nurse, a medical librarian, or someone affiliated with a hospital or library may have Medline access. The National Library of Medicine's Medline web address is *http://www4.ncbi.nlm.nih.gov/PubMed/*.

At most Medline sites you'll generally find a search engine that accepts keywords and returns summaries of the medical research publications that match your keywords. For example, if you key the terms "colorectal, treatment, 5-fluorouracil" and click on the search button, you'll receive in return the titles of a great many studies regarding treating colorectal cancer with 5-fluorouracil.

Note that the latest studies are displayed first. Clicking the mouse on each title will cause the summary (abstract) of the study's results to display on your screen. After you've read a few of these abstracts the terminology is likely to become more familiar, and you can repeat the search again, using additional keywords to narrow the number of studies returned to a reasonable number for a more incisive review. You can reinitiate searches in the following days or months using other keywords to build your knowledge base about your illness.

Almost all of the Web-based Medline search engines use an organizational hierarchy called MEdical Subject Headings (MESH). MESH terms group references by category so that you'll get more specific research papers returned for your searching efforts, even if you're not familiar with the right medical terms or if you misspell a word slightly. Some Medline search tools invoke MESH terms behind the scenes when you enter a keyword; others, like PaperChase, will prompt you to pick a MESH term from a list that they produce that is associated with the keyword you entered. Still others have advanced searches you can invoke using MESH terms explicitly.

Here is a partial list of MESH terms that might be used behind the scenes, or offered to you as a choice, when the word "mucinous" is the keyword used in a Medline search:

- Mucin

- Carcinoma, Mucinous

- Colitis, Mucous

- Mucinoses

- Colon

- Muci Mucin

- Cystadenoma, Mucinous

- Cystadenocarcinoma, Mucinous

A good way to get background information on any medical topic is to seek out the review articles in Medline. Enter various search terms, like:

- "infusion pump," "colorectal cancer," review

- "colon cancer," vaccine, review

- "rectal cancer," "signet-ring cell," review

Note that placing quotes around search terms causes the search engine to treat these words as a single search term.

Including the word "review" will retrieve abstracts of review articles that are geared to physicians who might not be specialists, articles appearing in more generalized publications such as *Family Practitioner* or *Nature*, that may contain more explanatory material and make fewer assumptions.

If you need help with searching, you can call the National Library of Medicine at (800) 272-4787 or (301) 496-6308.

If the Medline summaries (abstracts) you read are more tantalizing than edifying, you can order the full text of any research paper from companies that specialize in this service. Some of these companies, such as InfoTrieve, are Web-based; others can be found by calling a medical school library and getting recommendations from a librarian. Unfortunately, at the time of this writing, the National Library of Medicine's service does not offer full text retrieval to those not associated with an academic library. Those who are, however, can use the Loansome Doc service to order full text of papers.

On the Internet, the Medline service providers HealthGate, Medscape, Helix, PhyNet, PDRnet.Com, SilverPlatter, Ovid On Call, Infotrieve, PaperChase, and others offer full-text services for a fee.

By using medical libraries

Another way to find articles in medical journals is to visit a medical or university library and examine their journals and recent texts, borrowing or photocopying what you find most useful. Copyright law permits photocopying one copy of a journal article if it's for your own immediate use. Avoid relying solely on textbooks that are older than two years, as the time it takes to bring a text to print makes the source material used to prepare a text quickly out of date.

Note that some university and medical libraries restrict entry to those affiliated with the institution is some way. You can find the nearest medical library open to the public by calling the National Network of Libraries of Medicine at (800) 338-7657.

Your local hospitals also may have medical libraries.

To find articles in medical journals, ask the main information desk where periodicals are stored, and how to search them by subject. There's some variety in how different libraries store, search, and retrieve journal articles. Some academic libraries have all periodicals stored on CD-ROM, for example, but others are still stored as paper copy in the stacks. Regardless of these differences, there's always a way to search by subject, and this should be your starting point. The library you visit may also have access to Medline or Index Medicus.

Often the periodicals section of a medical or academic library will have staff devoted to helping you. All should have material you can read at your leisure describing how to search their collection. Don't be shy about asking for help. Most librarians are proud of their ability to root out obscure references and are in that field because they want to connect people to information.

Arrive prepared to pay photocopy fees and with coins for photocopy machines.

By hiring a search firm

Before hiring a commercial firm to do a search of the medical literature, you might want to call the National Library of Medicine's Management Desk at (800) 638-8480 and ask for whatever help they can provide.

You might choose to pay a search fee to one of a number of companies who provide this service. Tell them what topic you're interested in, but keep in mind that the more specific you can be, the better: treatments for stage II sigmoid colon cancer for those under age 50, rather than just "colorectal cancer," for instance, will yield more useful material on this topic. The search firm will locate and mail to you copies of articles from medical journals.

Here's a partial list of such companies. Their being included here does not imply an endorsement of their service:

- The Health Resource, Inc., (501) 329-5272
- Can Help, (360) 437-2291
- Schine On-Line Services, (800) FIND-CURE

How to obtain medical textbooks

Texts on cancer, immunology, and surgery for colorectal cancer can provide you with the foundation for understanding more timely sources such as the papers published in medical journals. In general, the more recent the text, the better.

A source of background information might be an oncology text aimed at pre-med college students or first-year medical students. The terminology might be a notch higher than many people are comfortable with, but not nearly as difficult as that found in medical journals, and definitely geared to providing broad, fundamental information.

Using the list of books in the bibliography as a guide to reliable texts, visit your local public or academic library or a medical bookstore.

You can also buy textbooks. They'll probably range in price from $40 to $200, but it's fairly easy to get used copies at college and university bookstores. Medical bookstores usually are found near medical schools. Some of the largest well-known bookstore chains also carry hard-to-find textbooks, or they can order them for you. Several bookstores have web sites that greatly facilitate ordering books, especially if you're not feeling well enough to drive, park, browse, and lug heavy texts home.

Because of the high cost of textbooks, borrowing texts is an attractive alternative for most people.

If you haven't used a public library lately to search for holdings, you might be pleasantly surprised to find that, in many cases, the old card catalogs are gone, replaced by fast and easy-to-use computer workstations. Their databases can tell you within a few minutes how many copies of a book are in their system, which branches of the library own the book, whether another borrower has taken it out, and when it's due back.

If your public library is in a large urban area, the materials you need may be readily accessible, but if not, your library system may be able to borrow the materials you need even if they are not in their holdings. As with searching for medical research papers, it pays to ask for help. You may have to wait longer for an interlibrary loan, but it can save you the cost of an expensive text.

How to find clinical trials

New and possibly better treatments are available to colorectal cancer patients in carefully controlled settings called clinical trials, which are described in depth in Chapter 20, *Clinical Trials*. You should become familiar with the trials that are available before you need one, for frequently trials are needed when events have reached crisis level and time is running low.

In order to choose the best from among several clinical trials, it's necessary to be familiar with the track record, if any, of the treatments being used in each trial. Each of the drug names or surgical techniques appearing in a trial's title can be used as a keyword to search medical journals (as described earlier in the section called "How to obtain medical research papers") for any previous research studies published. This is a daunting task: do not expect to finish it in one sitting, or even in a few days. Once it's done, however, you only need to search for new treatments as they first appear in the clinical trials database or among your other sources of information.

You can use several methods to find clinical trials: asking your oncologist, calling NCI, hiring a search firm, or searching on a computer.

By asking your oncologist

Ask your oncologist which trials would suit your medical circumstances. This has its advantages and disadvantages, one advantage being that you need do very little except trust.

By calling the National Cancer Institute

Call NCI at (800) 4-CANCER and ask about trials for colorectal cancer, being sure to specify whether you're willing to travel—otherwise they'll send you local trials only. Be sure to ask for the full document, not the summary. Be warned that if you call often with this request (which is not an unreasonable thing to do, because new trials are added every month), eventually they may decline to send you any more listings. This has been the experience of some cancer survivors who've used this service, which is provided by various regional cancer care centers under the auspices of NCI.

By hiring a search firm

Commercial firms exist that can do a medical literature search for you. A partial list of such companies appears earlier in the section called "How to obtain medical research papers."

By personal computer

You can use a computer to research US and international clinical trials at the NCI's web site (*http://cnetdb.nci.nih.gov/trialsrch.shtml*). This, in conjunction with learning to use Medline, is by far the most comprehensive way to check on new treatments being tested. Once available only to those who sub-scribed to the NCI's Information Associates' program for $100 per year, this tool is now provided free of charge by the NCI on the Internet. We strongly suggest that you examine all trials available for colorectal cancer, not just those in your area.

When you visit this site, you'll be presented with a menu of choices for find-ing trials by cancer type, location of trial, kind of trial, and so on. Use the down arrow next to Diagnosis to expand the list of cancers, then scroll down and click on one of these:

- Colon cancer

- Rectal cancer

- Metastatic cancer, to liver (or to lung, etc.)

- Solid tumor, unspecified, adult

If you're using this search engine for the first time, it's a good idea to view all colorectal cancer trials available. Use the down arrow next to Trial Type to select the word "treatment," then click the search button. The result will be a large list of all trials for colorectal cancer that focus on treatment.

You can repeat the search using the City and State fields to see trials only in your own area, or with the Phase field to see only phase I, phase II, or phase III trials, which are explained in Chapter 20.

If you're interested in a particular kind of drug or method, you can use the Modality field to select only trials using this technology, such as monoclonal antibodies, which are categorized as such, and also as "antibody therapy."

Other means of finding clinical trials include:

- CenterWatch's site on the Internet to track new cancer treatment trials, *http://www.centerwatch.com.*

- Commercial Internet service providers such as America Online (AOL) to receive email press releases from pharmaceutical companies concerning new products in development.

- The National Childhood Cancer Foundation site to find trials specifi-cally for children, *http://www.nccf.org* or (800) 458-6223.

How to find support groups

Local hospitals, a local branch of the national Wellness Community, the American Cancer Society, and the Internet offer solid information and access to others who have been through it, too—their help and comfort is beyond estimation. The American Cancer Society can be reached at (800) ACS-2345; ask for their *I Can Cope* program. The Wellness Community in your area is listed in the phone book.

If you have Internet access, the Association of Cancer Online Resources (ACOR) has pointers to all of the Internet cancer email discussion groups. Highly recommended is the COLON list for emotional support and medical information. For this and other Internet discussion groups, ACOR (*http://www.acor.org*) offers a handy automatic subscription feature for these discussion mailing lists.

Several of the groups listed in the following section, "Groups for curing colorectal cancer," also offer one-on-one phone support for those with colorectal cancer.

Groups for curing colorectal cancer

These nonprofit groups specialize in helping those with colorectal cancer and in supporting research. Complete contact information can be found in Appendix A.

- Colon Cancer Alliance: *http://www.ccalliance.org/index.html*
- Hereditary Cancer Institute: (402) 280-1746
- Hereditary Colorectal Cancer Polyposis Registry: (410) 955-3875
- Intestinal Multiple Polyposis and Colorectal Cancer (IMPACC): (717) 788-1818
- National Lymphedema Network: (800) 541-3259
- The American Cancer Society: (800) ACS-2345, *http://www.cancer.org*

How to verify drug information

Pharmaceutical information tools are useful for finding drug side effects, mode of action, and marketing names. Your pharmacist, your library or bookstore, your computer, and the FDA can be sources of information.

You can call your pharmacist for information about drugs, or ask for the foldout paper of small print that comes from the drug manufacturer but is seldom included with your prescription unless you ask for it.

The Physician's Desk Reference (PDR), a compendium of information about drugs, is now reprinted in versions that are easier for the general public to understand, but you might appreciate the learning experience gained from reading the original PDR. In addition to the PDR, many other drug encyclopedias are available for the general public.

The Food and Drug Administration is a good means for verifying drug information. Call (888) 332-4543, (800) 532-4440, or visit online at *http://www.fda.gov*.

You can report adverse effects of drugs to the FDA, too, or use their Med-Watch web site: *http://www.fda.gov/medwatch/how.htm*.

The following Web sites have search engines requiring only the drug name:

* Rxmed, *http://www.rxmed.com*
* Clinical Pharmacology Online, *http://www.cponline.gsm.com*
* PharmInfoNet, *http://pharminfo.com/drg_mnu.html*
* DrugInfoNet, *http://www.druginfonet.com*
* HealthTouch, *http://www.healthtouch.com/level1/p_dri.htm*
* PlanetRx, *http://www.planetrx.com*
* Mythos Pharmacy Online, *http://www.mythos.com/pharmacy*

How to verify your chemotherapy dose

For most drugs, you can use a general formula for calculating dosages of your chemotherapy drugs, and can compare it to the amount that is recommended for you in your medical records. Keep in mind, though, that your doctor may be using a different dose for very good reasons, or that your regimen might include drugs that are not given based on body surface area, but instead on renal function, for example.

Glaxo's DoseCalc site at *http://www.meds.com/DChome.html* deserves special mention as a user-friendly research site because it's a great way to verify your chemotherapy dosage. Enter your height, weight, and a drug name. Behind the scenes, it calculates your square feet per meter (yes, square, not cubic, feet per meter—the basis for most chemotherapy dosages) and gives you the standard dose administered for a person your size.

You can also do this calculation using your body surface area and the standard recommended dose for your body surface area. Appendix C is a chart of heights, weights, and body surface areas. If your height or weight fall outside the ranges of this chart, you can use one of the following web sites to calculate your body surface area:

- Cornell University, *http://www-users.med.cornell.edu/~spon/picu/bsacalc.htm*
- Medical College of Wisconsin, *http://www.intmed.mcw.edu/clincalc/body.html*
- Martindale's HS Guide, *http://www-sci.lib.uci.edu/HSG/Pharmacy.html*

Or try a Web search on the phrase "body surface area." Note that some of these sites use a slightly different formula and so the results will differ slightly.

For the truly dedicated, calculation of body surface area can be done by hand. One formula for calculating your body's surface area in square meters is the DuBois & DuBois formula:

$$(kg^{0.425}) \times (cm^{0.725}) \times (0.007184)$$

This formula is equivalent to: (your weight in kilograms raised to power 0.425) x (your height in centimeters raised to power 0.725) x (0.007184).

First convert your weight to kilograms and your height to centimeters. One pound = 0.45 kilogram; one inch = 2.54 centimeters. For example, if your weight is 140 lbs, multiply 140 by 0.45 to get 63 kg. If your height is 5'6", multiply 66 by 2.54 to get 167.64 cm.

To raise a number to a power in Windows 95, click Start, Program, Accessories, Calculator. Click View; click Scientific. Using our example above, enter 63, then click the X^Y key and enter .425; finally, click equal. Do the same for height, for example:

63 kg to the power 0.425 = 5.817

167.64 cm to the power 0.725 = 40.9896

Then multiply 5.817 × 40.9896 × 0.007184 = 1.713

Thus, 1.71 rounded is your body surface in square meters if you're 5'6" tall and weigh 140 pounds.

Once you've calculated your body surface area, you need to know the recommended dose per square meter for each of the drugs you're getting. You can ask your doctor's staff for this information, or use Glaxo's site, listed earlier. If you notice a substantial difference between the calculated and actual dose given, ask your doctor why. Often there are very good reasons for differences.

How to interpret test results

Here are a few ways to find the normal values of tests that you can compare to your own test results. Please note that a value outside of the normal range does not always indicate a problem. Your doctor is generally the best person to tell you how to interpret test results, but for your background information, there are several references available for comparing your test results to normal values.

Appendix B, *Blood Test Values*, lists the normal adult values for a variety of blood tests.

The *Merck Manual*, either the paper version or their web site, has a section devoted to laboratory pathology. Many public libraries have a copy of the Merck Manual in their non-circulating reference section. At Merck's web site, just enter the test name and click on the search button. *http://www.merck.com* is the home page from which you can find the search facility.

Each of the following web sites has a search engine for finding the normal values of various test results:

- The University of Michigan Pathology Laboratories Handbook. Enter the test name and click search: *http://po.path.med.umich.edu/handbook/*.

- The Lupus Lab Tests web site has tests commonly done for lupus, but many of these are also done for various cancers such as colorectal cancer: *http://www.mtio.com/mclfa/lfalt1.htm*.

- HealthGate's BeWell site for medical consumers: *http://bewell.com/symtests/index.asp*.

How to assess unproven remedies

If your treatment isn't giving you good results, you may become vulnerable to claims for a quick cure made by certain practitioners. While some of these treatments may have merit, others are simply the means by which charlatans realize financial gain. How can you separate treatments that may have unrecognized medical potential from those that have been tried and discarded by reputable researchers, and those that are or were the focus of legal action?

- QuackWatch on the Internet gives the medical scientist's evaluation of those unusual remedies you've been hearing about: *http://www.quackwatch.com*.

- The National Cancer Institute publishes a great deal of information on untested remedies. Call (800) 4-CANCER.

- The American Cancer Society has a list of questions you should ask before becoming involved with unusual remedies. Call (800) ACS-2345, or visit their web site at *http://www.cancer.org*.

- The Consumer Health Information Research Institute provides an integrity index, a credibility of publication index, including one that rates cancer books: (816) 228-4595 or *http://www.reutershealth.com*.

Unique web resources

If you don't have a computer yet, or if the kids won't let you near it, this section may convince you how easily and quickly you can get the answers you've been looking for:

Please note that web sites may be inaccessible occasionally owing to data reorganization or maintenance, and that web site addresses can change:

- The American Medical Association has a doctor locator and other useful features: *http://www.ama-assn.org*.

- Steve Dunn's CancerGuide is an excellent source of information on clinical trials and researching your illness: *http://cancerguide.org*.

- Oncolink, sponsored by the University of Pennsylvania, is a highly reliable source of cancer information: *http://www.oncolink.upenn.edu*.

- The *Merck Manuals* online are an indispensable source of medical information: *http://www.merck.com.*

- Cancer News has links to several sites containing press releases: *http://www.cancernews.com.*

- Mid-South Therapeutics, Inc, hosts a web site with information for patients about tests and procedures: *http://www.msit.com/patients.htm.*

- HealthAnswers offers a web site with a search engine that can supply information about how to prepare for tests, and so on: *http://www.health-answers.com.*

- The Thrive Health Library is a good general site for questions and answers: *http://www.thriveonline.com.*

- HealthGate's BeWell site for diagnostic tests: *http://bewell.com/symtests/index.asp.*

What next?

Think of researching your condition as a cyclical activity. Although you can accumulate and absorb the basic facts about colorectal cancer in a burst of initial activity, certain parts of the literature search process should be repeated about once a month in order to stay in touch with improvements in care. Three areas in particular should be revisited on a regular schedule:

- NCI updates the physician's state-of-the-art treatment statements as new standards of care are chosen. If the treatises on colon or rectal cancers are modified, NCI can notify you via email, or you can call NCI at (800) 4-CANCER each month and ask them to check the date of the last update on the colorectal cancer physician's statement. NCI classifies changes to these documents as either substantial or editorial. Editorial changes might include replacing one citation with a better one.

- Every month, new research papers on colorectal cancer are published in many medical journals, and their summaries (abstracts) are collected in Medline and in Cancerlit, which is a subset of Medline consisting of cancer literature only.

- New clinical trials for treatment are added to the NCI database every month.

Summary

This chapter describes three critical techniques for researching your illness: tapping National Cancer Institute information repositories, accessing medical research papers, and locating clinical trials. Supplementary resources such as finding medical textbooks, verifying test results, locating information on drug side effects, and locating support groups, are also discussed.

Your approach to learning can make a difference, and the learning experience is a continuous one. It's best to keep an open mind, and to repeat your search efforts from time to time.

Resources

THE LISTS THAT FOLLOW REITERATE THE VARIOUS GROUPS, publications, services, and web tools discussed throughout this book, and include additional resources that also may serve your needs. All entries in each category are listed in alphabetic order, not by importance.

Key colorectal cancer resources

This first category includes resources you're likely to use most often, those that are the richest sources of colorectal cancer-specific information.

Colorectal cancer organizations

Colon Cancer Alliance
ACOR/CCA
c/o Julian Sheffield, Treasurer CCA
175 Ninth Avenue
New York, NY 10011
Email: *ccalliance@acor.org*
http://www.ccalliance.org

The Colon Cancer Alliance brings the voice of survivors to battle colorectal cancer through patient support, education, research and advocacy.

Hereditary Cancer Institute
Creighton University
2500 California Plaza
Omaha, NE 68178
(402) 280-2942

Hereditary Cancer Institute provides educational material and can help evaluate families for possible hereditary cancers.

Hereditary Colorectal Cancer Polyposis Registry
Johns Hopkins Hospital
550 North Broadway, Suite 108
Baltimore, MD 21205
(410) 955-3875

Hereditary Colorectal Cancer Polyposis Registry provides an opportunity to participate in research on hereditary colorectal cancer.

IMPACC
Box 908
Conynghan, PA 18219
(570) 788-1818

Intestinal Multiple Polyposis and Colorectal Cancer (IMPACC) is a clearinghouse for information about polyposis.

National Lymphedema Network
2211 Post Street, Suite 404
San Francisco, CA 94115
(800) 541-3259

Provides information on swollen limbs which may occur soon or many years after treatment.

Ostomy assistance

International Ostomy Association
c/o British Colostomy Association
15 Station Road, Reading, Berks
England RG1 1LG
Email: *ioa@ostomyinternational.org*
http://www.ostomyinternational.org

Ostomy Rehabilitation Program
American Cancer Society
(800) ACS-2345

United Ostomy Association
19772 MacArthur Boulevard, Suite 200
Irvine, CA 92612-2405
(800) 826-0826
Email: *uoa@deltanet.com*
http://www.uoa.org

Holds in-person support groups throughout the US.

Wound Ostomy and Continence Nurses Society
2755 Bristol Street, Suite 110
Costa Mesa, CA 92626
(714) 476-0268

Can refer you to an enterostomal therapy nurse in your area.

Colorectal cancer support groups

A list of colorectal cancer-related internet support groups follows. Because the Internet is a dynamic resource, this list may not be comprehensive. The number of subscribers given was approximate at the time of writing, and will vary over time. The Association of Cancer Online Resources (ACOR) at *http://www.acor.org* has pointers to cancer email discussion groups. ACOR offers a handy automatic subscription feature for these and other discussion mailing lists.

- COLON, run by Bill Glenning and Gilles Frydman, offers medical discussion and emotional support for all colorectal cancer survivors and their loved ones. COLON has about 500 subscribers.

- Cancer-Pain, Cancer-Sexuality, and Cancer-Fatigue are ACOR discussion groups for those with cancer-related side effects and long-term effects. These groups were formed in early 1999. See ACOR's site: *http://www.acor.org*.

- YAP, a discussion group for young adults age 18–25, dealing with their own illness or that of a loved one.

Colorectal cancer reading and reference material

Reference material

The National Library of Medicine's MEDLINE database at *http://www4.ncbi.nlm.nih. gov/PubMed/* is the best place to find the published results of studies on cancer treatment and care. It houses more than 9 million research papers. If you need help with searching, you can call the National Library of Medicine at (800) 272-4787 or (301) 496-6308.

The US National Cancer Institute (NCI), a division of the National Institutes of Health, has a hotline; an enormous web site; and numerous tracts, statements, booklets, and books about cancer treatment and care. Many of the statements about cancer come in two versions: for patients and for physicians. You might prefer to start with the patients' versions, but it's likely that, as you learn more, the physicians' statements will provide better, more detailed answers to your questions. The physicians' information is often part of PDQ, Physicians' Data Query.

NCI
Bethesda, MD 20892
(800) 4-CANCER
http://cancernet.nci.nih.gov

Books

Beck, G., ed. *Handbook of Colorectal Surgery.* Louis, Missouri: Quality Medical Publishing, 1997.

Cohen, A., and S. Winawer, eds. *Cancer of the Colon, Rectum, and Anus.* New York: McGraw-Hill, Inc., 1995. As of this writing, this is the most current and comprehensive textbook available that is specifically devoted to colorectal cancer. You might be able to find a copy in your doctor's office, a hospital library, or a university library. It can be purchased through any bookstore, including web-based bookstores, by ordering it from the publisher.

Levin, B. *Colorectal Cancer: A Thorough and Compassionate Resource for Patients and Their Families.* New York: American Cancer Society/Random House, 1999.

Miscovitz, P., and M. Betancourt. *What to Do If You Get Colon Cancer.* New York: John Wiley and Sons, 1997.

Mullen, B., and K. McGinn. *The Ostomy Book.* Palo Alto, California: Bull Publishing, 1992.

Pezim, M. *Colon and Rectal Cancer: All you need to know to take an active part in your treatment.* Vancouver, British Columbia: Intelligent Patient Guide, Ltd., 1992.

Phillips, Robert. *Coping with an Ostomy.* Wayne, New Jersey: Avery Publishing, 1986.

Phillips, Robin, ed. *Colorectal Surgery.* London: W. B. Saunders Co. Ltd., 1998.

Wanebo, H., ed. *Surgery for Gastrointestinal Cancer: A Multidisciplinary Approach.* Philadelphia: Lippincott-Raven, 1997. Another comprehensive textbook.

Document retrieval services

Document retrieval services can fax or mail you the full text of any published research paper. On the Internet, the Medline service providers HealthGate, Medscape, Helix, PhyNet, PDRnet.Com, SilverPlatter, Ovid On Call, Infotrieve, PaperChase, and others offer full-text services for a fee. Do a Web search on any of these names.

Companies that will do medical information searches for you for a fee are:

Can Help
(360) 437-2291

The Health Resource, Inc.
(501) 329-5272

Schine On-Line Services
(800) FIND-CURE

General cancer reading

The Alpha Book on Cancer and Living. Alameda, California: The Alpha Institute, 1993.

Altman, R., and M. Sarg. *The Cancer Dictionary.* New York: Facts On File, 1992. A good medical dictionary specifically for cancer survivors.

Brenner and Hall. *Making the Radiation Therapy Decision.* RGA Publishing Group, 1996.

Cancer Rates and Risks, 1996. The National Cancer Institute. (800) 4-CANCER.

Crane, Judy B. *How to Survive Your Hospital Stay.* Westlake Village, California: The Center Press, 1997.

Cukier, Daniel, and Virginia McCullough. *Coping with Radiation Therapy: A Ray of Hope.* Los Angeles: Lowell House, 1996.

Dollinger, Rosenbaum, and Cable. *Everyone's Guide to Cancer Therapy.* Andrews & McMeel, 1994.

Drum, D. *Making the Chemotherapy Decision.* Los Angeles: Lowell House, 1997.

Dunn, Steve. *CancerGuide.* Available online at *http://www.cancerguide.org/sdunn_story. html.*

Friedman, A., T. Klein, and H. Friedman. *Psychoneuroimmunology, Stress, and Infection.* New York: CRC Press, 1996.

Glaser, Ronald, and Janice Kiecolt-Glaser. *Handbook of Human Stress and Immunity.* New York: Academic Press, 1994.

Harpham, Wendy. *After Cancer: A Guide to Your New Life.* New York: W. W. Norton, 1994.

Harpham, Wendy. *Diagnosis: Cancer.* New York: W. W. Norton, 1998.

Harpham, Wendy. *When a Parent Has Cancer: A Guide to Caring for Your Children.* New York: HarperCollins, 1997.

Hoffman, Barbara, ed. *A Cancer Survivor's Almanac.* Minneapolis: The National Coalition for Cancer Survivorship/Chronimed, 1996.

Inlander, Charles, B., ed. *People's Medical Society Health Desk Reference: Information Your Doctor Can't or Won't Tell You.* New York: Hyperion, 1996.

Johnson, J., and L. Klein. *I Can Cope: Staying Healthy with Cancer.* Minneapolis: Chronimed, 1994.

Keene, Nancy. *Working with Your Doctor: Getting the Healthcare You Deserve.* Sebastopol, California: O'Reilly & Associates, 1997.

Keene, Nancy. *Your Child in the Hospital: A Practical Guide for Parents.* Sebastopol, California: O'Reilly & Associates, 1997.

Lerner, Michael. *Choices in Healing: Integrating the Best of Conventional and Complementary Approaches to Cancer.* Cambridge, Massachusetts: The MIT Press, 1996.

McKay, J., N. Hirano, and M. Lampenfeld. *The Chemotherapy & Radiation Therapy Survival Guide.* New Harbinger Publications, 1998.

The Merck Manual, available in either the paper version or at their web site, is a vast resource. Many public libraries have a copy of the Merck Manual in their non-circulating reference section. *http://www.merck.com*

Murphy, G., L. Morris, and D. Lange, eds. *Informed Decisions—The Complete Book of Cancer Diagnosis, Treatment and Recovery.* The American Cancer Society/Viking, 1997. A comprehensive guide to the care and treatment of all aspects of all cancers; has an extensive list of organizations that help cancer survivors.

Niebuhr, Bruce. *Handbook of Clinical Trial and Epidemiological Research Designs.* Available online at *http://www.sahs.utmb.edu/sahs/oret/intro_to_research/clintrls.htm.*

Olson, Kaye, RN. *Surgery and Recovery: How to Reduce Anxiety and Promote Healthy Healing.* Traverse City, Michigan: Rhodes and Easton, 1998.

Radiation Therapy and You. A 50-page booklet available from the National Cancer Institute, (800) 4-CANCER.

Schover, L. *Sexuality and Fertility after Cancer.* New York: John Wiley & Sons, 1997.

Spiegel, David. *Living Beyond Limits: New Hope and Health for Facing Life-Threatening Illness.* Fawcett Books, 1994.

Youngson, Robert, with the Diagram Group. *The Surgery Book.* New York: St. Martin's Press, 1993.

Zakarian, Beverly. *The Activist Cancer Patient.* New York: John Wiley & Sons, 1996.

Zukerman, Eugenia, and Julie Ingelfinger. *Coping with Prednisone—and other cortisone-related medicines.* New York: St. Martin's Press, 1997.

General cancer organizations

Agency for Health Care Policy and Research
P.O. Box 8547
Silver Spring, MD 20907-8547
(800) 358-9295

American Cancer Society National Office
1599 Clifton Road NE
Atlanta, GA 30329-4251
(800) ACS-2345
http://www.cancer.org

The American Cancer Society has many national and local programs, as well as a 24-hour support line, to help cancer survivors with problems such as travel, lodging, and emotional issues.

American Red Cross
430 17th Street NW
Washington, DC 20006
(202) 737-8300

The American Self-Help Clearinghouse
25 Pocono Road
Denville, NJ 07834
(973) 625-7101

Publishes a national directory of self-help groups.

Burger King Cancer Caring Center
4117 Liberty Avenue
Pittsburgh, PA 15224
(412) 622-1212

Provides counseling and a hotline service for those with cancer.

Cancer Family Care
7162 Reading Road, Suite 1050
Cincinnati, OH 45237
(513) 731-3346

Offers counseling to families affected by cancer.

Cancer Research Institute
681 Fifth Avenue
New York, NY 10022
(800) 99-CANCER

Offers services such as PDQ searches for clinical trials and free literature on cancer.

Cancervive
6500 Wilshire Boulevard, Suite 500
Los Angeles, CA 90048
(213) 655-3758

Offers many services to cancer survivors.

Center for Medical Consumers
237 Thompson Street
New York, NY 10012
(212) 674-7105

Provides information referrals to other organizations, and maintains a medical consumer's library.

Consumer Health Information Research Institute
300 East Pink Hill Road
Independence, MO 64057
(816) 228-4595
http://www.reutershealth.com

Provides an integrity index, and a credibility of publication index, including one that rates cancer books.

Hereditary Cancer Institute
2500 California Plaza
Omaha, NE 68178
(402) 280-1746 or (402) 280-2942

Evaluates families for risk, and furnishes educational material to families with hereditary cancers.

Make Today Count
1235 East Cherokee
Springfield, MO 65804
(800) 432-2273

Offers peer support via local chapters for those with life-threatening illnesses.

Mautamar Project
1707 L Street NW, Suite 1060
Washington, DC 20036
(202) 332-5536

Offers support to lesbians with cancer and their families.

National AIDS Hotline
(800) 342-2437

Furnishes assistance to those with AIDS, including AIDS-related colorectal cancer.

National Cancer Care Foundation
1180 Avenue of the Americas
New York, NY 10036
(212) 382-2078 or (800) 813-HOPE

Provides information, support, and counseling for those affected by cancer.

National Coalition for Cancer Research
426 C Street NE
Washington, DC 20002
(202) 544-1880

An activist group that monitors government spending on cancer.

National Coalition for Cancer Survivorship
1010 Wayne Avenue, 5th Floor
Silver Spring, MD 20910
(301) 650-8868

Formed by cancer survivors to offer support and to effect change in progress against cancer through legislative efforts, they have published the Cancer Survivor's Almanac, a good reference for any cancer survivor.

National Family Caregivers Association
9621 East Bexhill Drive
Kensington, MD 20895
(800) 896-3650

Provides a variety of services to caregivers.

People Living Through Cancer, Inc.
323 Eighth Street, SW
Albuquerque, NM 87102
(505) 242-3263
Email: *cancerhope@aol.com*

Offers many services to cancer survivors.

PWA Coalition Hotline
50 West 17th Street, 8th Floor
New York, NY 10011
(800) 828-3280

Furnishes assistance to those with AIDS, including AIDS-related colorectal cancer. A really nice group of people.

R. A. Bloch Cancer Foundation
4410 Main Street
Kansas City, MO 64111
(816) 932-8453

Offers a variety of services to cancer patients and survivors, such as telephone-based second medical opinions and one-on-one phone contact between cancer survivors.

Well Spouse Foundation
610 Lexington Avenue, Suite 814
New York, NY 10022
(800) 838-0879

Offers support to those whose spouses are chronically ill.

Wellness Community
2716 Ocean Park Boulevard, Suite 1040
Santa Monica, CA 90405
(310) 314-2555

Has branches throughout the US, check your local phone book for the chapter nearest you.

Children's cancer resources

Included below are organizations and reading material specifically for children.

Organizations that help children with cancer

Association for the Care of Children's Health
7910 Woodmont Avenue, Suite 300
Bethesda, MD 20814
(800) 808-ACCH
(609) 224-1742

Provides information for making informed decisions about care.

Candlelighters Foundation
7910 Woodmont Avenue, Suite 460
Bethesda, MD 20814
(800) 366-2223

Provides information and support for parents of children with cancer.

Chai Lifeline/Camp Simcha
48 West 25th Street
New York, NY 10010
(800) 343-2527

Provides a free kosher camp for children of any religion with cancer, including transportation from anywhere in the world.

Children's Hospice International
1850 M Street NW, Suite 900
Washington, DC 20036
(800) 242-4453

Provides many types of assistance to children with cancer and their families.

Federation for Children with Special Needs
95 Berkeley Street, Suite 104
Boston, MA 02116
(617) 482-2915

Provides support for parents regarding educational and healthcare rights.

Hole in the Wall Gang Camp
565 Ashford Center Road
Ashford, CT 06278
(860) 429-3444

A free ten-day summer camp for children ages seven through fifteen with cancer.

Make-A-Wish Foundation
100 W. Clarendon, Suite 2200
Phoenix, AZ 85013
(602) 279-9474

Offers sick children ages two through eighteen an opportunity for an adventure.

Sibling Information Network
A. J. Papanikou Center
University of Connecticut
249 Glenbrook Road, Box U64
Storrs, CT
(860) 486-4985

Publishes a newsletter of interest to those who have children with developmental disabilities.

Special Love, Inc. (Camp Fantastic)
117 Youth Development Court
Winchester, VA 22602
(540) 667-3774

Offers recreational programs for children with cancer and their families.

Starlight Foundation International
12424 Wilshire Boulevard, Suite 1050
Los Angeles, CA 90025
(800) 274-7827

Provides entertainment for sick children between ages four and eighteen.

Sunshine Foundation
P.O. Box 255
Loughman, FL 33858
(800) 767-1976

Grants wishes to sick children.

Sunshine Kids
2902 Ferndale Place
Houston, TX 77098
(800) 594-5756

Offers sports, cultural events and group activities for children being treated for cancer.

Vital Options
(818) 508-5657

A group dedicated to providing support to young adults with cancer and other serious illnesses.

Books about cancer for children

Clifford, Christine. *Our Family Has Cancer, Too!* Pfeifer-Hamilton Publishing, 1997.

Fromer, Margot Joan. *Surviving Childhood Cancer: A Guide for Families.* American Psychiatric Press, 1995. Written for children.

Harpham, Wendy Schlessel. *Becky and the Worry Cup: A Children's Book about a Parent's Cancer.* HarperCollins, 1997.

Kohlenberg, Sherry. *Sammy's Mommy Has Cancer.* Magination, 1993. For preschoolers.

Martin, Ann M. *Jessi's Wish (Baby-Sitters Club No. 48).* Apple, 1991. Through Danielle, who has cancer, Jessi learns new things about herself.

Trillin, Alice. *Dear Bruno.* New Press, 1996. A cartoon book about adjusting to cancer, primarily but not exclusively, for children.

Books about dying for children

Buscaglia, Leo. *The Fall of Freddie the Leaf.* New York: C.B. Slack, 1982.

Hitchcock, R. *Tim's Dad: A Story about a Boy Whose Father Dies.* Springfield, Illinois: Human Services, 1988.

Holden, L. D. *Gran-Gran's Best Trick: A story for children who have lost someone they love.* New York: Magination, 1989.

Krementz, Jill. *How It Feels When a Parent Dies.* New York: Alfred A. Knopf, 1981.

LeShan, Ed. *Learning to Say Good-bye: When a Parent Dies.* New York: Macmillan, 1976.

O'Toole, Donna. *Aarvy Aardvark Finds Hope.* Burnsville, North Carolina: Celo Press, 1988.

Vigna, J. *Saying Good-Bye to Daddy.* Morton Grove, Illinois: Albert Whitman, 1991.

White, E.B. *Charlotte's Web.* New York: Harper & Row, 1952.

Cancer magazines

Cancer Communication, **published by PAACT**
Patient Advocates for Advanced Cancer Treatments
1143 Parmelee, NW
Grand Rapids, MI 49504
(616) 453-1477

Coping
PO Box 682268
Franklin, TN 37068
(615) 790-2400

Living Through Cancer
323 Eighth Street, SW
Albuquerque, NM 87102
(505) 242-3263

Medical resources

Medical information targeted to special topics is available through the resources
listed in these categories.

Verifying doctor and hospital credentials

The ABMS Public Education Program
47 Perimeter Center East, Suite 500
Atlanta, GA 30346
(800) 733-2267
http://www.certifieddoctor.org

They publish *The Official ABMS Directory of Board Certified Medical Specialists,* a
directory of board-certified physicians who have chosen to specialize in a particular
area of medicine.

The American College of Surgeons
633 North Saint Clair Street
Chicago, IL 60611
(312) 202-5000

They can verify whether your surgeon is board-certified in a surgical specialty.

American Medical Association
http://www.ama-assn.org/aps/amahg.htm

The AMA publishes the *Directory of Physicians in the US* that can help you verify your
doctor's credentials. Their *Physician Select* web site is also an excellent means to
check your doctor's education and board certification.

The American Society of Pediatric Hematology/Oncology (ASPH/O) established standard requirements for programs treating children with cancer and blood disorders.

Center for Medical Consumers
237 Thompson Street
New York, NY 10012
(212) 674-7105

Provides information referrals to other organizations, and maintains a medical consumer's library.

College of American Pathologists
325 Waukegan Road
Northfield, IL 60093-2750
(800) 323-4040

The Consumer Health Information Research Institute
(816) 228-4595
http://www.reutershealth.com

Provides an integrity index, a credibility of publication index.

The Joint Commission on Accreditation of Health Care Organizations (JCAHO)
1 Renaissance Boulevard
Oakbrook Terrace IL 60181
(630) 792-5800

National Council Against Health Fraud
P.O. Box 1276
Loma Linda, CA 92354
(909) 824-4690

Medi-net
http://www.askmedi.com

Provides information on every doctor licensed in the US.

QuackWatch
http://www.quackwatch.com

Gives the medical scientist's evaluation of those unusual remedies you've been hearing about.

U.S. News and World Report
"Best Hospitals" annual edition
2400 N Street N.W.
Washington, DC 20037-1196
(202) 955-2000
http://www.usnews.com/usnews/nycu/health/hosptl/tophosp.htm

Drug and dosage information

Clinical Pharmacology Online
http://www.cponline.gsm.com

DrugInfoNet
http://www.druginfonet.com

Glaxo's DoseCalc
http://www.meds.com/DChome.html

HealthTouch
http://www.healthtouch.com/level1/p_dri.htm

PharmInfoNet
http://pharminfo.com

PlanetRx
http://www.planetrx.com

Mythos Pharmacy Online
http://www.mythos.com/pharmacy/

Physician's Desk Reference

The *Physician's Desk Reference* (PDR), a compendium of information about drugs, is now reprinted in versions that are easier for the general public to understand, but you might appreciate the learning experience gained from reading the original PDR. In addition to the PDR, there are many other drug encyclopedias available for the general public. Available through bookstores or in libraries.

RxMed
http://www.rxmed.com/prescribe.html

US Food and Drug Administration (FDA)
5600 Fishers Lane
Rockville, MD 20857
(301) 827-4420
(888) 332-4543
(800) 532-4440
http://www.fda.gov

You can report adverse effects of drugs to the FDA, too, or use their MedWatch web site: *http://www.fda.gov/medwatch/how.htm*.

Calculating body surface area

Cornell University
http://www-users.med.cornell.edu/~spon/picu/bsacalc.htm

Martindale's HS Guide
http://www-sci.lib.uci.edu/HSG/Pharmacy.html

Medical College of Wisconsin
http://www.intmed.mcw.edu/clincalc/body.html

Tests and procedures

These resources can help you learn how tests are done, and what the results mean.

Information on how tests are done

Andrews, Maraca, and Michael Shaw. *Everything You Need to Know About Medical Tests*. Springhouse, 1996. An excellent comprehensive reference written for the patient in a readable and respectful style.

Barry, L., ed. *The Patient's Guide to Medical Tests*. Houghton Mifflin Co., 1997.

The Biology Project. University of Arizona: *http://www.biology.arizona.edu*.

Brodin, Michael B. *The Encyclopedia of Medical Tests*. Pocket Books, 1997. A 1982 book with the same title written by Pinckney and Pinckney should be passed over in favor of this newer book.

Department of Pathology, University of Washington, Seattle: *http://www.pathology.washington.edu*.

The Family Internet site: *http://familyinternet.com*.

HealthGate: *http://bewell.com*.

Keene, Nancy. *Your Child in the Hospital*. Sebastopol, California: O'Reilly and Associates, 1997. Covers all aspects of the child's experiences with hospitalization, from tests and treatment to emotional issues such as sibling reactions.

Mid-South Imaging & Therapeutics, P.A.: *http://www.msit.com*.

Pagana, Kathleen, and Timothy Pagana, eds. *Mosby's Diagnostic and Laboratory Test Reference*, 1992.

Shtasel, Philip. *Medical Tests and Diagnostic Procedures—A Patient's Guide to Just What the Doctor Ordered*. Harper and Row, 1990.

Stauffer, Joseph, and Joseph C. Segen. *The Patient's Guide to Medical Tests: Everything You Need to Know About the Tests Your Doctor Prescribes*, 4th ed. Facts on File, 1997.

ThriveOnline: *http://www.thriveonline.com*.

Normal values of tests

The University of Pennsylvania Cancer Center. Enter the test name and click search: *http://www.oncolink.upenn.edu*.

The University of Michigan Pathology Laboratories Handbook. Enter the test name and click search: *http://po.path.med.umich.edu/handbook/*.

Clinical trials and investigational new substances

The Food and Drug Administration (*http://www.fda.gov*) contains regulations for investigational new drugs and for importing foreign drugs for single-patient use. (800) 532-4440.

The book *Intuitive Biostatistics,* by Harvey Motulsky, can help you understand published results of clinical trials, and can help you assess trial design if you're planning to enroll in a trial.

The National Cancer Institute Clinical Trials web site is the most comprehensive way to locate trials of new substances and treatments: *http://cnetdb.nci.nih.gov/trialsrch.shtml.*

QuackWatch on the Internet gives the medical scientist's evaluation of those unusual remedies you've been hearing about: *http://www.quackwatch.com.*

Niebuhr, Bruce. *Handbook of Clinical Trial and Epidemiological Research Designs.* January 1998. *http://www.sahs.utmb.edu/sahs/oret/intro_to_research/clintrls.htm.*

Steve Dunn's Cancerguide is an excellent resource for learning how to assess clinical trials and how to research your illness: *http://www.cancerguide.org.*

Resources for pain and other side effects

The American Cancer Society has many programs to help cancer survivors with problems such as pain. Dial (800) ACS-2345 or check your local phone directory for the office nearest you.

American Society of Anesthesiologists
515 Busse Highway
Park Ridge, IL 60068
(847) 825-5586

American Society of Clinical Hypnosis
2200 East Vine Avenue, Suite 291
Des Plaines, IL 60018
(847) 297-3317

National Chronic Pain Outreach Association
7979 Old Georgetown Road, Suite 100
Bethesda, MD 20814-2429
(301) 652-4948

Educates families, patients, and caretakers about chronic pain and the choices of treatment.

National Lymphedema Network
2211 Post Street, Suite 404
San Francisco, CA 94115
(800) 541-3259

Provides information on swollen limbs which may occur soon or many years after treatment.

Cancer-Pain is an ACOR discussion group for those with cancer-related pain. This group was formed in early 1999. See ACOR's site: *http://www.acor.org.*

Acupuncture and massage

American Association of Oriental Medicine
433 Front Street
Catasauqua, PA 18032-2506
Phone: (610) 266-1433
Fax: 264-2768
Email: *AAOM1@aol.com*

National Acupuncture and Oriental Medicine Alliance
PO Box 77511
Seattle, WA 98177-0531
(206) 524-3511
Email: *76143.2061@compuserve.com*

National Acupuncture Foundation
1718 M Street, Suite 195
Washington, DC 20036
Phone: (202) 332-5794

The following two web sites have useful information about acupuncture:

http://www.acupuncture.com/Referrals/ref2.htm
http://www.acupuncture.com/StateLaws/StateLaws.htm

American Massage Therapy Association
820 Davis Street, Suite 100
Evanston, IL 60201-4444
Phone: (847) 864-0123
Fax: (847) 864-1178
http://www.amtamassage.org

Legal, financial, employment, and insurance resources

Beyond the physical aspects of cancer lie its effects on our careers and finances. The following resources can offer guidance and aid.

Organizations that help with legal and financial issues

The Center for Medical Consumers
237 Thompson Street
New York, NY 10012
(212) 674-7105

Provides information referrals to other organizations and maintains a medical consumer's library.

Consumer Credit Counseling
(800) 388-2227

Provides help getting expenses under control.

The Federal Trade Commission
(202) 326-3650

Provides information about the Federal Consumer Credit Protection Act, a landmark series of laws passed in 1968 to protect debtors.

Health Care Cost Hotline
(900) 225-2500

Can furnish the median fee and range of fees charged by doctors for various services and procedures. The call is $2.00 to $4.00 per minute.

Health Insurance Association of America (HIAA)
555 13th Street NW
Washington, DC 20004
(202) 824-1600
http://www.hiaa.org/index.html

Has more than 250 members consisting of insurers and managed care companies. HIAA can supply booklets on disability income, health insurance, long-term care, medical savings accounts, and general insurance information, including a directory of state insurance departments.

Lexis Law Publishing
(800) 542-0957

This group can send you a copy of any law.

The Medical Information Bureau (MIB)
P.O. Box 105, Essex Station
Boston, MA 02112
(617) 424-3660

Records all entries made by insurance companies about your health, and will send a copy of this information to your physician if you request it. If you find an error in these files, you can contact the Bureau for the procedures necessary to correct errors.

Magazines for legal and financial issues

Health Pages
(212) 929-6131

Medical Economics
(201) 945-9058

Both report on ranges and norms of doctor's fees.

Social Security Administration bulletins

The chief resource in this category is the 1997 Social Security Handbook, 13th edition: *http://www.ssa.gov/OP_Home/ handbook/ssa-hbk.htm*.

Other, more specific SSA bulletins include:

Social Security: "What You Need to Know When You Get Disability Benefits" (6/96; Pub. No. 05-10153).

"Social Security Disability Programs" (5/96; Pub. No. 05-10057).

"A Guide to Social Security and SSI Disability Benefits for People with HIV Infection" (6/95; Pub. No. 05-10020).

"How We Decide If You Are Still Disabled" (4/96; Pub. No. 05-10053).

"How Social Security Can Help with Vocational Rehabilitation" (9/94; Pub. No. 05-10050).

"Working While Disabled...How We Can Help" (1/96; Pub. No. 05-10095).

"Red Book on Work Incentives for People with Disabilities" (8/95; Pub. No. 64-030).

Free treatment resources

The National Cancer Institute
Bethesda, MD
(800) 4-CANCER

The St. Jude Children's Research Hospital
(901) 495-3300

Free travel and lodging for care

See Chapter 21, *Traveling for Care*, which consists of too many resources to duplicate here.

Air Care Alliance
(888) 662-6794
(757) 318-9145
Helps cancer patients travel to distant health centers for care.

American Cancer Society (ACS)
http://www.cancer.org
Sponsors Hope Lodges, which provide free lodging for those who travel to receive cancer care.

The Candlelighters Childhood Cancer Foundation
(301) 657-8401 or (800) 366-CCCF (United States)
(800) 363-1062 (Canada)
http://www.candlelighters.org
Can help you make travel arrangements.

Corporate Angel Network
(914) 328-1313
http://www.corpangelnetwork.org

Helps cancer patients travel to distant health centers for care.

Mercy Medical Airlift
(800) 296-1191
http://www.mercymedical.org

Helps cancer patients travel to distant health centers for care.

National Association of Hospital Hospitality Houses (NAHHH)
(301) 961-3094, (317) 883-2226, or (800) 542-9730

Can recommend nearby hotels with reduced rates for cancer patients.

The National Cancer Institute
Bethesda, MD
(800) 4-CANCER

In some cases, will help pay for the travel and lodging expenses of those being treated at NCI.

Ronald McDonald House Coordinator
c/o McDonalds Corporation
(630) 623-7048
http://www.rmhc.com

Provides free lodging for children who are being treated for cancer.

End-of-life resources

Resources for increasing comfort and serenity in the last stage of life are included in this category.

Home and hospice care

Community Health Accreditation Program, Inc.
350 Hudson Street
New York, NY 10014
(800) 669-9656

Provides a list of accredited home care organizations.

National Association for Home Care
519 C Street, NE
Washington, DC 20002
(202) 547-7424

Represents all home healthcare agencies in the US. They offer publications on selecting home care.

National Hospice Organization
1901 North Moore Street, Suite 901
Arlington, VA 22209
(800) 658-8898

Offers information on the goals of hospice and how to choose a hospice.

Oley Foundation
214 Hun Memorial
Albany Medical Center A-23
Albany, NY 12208
(800) 776-OLEY

Offers help with parenteral or enteral nutrition—that is, feeding by IV or stomach tube.

Olsten Health Services National Resource Center
175 Broadhollow Road
Melville, NY 11747
(800) 66-NURSE

Offers help with all home healthcare services.

Visiting Nurse Associations of America
3801 East Florida Avenue, Suite 900
Denver, CO 80210
(800) 426-2547

Provides skilled nurses, aides, and therapists for home care.

Reading material about dying

Basta, Lofty. *A Graceful Exit: Life and Death on Your Own Terms.* New York: Plenum Press, 1996.

Bernard, Jan, and Miriam Schneider. *The True Work of Dying.* New York: Avon Books, 1996.

Callanan, Maggie, and Patricia Kelley. *Final Gifts: Understanding the Special Awareness, Needs, and Communications of the Dying.* New York: Bantam Books, 1996.

Furman, Joan, and David McNabb. *The Dying Time: Practical Wisdom for the Dying.* New York: Bell Tower, 1997.

Groopman, Jerome. *The Measure of Our Days.* New York: Viking (Penguin), 1997.

Humphry, Derek. *Final Exit: The Practicalities of Self-Deliverance and Assisted Suicide for the Dying.* The Hemlock Society, 1997.

Kramp, Erin Tierney, Douglas H. Kramp, and Emily P. McKhann. *Living with the End in Mind: A Practical Checklist fort Living Life to the Fullest by Embracing Your Mortality.* Three Rivers Press, 1998.

Kubler-Ross, Elisabeth. *On Death and Dying.* New York: Macmillan Publishing, 1969.

Kubler-Ross, Elisabeth. *Death: The Final Stage of Growth.* New York: Simon and Schuster, 1975.

Kubler-Ross, Elisabeth. *To Live Until We Say Good-bye.* New York: Fireside (Simon and Schuster), 1978.

Kubler-Ross, Elisabeth. *Living with Death and Dying*. New York: Touchstone (Simon and Schuster), 1981.

Lattanzi-Licht, Marcia, John Mahoney, and Galen Miller. *The Hospice Choice: In Pursuit of a Peaceful Death*. New York: Fireside (Simon and Schuster), 1998.

McPhelimy, Lynn. *In the Checklist of Life: A Working Book to Help You Live & Leave Life*. A. A. I. P. Pub. Co., 1998.

Nuland, Sherwin. *How We Die: Reflections on Life's Final Chapter*. New York: Alfred A. Knopf, 1993.

Ray, M. Catherine. *I'm With You Now: A Guide Through Incurable Illness for Patients, Families, and Friends*. New York: Bantam Books, 1997.

Weenolsen, Patricia. *The Art of Dying*. New York: St. Martin' s Press, 1996.

Blood Test Values

THE FOLLOWING TABLES WILL PROVIDE YOU WITH approximate quantitative information about certain blood test results. Test results can be influenced by many things, such as how the blood was drawn and stored, whether the patient exercised recently or was dehydrated, how tight the tourniquet was, medications taken by the patient, and so on. Your lab will display its own norms alongside your test results. These norms may differ from other sources, as each lab recalculates their norms as their data accumulate.

Carcinoembryonic antigen (CEA) in particular is subject to differing assay calibrations by different labs, and is known to fluctuate throughout the day and in response to noncancerous conditions such as pregnancy, infections that affect the liver, and changes in smoking or alcohol consumption habits. CA19-9 and TPA are of limited usefulness because their sensitivity and specificity for colorectal cancers still are being scrutinized.

In order to evaluate correctly any cancer antigen test results you receive, you and your doctor should verify what range of values your laboratory is using, and note previous values among your own medical records to detect a trend, which may be more meaningful than an absolute value.

Table B-1. Cancer Antigens

Test Name	Low Normal	High Normal, Nonsmoker	High Normal, Smoker
CEA	0	3.0 ng/ml	5.0 ng/ml
CA19-9	0	37 U/ml[1]	N/A
TPA	0	187,000 U/ml[2]	N/A
CA 15-3	0	25 U/ml – 40 U/ml[3]	N/A

Table B-2. Complete Blood Counts in Normal Adults

Test Name	Low	High
White cell count (WBC) x 10^9/liter blood	3.9	11.3
White Cell Differentials (percents)		
Polys	42%	78%
Bands	0%	4%
Lymphocytes	15%	45%
Monocytes	0%	12%
Eosinophils	0%	7%
Basophils	0%	2%

Table B-2. *Complete Blood Counts in Normal Adults (continued)*

Test Name	Low	High
Atypical lymphocytes	0%	4%
Platelet count (PLT) x10⁹/liter blood	140	450
Mean platelet volume (MPV)	6.3	10.3
Mean corpuscular volume, fl/red cell (MCV)	80.0	100
Mean corpuscular hemoglobin, pg/red cell (MCH)	26.4	34.0
Mean corpuscular hemoglobin conc., g/dl red cells (MCHC)	31.0	36.0
Red cell distribution width (RDW), CV (%)	11.5%	14.5%

Table B-3. *Complete Blood Counts in Normal Adults: Red Cell Counts by Gender*

Test Name	Men		Women	
	Low	High	Low	High
Red cell count (RBC) x 10¹²/liter blood	4.52	5.90	4.1	5.10
Hemoglobin (HB) g/dl blood	14.0	18.0	12.3	15.3
Hematocrit (HCT)	0.40	0.52	0.36	0.45

Table B-4. *Other Blood Values in Normal Adults*

Test Name	Low	High
Direct bilirubin, mg/dl (Bili)	0	0.4
Total bilirubin, mg/dl (Bili)	0	1.0
Blood urea nitrogen, mg/dl (BUN)	8	25
Cholesterol	130	200
Creatinine, mg/dl (CRT)	0.6	1.5
Calcium mg/dl (Ca)	8.5	10.5
Chlorine mEq.l (Cl)	95	100
Potassium, mEq/l (K)	3.5	5.0
Phosphate mg/dl (P)	2.5	4.5
Sodium, mEq/l (Na)	135	145
Magnesium, mEq/l (Mg)	1.5	2.5
Erythrocyte Sedimentation Rate mm/hr (ESR)	0	20
Glucose, mg/dl	65	100
Lactate Dehydrogenase u/l (LDH)	100	190
Albumin gm/dl (Alb)	3.5	5.0
Alkaline Phosphatase (AlkP) u/l	50	135
(ALT, formerly SGPT) u/l	5	40
(AST, formerly SGOT) u/l	10	50
Thyroid TSH	0.5	5.0
Thyroid free T4	1	4
Uric acid, mg/dl	2.5	8.0

Body Surface Area in Square Meters

THE CHART ON THE FOLLOWING PAGE SHOWS BODY SURFACE AREA for typical heights and weights. Calculations were made using the DuBois & DuBois formula:

$$kg^{0.425} \times cm^{0.725} \times 0.007184$$

Weight is the horizontal axis, first in pounds, then in kilograms. Height is the vertical axis, first in inches, then in centimeters. Results are body surface areas in square meters.

If your height or weight falls between or outside the ranges of this chart, you can use one of the following web sites to calculate body surface area:

- Cornell University: *http://www-users.med.cornell.edu/~spon/picu/bsacalc.htm*
- Medical College of Wisconsin: *http://www.intmed.mcw.edu/clincalc/body.html*
- Martindalee's HS Guide: *http://www-sci.lib.uci.edu/HSG/Pharmacy.html*

Or, try a web search on the phrase "body surface area." Note that some of these sites use slightly different formula, so the results will differ slightly.

Note that certain drugs are not dosed based on body surface area, but on other parameters such as renal function.

Lbs/Kg → In/Cm ↓	100/45	110/49.5	120/54	130/58.5	140/63	150/67.5	160/72	170/76.5	180/81	190/85.5	200/90	210/94.5	220/99	230/103.5	240/108	250/112.5	260/117	270/122.5
60/152.4	1.38	1.44	1.50	1.55	1.60	1.65	1.69	1.74	1.78	1.82	1.86	1.90	1.94	1.97	2.01	2.04	2.08	2.11
61/154.9	1.40	1.46	1.52	1.57	1.62	1.67	1.71	1.76	1.80	1.84	1.88	1.92	1.96	2.00.	2.03	2.07	2.11	2.14
62/157.5	1.42	1.48	1.53	1.59	1.64	1.69	1.73	1.78	1.82	1.86	1.91	1.94	1.98	2.02	2.06	2.09	2.13	2.16
63/160.0	1.43	1.49	1.55	1.61	1.66	1.71	1.75	1.80	1.84	1.88	1.93	1.97	2.01	2.04	2.08	2.12	2.16	2.19
64/162.6	1.45	1.51	1.57	1.62	1.68	1.73	1.77	1.82	1.86	1.91	1.95	1.99	2.03	2.07	2.11	2.14	2.18	2.21
65/165.1	1.47	1.53	1.59	1.64	1.70	1.74	1.79	1.84	1.88	1.93	1.97	2.01	2.05	2.09	2.13	2.17	2.20	2.24
66/167.6	1.48	1.55	1.60	1.66	1.71	1.76	1.81	1.86	1.90	1.95	1.99	2.03	2.08	2.11	2.15	2.19	2.23	2.26
67/170.2	1.50	1.56	1.62	1.68	1.73	1.78	1.83	1.88	1.93	1.97	2.02	2.06	2.10	2.14	2.18	2.21	2.25	2.29
68/172.7	1.52	1.58	1.64	1.70	1.75	1.80	1.85	1.90	1.95	1.99	2.04	2.08	2.12	2.16	2.20	2.24	2.28	2.31
69/175.3	1.53	1.60	1.66	1.72	1.77	1.82	1.87	1.92	1.97	2.01	2.06	2.10	2.14	2.18	2.22	2.26	2.30	2.34
70/177.8	1.55	1.61	1.67	1.73	1.79	1.84	1.89	1.94	1.99	2.03	2.08	2.12	2.17	2.21	2.25	2.29	2.33	2.36
71/180.3	1.56	1.63	1.69	1.75	1.81	1.86	1.91	1.96	2.01	2.05	2.10	2.15	2.19	2.23	2.27	2.31	2.35	2.39
72/182.3	1.58	1.64	1.71	1.76	1.82	1.87	1.93	1.98	2.02	2.07	2.12	2.16	2.21	2.25	2.29	2.33	2.37	2.41
73/185.4	1.60	1.66	1.73	1.79	1.84	1.90	1.95	2.00	2.05	2.10	2.14	2.19	2.23	2.27	2.32	2.36	2.40	2.44
74/188.0	1.61	1.68	1.74	1.80	1.86	1.92	1.97	2.02	2.07	2.12	2.17	2.21	2.26	2.30	2.34	2.38	2.42	2.46
75/190.5	1.63	1.70	1.76	1.82	1.88	1.94	1.99	2.04	2.09	2.14	2.19	2.23	2.28	2.32	2.36	2.40	2.45	2.48
76/193.0	1.64	1.71	1.78	1.84	1.90	1.95	2.01	2.06	2.11	2.16	2.21	2.25	2.30	2.34	2.38	2.43	2.47	2.51
77/195.6	1.66	1.73	1.79	1.86	1.92	1.97	2.03	2.08	2.13	2.18	2.23	2.28	2.32	2.36	2.41	2.45	2.49	2.53
78/198.0	1.67	1.74	1.81	1.87	1.93	1.99	2.05	2.10	2.15	2.20	2.25	2.30	2.34	2.39	2.43	2.47	2.52	2.56

Staging System Equivalents

OVER TIME, VARIOUS SYSTEMS HAVE BEEN DEVISED to describe the spread of colorectal cancer. The most recent staging system developed, the TNM system, is now the most commonly used in the US, as it is considered the most accurate and detailed.

Approximate TNM equivalents to older staging systems, the Dukes and Astler-Coller systems, are shown in the table below, although experts caution that the translation is not exact. A description of the terms used in the TNM system is included following the table.

In the TNM system, the terms and criteria for staging colon and rectal cancers are the same.

TNM Stage	TNM Characteristics	Dukes Equivalent	Astler-Coller Equivalent
0	Tis, N0, M0	—	—
I	T1, N0, M0 T2, N0, M0	A	A and B1
II	T3, N0, M0 T4, N0, M0	B	B2 and B3
III	Any T, N1, M0 Any T, N2, M0	C	C1 – C3
IV	Any T, Any N, M1	D	D

T: assessment of primary tumor

The following criteria are used by the National Cancer Institute to evaluate the extent of spread of the original tumor. At this point it might be useful to refer to Figure 1-1, "Cross section of the colon," in Chapter 1. Going outward, the layers of the bowel are mucosa (comprised of epithelium, basement membrane, lamina propria, muscularis mucosae), submucosa, muscularis propria, subserosa. The serosa is an additional outer layer in areas of the peritoneal cavity where the bowel is freely moving:

- TX: The primary tumor cannot be evaluated.

- T0: The existence of a primary tumor cannot be ascertained.

- Tis: Carcinoma in situ (tumor in place): an intraepithelial tumor or an invasion of the lamina propria. Tis includes cancer cells entirely contained within the glandular basement membrane (intraepithelial) or lamina propria (intramucosal) with no breach through the muscularis mucosae into the submucosa.

- T1: The tumor invades the submucosa, the second layer of the large intestine.

- T2: The tumor invades the muscularis propria.
- T3: The tumor invades through the muscularis propria into the subserosa, or into nonperitonealized pericolic or perirectal tissues.
- T4: The tumor directly invades other organs or structures, and/or penetrates the visceral peritoneum. In T4, the term "direct invasion" includes invasion of other sections of colon or rectum by way of the serosa; for instance, invasion of the sigmoid colon by a carcinoma of the cecum.

N: assessment of regional lymph nodes

The following terms describe the criteria used to evaluate the degree to which lymph nodes have been invaded by cancerous cells:

- NX: Regional lymph nodes cannot be evaluated.
- N0: No invasion of regional lymph nodes (metastasis) is apparent.
- N1: Invasion of one to three regional lymph nodes has been found.
- N2: Invasion of four or more regional lymph nodes has been found.

M: assessment of distant metastasis

The following terms describe the criteria used to rank the spread of disease, if any, to distant organs:

- MX: Distant metastasis cannot be determined.
- M0: No distant metastasis is apparent.
- M1: Distant metastasis is apparent.

Notes

Chapter 3: *What Is Colorectal Cancer?*

1. R. L. Nelson et al., "Determination of factors responsible for the declining incidence of colorectal cancer," *Diseases of the Colon and Rectum* 42, no. 6 (June 1999): 741-52.
2. T. Naoe et al., "Molecular analysis of the t(15;17) translocation in de novo and secondary acute promyelocytic leukemia," *Leukemia*, Supplement 3 (11 April 1997): 287-8.
3. J. Lennard-Jones and W. Connell, "Surveillance–Inflammatory Bowel Disease," *Cancer of the Colon, Rectum, and Anus*, A. Cohen, ed. (1995), Chapter 34.
4. C. S. Fuchs et al., "Dietary fiber and the risk of colorectal cancer and adenoma in women," *New England Journal of Medicine*, 340, no. 3 (21 January 1999): 169-76.
5. G. A. Colditz et al., "Physical activity and reduced risk of colon cancer: implications for prevention," *Cancer Causes and Control*, 8, no. 4 (July 1997): 649-67.
6. A. I. Neugut, "Leisure and occupational physical activity and risk of colorectal adenomatous polyps," *International Journal of Cancer* 68, no. 6 (11 December 1996): 744-8.
7. I. Thune and E. Lund, "Physical activity and risk of colorectal cancer in men and women," *British Journal of Cancer* 73, no. 9 (May 1996): 1134-40.

Chapter 4: *Prognosis*

1. R. Pazdur et al., "The oral fluorouracil prodrugs," *Oncology (Huntington)* 10, Supplement 7 (12 October 1998):48-51.
2. P. H. Sugarbaker et al., "Peritoneal carcinomatosis from adenocarcinoma of the colon," *World Journal of Surgery* 5 (20 June 1996): 585-91; discussion 592.
3. S. Y. Hsieh et al., "A clinical study on pseudomyxoma peritonei," *Journal of Gastroenterology and Hepatology* 10, no. 1 (January-February 1995): 86-91.
4. S. R. Harris and U. P. Thorgeirsson, "Tumor angiogenesis: biology and therapeutic prospects," *In Vivo* 12, no. 6 (November-December 1998): 563-70.
5. S. Hamilton, "Pathologic Features of Colorectal Cancer," *Cancer of the Colon, Rectum, and Anus*, Chapter 18.
6. G. B. Secco, "Primary mucinous adenocarcinomas and signet-ring cell carcinomas of colon and rectum," *Oncology* 51, no. 1 (January-February 1994): 30-4.
7. T. Anthony et al., "Primary signet-ring cell carcinoma of the colon and rectum," *Annals of Surgical Oncology* 3, no. 4 (July 1996): 344-8.
8. G. Li Destri et al., "Monitoring carcinoembryonic antigen in colorectal cancer: is it still useful?" *Surgery Today* 28, no. 12 (1998): 1233-6.

9. F. A. Sinicrope et al., "Relationship of P-glycoprotein and carcinoembryonic antigen expression in human colon carcinoma to local invasion, DNA ploidy, and disease relapse," *Cancer* 74, no. 11 (1 December 1994): 2908-17.

10. S. Braun and K. Pantel, "Immunodiagnosis and immunotherapy of isolated tumor cells disseminated to bone marrow of patients with colorectal cancer," *Tumori* 81, 3 Supplement (May-June 1995): 78-83.

11. D. Nori, "Tumor ploidy as a risk factor for disease recurrence and short survival in surgically treated Dukes' B2 colon cancer patients," *Tumour Biology* 17, no. 2 (1996): 75-80.

12. S. Hamilton, "Pathologic Features of Colorectal Cancer."

Chapter 6: *Modes of Treatment*

1. E. Mamounas et al., "Comparative efficacy of adjuvant chemotherapy in patients with Dukes' B versus Dukes' C colon cancer: results from four National Surgical Adjuvant Breast and Bowel Project adjuvant studies (C-01, C-02, C-03, and C-04)," *Journal of Clinical Oncology* 17, no. 5 (May 1999): 1349-55.

2. K. Ghoshal and S. T. Jacob, "An alternative molecular mechanism of action of 5-fluorouracil, a potent anticancer drug," *Biochemical Pharmacology* 53, no. 11 (1 June 1997): 1569-75.

Chapter 12: *Stress and the Immune System*

1. W. Neuhaus et al., "A prospective study concerning psychological characteristics of patients with breast cancer," *Archives of Gynecology and Obstetrics* 255, no. 4 (1994): 201-9.
R. Schwarz and S. Geyer, "Social and psychological differences between cancer and noncancer patients: cause or consequence of the disease?" *Psychotherapy and Psychosomatics* 41, no. 4 (1984): 195-9.

Chapter 14: *Getting Support*

1. Ellen E. Schultz, "If You Use Firm's Counselors, Remember Your Secrets Could Be Used Against You," *Wall Street Journal*, 26 May 1994.

Chapter 19: *Recurrence of Disease*

1. G. Li Destri, "Monitoring carcinoembryonic antigen," 1233-6.

Chapter 20: *Clinical Trials*

1. Bruce Niebuhr, "Handbook of Clinical Trial and Epidemiological Research Designs," January 1998, *http://www.sahs.utmb.edu/sahs/oret/intro_to_research/clintrls.htm*.

2. See trials MSKCC-95021A4 and NCCTG-984652, for example.

3. Bruce Niebuhr, "Handbook."

Appendix B: *Blood Test Values*

1. S. Eda et al., "Clinical evaluation of latex photometric immunoassay for serum CA19-9," *Rinsho Byori* 43 no. 3 (March 1995): 257-62.
2. P. Polterauer, E. Legenstein, and M. Muller, "Serum concentrations of tissue polypeptide antigen and alpha 1-fetoprotein in patients with primary liver cancer, liver metastasis and liver cirrhosis," *Wien Klin Wochenschr* 97, no. 9 (26 Apr 1985): 417-20.
3. E. Fritsche and J. Benz, "Is follow-up of breast cancer with CEA and CA 15-3 justified?" *Helv Chir Acta* 59, no. 1 (May 1992): 225-9.

Glossary

THIS GLOSSARY LISTS ONLY TERMS SPECIFIC TO COLORECTAL CANCERS. For a comprehensive glossary of cancer medical terminology, see Roberta Altman's and Michael Sarg's *The Cancer Dictionary*. For more general medical terms, any one of several inexpensive medical dictionaries available in bookstores and libraries should suffice.

Guides to pronunciation are included.

But first—unusual phrases

Before we list terms you may find when reading about colorectal cancers, we must point out that there are a few specific words and phrases that may be jarring because they mean something other in medicine than they do in everyday usage:

Anecdotal
> When used in a medical context does not mean a funny story. It means a single case report not yet substantiated by studies using large numbers of people.

Impressive or not impressive
> When used in a medical context does not mean anything derogatory. It means that, when the patient was examined, a particular feature did not strike the examiner as overwhelmingly unusual. For instance, after palpating your abdomen, the doctor may note in your medical record that your spleen was "not impressive." This means it did not feel enlarged, and that you did not report pain when she pressed on it.

Morbid or morbidity
> Does not mean that you have a neurotic outlook. These words simply mean illness, and are somewhat the opposite of mortality. You might read, for example, that a treatment resulted in 20 percent low-level morbidity but only 2 percent mortality. Likewise, comorbidity means the illnesses a person has in addition to cancer, such as high blood pressure or diabetes.

"The patient denies..."
> Does not mean that the doctor thinks you're lying. It's just used as the opposite of "the patient reports..." For instance, your medical record might read, "The patient reports frequent morning cough, but denies the presence of phlegm."

Pathological
> In the context of tissue studies means the study of the appearance of healthy cells, cancerous cells, and affected organs. It does not mean mental or emotional illness, such as would be meant by the phrase "pathological liar" or the word psychopath.

Tolerable

A word often used by medical staff to describe the side effects of treatment. Your idea of what is tolerable may be much lower than their definition, because medicine defines a tolerable side effect as one that can be ameliorated with supportive care and that does not result in permanent organ damage. For you, these side effects may be intolerable.

Colorectal cancer terminology

Absolute neutrophil count (NEW tro fil) or ANC

The total number of neutrophils in the blood, a measure of one's ability to fight infection. Also called absolute granulocyte count. ANC can be suppressed by chemotherapy.

Adenoma (ad en OH muh)

A polyp; an initially benign growth that forms in the colon from the innermost layer of mucin-producing epithelial cells.

Adenopathy (ad en AH path ee)

The enlargement of lymph glands. Its presence in a colorectal cancer survivor might suggest the spread of cancer to the lymphatic system.

Anastomosis (eh nas teh MOW sis)

The rejoining of two ends of tissue after a portion of the tissue between them has been removed.

Anemia (an KNEE me uh)

A lack of adequate numbers of oxygen-carrying red blood cells.

Apoptosis (app uh TOE sis; variant: a pup TOE sis)

Orderly cell death characterized by slow dissolving and reuse of cell parts by neighboring tissue. Some chemotherapy drugs induce apoptosis; others cause cell lysis or bursting.

Ascending colon

The portion of colon that begins in the lower right part of the abdomen, departing from the end of the small intestine. It rises on the right side up to the rib cage, where it turns to cross under the liver as the transverse colon.

Bulky disease

Any cancer that measures greater than ten centimeters in any dimension.

Carcinoma in situ (kar sih NO ma in SEE tyoo ; in SIGH tyoo)

A tumor that is still confined to the mucosa.

Cecum (SEE come)

The beginning of the large intestine where the small intestine empties into it. The cecum is located in the lower right abdomen.

Centigrey or cGy

A measurement of radiation dose absorbed by the body.

Clear margins

The desirable result of surgery for colorectal cancer. All tissue samples should have clear margins on all edges.

Colectomy (coal EK tow mee)

The removal of part or all of the colon.

Colonoscopy (coal un OSS kow pee)
> The examination of the entire length of the colon, up to its juncture with the small intestine, using a flexible tube that has a camera and a light source attached.

Colostomy (coal OSS tow mee)
> The temporary or permanent channeling of the remaining open end of colon through the stomach wall and skin, where an ostomy appliance will attach to capture waste.

Complete blood count or CBC
> A count of the red, white, and platelet cells in peripheral blood.

Complete remission
> The disappearance of all signs of disease for one month or longer.

Cytotoxic (sigh toe TOX ic)
> A term for anything that kills cells. Many chemotherapy and radiotherapy regimens are cytotoxic to both healthy and cancerous cells.

Descending colon
> The portion of colon that continues down from the upper left part of the abdomen. It descends from the transverse colon at the splenic flexure. It descends on the left side of the abdomen, where it turns inward to become the sigmoid colon.

Differentiation (diff er en she A shun)
> The term used to describe the process of cells maturing and developing for a particular task. In general, normal young cells of most organs are undifferentiated and very similar to each other. They differentiate into functional cells of their respective organ types as they age. Cancer cells that fail to differentiate often are characterized as very aggressive, not functional for their organ type, and hard to identify as belonging to a particular type of tissue.

Distal (DISS tul)
> The portion of the colon that is closest to the rectum and anus.

Enterostomal therapist (enter OSS tow mull)
> A specialist, often an RN, who is trained to help colostomates care for their stoma and ostomy appliances.

Erythrocyte (eh REETH ro site)
> A red blood cell. Red blood cells are responsible for carrying oxygen to body tissues.

Erythropenia (eh REETH ro PEA' nee uh)
> The condition of having abnormally low numbers of red blood cells.

Event-free survival
> The total amount of time that a patient survives, without relapse, following treatment. See Overall survival.

Familial adenomatous polyposis (FAP)
(fum ILL yull add eh KNOW muh tus poll ip OH sis)
> An inherited condition characterized by the development of many intestinal polyps, often early in life. FAP can lead to colonic malignancies if the entire colon is not removed. Removal of all polyps with a colonoscope is not possible because they are too numerous and are likely to recur.

Fecal occult blood test (FOBT)
  A test using agents that can detect certain components of blood (often iron metabolites) in fecal samples. Some oncologists recommend this testing as part of a constellation of follow-up care after treatment for colorectal cancer. The general population is urged to have this testing yearly (in conjunction with other tests) as part of screening for detection of early colonic cancers. See the tear-out page at the back of this book and Chapter 3 for more information on screening.

Fluorouracil (5-FU) (floor oh YOUR a sill)
  The drug most commonly used in the United States as first-line chemotherapy for several stages of colorectal cancer. 5-FU often is used along with leucovorin.

Granulocytes (GRAN you lo sites)
  Types of white blood cells that attack bacteria by engulfing them. Eosinophils, neutrophils, basophils, and mast cells are types of granulocytes.

Grey or Gy
  A measurement of radiation dose absorbed by the body.

Hematocrit or Hct (he MAH to crit)
  Describes the percentage by volume of red blood cells in whole blood drawn for a CBC.

Hemaglobin (HE muh glow bin)
  The iron-containing protein found in the center of a red blood cell that can bind to and transport oxygen.

Hemicolectomy (hem ee coal EK tow me)
  A partial colectomy, a partial removal of the colon.

Hepatic flexure (hep ATT ic FLEK sure)
  The point at which the ascending colon turns and crosses beneath the liver to the left side of the abdomen. Beyond the hepatic flexure the colon is called the transverse colon.

Ileostomy (ill ee OSS tow mee)
  The temporary or permanent channeling of the remaining open end of small intestine through the stomach wall and skin, where an ostomy appliance will attach to capture waste. Ileostomy is the correct term to use when all of the colon has been removed, although some colorectal cancer survivors use the terms colostomy and ileostomy interchangeably.

Ileum (ILL ee um)
  The small intestine, which empties into the large intestine or colon at the cecum, the beginning of the ascending colon.

J-pouch or ileoanal pouch
  Made by folding back on itself the end of the small intestine that remains after the entire colon has been removed. The two parallel folded pieces are stitched together, creating a reservoir that is twice the size of the original, unfolded tissue. A bottom opening in the J-pouch is surgically reconnected to the anus. The intention is to simulate the larger retention capacity of the colon and to preserve fecal continence.

Lamina propria (LAM ih nuh pro PREE uh)

The capillary-fed connective tissue beneath the basement membrane of the colon. It is a sublayer of the mucosa. Going outward, the layers of the bowel are mucosa, submucosa, muscularis propria, subserosa. Serosa is an additional outer layer in areas of the peritoneal cavity where the bowel is freely moving.

Left colon

Same as the descending colon.

Leucovorin (loo KAV uh rin)

A chemotherapy drug used along with fluorouracil to increase the effectiveness of 5-FU.

Leukocyte (LU ko site)

A general term for all white blood cells.

Leukopenia (LU ko PEA nee uh)

The condition of having abnormally low numbers of white blood cells. See also -penia.

Locus (LOW kus)

A position within a gene.

Loci (LOW sigh)

Multiple positions within a gene or genes.

Lumen (LOO men)

The empty interior of the colon through which food waste travels.

Lymphocytopenia (lim foe sit o PEA ne uh)

The condition of having abnormally low numbers of certain white blood cells called lymphocytes. See also -penia.

Mean

Same as an average.

Median

The midpoint. If 81 patients were treated with drug XYZ, and the time for white blood cell counts to recover following this treatment ranged from two to sixty days, after you rank the patients by the number of days required for their white blood cells to recover, the median is the number of days that it took patient number 41's white blood cells to recover.

Metachronous (meh TAH crow nis)

Second tumors that occur independently some time after the primary tumor, not as a result of spread of the first tumor, which is called metastasis.

Metastasis (me TAS te sis)

The spread of cancer to other tissues.

Micrometastasis (MY krow me TAS te sis)

Less than 2 millimeters of detectable cancer at a site other than the original tumor.

Mucosa (myew KO suh)

The inner lining of the colon containing epithelial cells that produce mucin. The mucosa is composed of several sublayers: the epithelium, the basement membrane, the lamina propria, and the muscularis mucosae. Going outward, the layers of the bowel are mucosa, submucosa, muscularis propria, subserosa. The serosa is an additional outer layer in areas of the peritoneal cavity where the bowel is freely moving.

Muscularis mucosa (mus kyew LAR is myew KO suh)
A sublayer of the mucosa, the innermost layer of the colon. Going outward, the layers of the bowel are mucosa, submucosa, muscularis propria, and subserosa. The serosa is an additional outer layer in areas of the peritoneal cavity where the bowel is freely moving.

Muscularis propria (mus kyew LAR is pro PREE uh)
The layer of the colon between the submucosa and the subserosa. Going outward, the layers of the bowel are mucosa, submucosa, muscularis propria, and subserosa. The serosa is an additional outer layer in areas of the peritoneal cavity where the bowel is freely moving.

Neutropenia (nu trow PEA nee uh)
The condition of having abnormally low numbers of one type of white blood cell called neutrophils.

NSAIDs
Nonsteroidal anti-inflammatory drugs, such as aspirin or ibuprofen.

Occult disease
Cancer not detectable by visual exam or by testing strategies such as imaging studies.

Overall survival
The total amount of time that a patient survives following treatment, including relapses that were successfully retreated. See Event-free survival.

Palliation (pal ee A shun)
The relief of pain without an intent to cure disease.

Partial response
Describes a tumor's response to treatment that is 50 percent smaller or more, but still remains. It's not unusual to see a partial response on imaging halfway through treatment, and a total response by the end of treatment. See Complete response.

Pedunculated (peh DUN kyew lay ted)
Describes a polyp on a stalk, the opposite of sessile.

-penia
A suffix denoting abnormally low numbers of blood cells: leukopenia, erythropenia, or thrombocytopenia.

Platelet
A blood cell called a thrombocyte, important in the blood clotting process.

Primary tumor
The original tumor. Metastases may spread from certain malignant primary tumors.

Proctocolectomy (prok tuh ko LEK tuh me)
The surgical removal of all of the colon and rectum.

Prognosis (prog KNOW sis)
The expected or probable outcome.

Proximal (PROX i mull)
   Portion of the colon that is closest to the juncture with the small intestine—that is, the portion farthest from the rectum and anus.

Rectum
   The last six inches of the colon, the portion just prior to the anus. Feces are stored in the rectum until they are voided. The boundary between the colon and the rectum is difficult to distinguish.

Remission
   The tumor-free time period, dated from the first, not the last, therapy session. Patients with tumors that recur within one month of treatment ending are considered to have had no remission. Disappearance of all disease is complete remission; reduction of tumor size by more than 50 percent is considered partial remission.

Right colon
   Same as the ascending colon.

Serosa (seer OH suh)
   The outermost layer of the bowel in areas where the bowel is freely moving (labile). Going outward, the layers of the bowel are mucosa, submucosa, muscularis propria, and subserosa, and serosa in areas of the peritoneal cavity where the bowel is freely moving.

Sessile (SESS isle or SESS ill)
   Describes a polyp or lesion that is lying flat—that is, not pedunculated.

Sigmoid colon (SIG moid)
   The portion of the colon on the lower left side of the abdomen between the descending colon and the rectum.

Sigmoidoscopy (sig moid OSS kuh pee)
   The examination of the rectum and the lower part of the colon using a flexible tube that has a camera and a light source attached.

Sphincter muscles (SFINK ter)
   Muscles that, when healthy and intact, are always somewhat contracted to keep an opening closed. For colorectal cancer survivors, the anal sphincter is the muscle most often mentioned.

Splenic flexure (SPLEN ik)
   The point at which the transverse colon turns and descends on the left side of the abdomen, beneath the spleen, becoming the descending colon.

Stable disease
   One or more tumors, still visible on imaging, that are not growing.

Stoma (STOW muh)
   Greek for mouth. When the context is colorectal surgery, stoma means an opening created in the wall of the abdomen through which a piece of the intestine passes in order to void fecal material.

Submucosa (sub myew KOW suh)
   Supportive tissue beneath the inner mucosal layer of the large intestine. Going outward, the layers of the bowel are mucosa, submucosa, muscularis propria, and subserosa. The serosa is an additional outer layer in areas of the peritoneal cavity where the bowel is freely moving.

Subserosa (sub seer OH suh)

The outermost layer of the colon in areas where the bowel is not freely moving (labile). In areas where the bowel is labile, the serosa is the outermost layer of the colon.

Synchronous (SINK run us)

Tumors that appear at the same time. See Metachronous.

Thrombocyte (THROM bow site)

A blood cell commonly called a platelet.

Thrombocytopenia (throm bi sigh toe PEA nee uh)

The condition of having abnormally low numbers of platelets.

Total response

Describes a tumor's response to treatment. The tumor has either completely disappeared, or is so small and stable it may just be scar tissue.

Transverse colon

The portion of horizontal colon between the ascending and descending colon. The transverse colon crosses the abdomen beneath the liver from the patient's right to the patient's left.

Tumor lysis syndrome

Arises from the death of certain large tumors, and may arise shortly after chemotherapy is started. It is characterized by symptoms of kidney failure owing to excessive amounts of calcium, phosphate, and potassium being released by dying tumors. See "Metabolic Imbalances" in Chapter 9, *Side Effects of Treatment*.

Vancomycin-resistant enterobacteria or VRE (van kow MY sin)

Intestinal bacteria that are no longer killed by one of the strongest antibiotics, Vancomycin.

Bibliography

The following list of reference materials does not include the many technical journal articles researched for this book. A complete bibliography, organized by chapter, can be found at *http://www.patientcenters.com/colorectal*.

Abromovitz, Les. *Family Insurance Handbook: The Complete Guide for the 1990s*. Blue Ridge Summit, Pennsylvania: TAB Books.

Alpha Book on Cancer and Living. Alameda, California: The Alpha Institute, 1993.

Altman, R., and M. Sarg. *The Cancer Dictionary*. New York: Facts on File, 1992.

American Medical Association Directory of Physicians in the US. Published by the American Medical Association, 1996.

Andrew, M., and M. Shaw. *Everything You Need to Know About Medical Tests*. Springhouse, 1996. An excellent comprehensive reference written for the patient in a readable and respectful style.

Barry, L., ed. *The Patient's Guide to Medical Tests*. Houghton Mifflin Co., 1997.

Basta, Lofty. *A Graceful Exit: Life and Death on Your Own Terms*. New York: Plenum Press, 1996.

Beck, G., ed. *Handbook of Colorectal Surgery*. St. Louis, Missouri: Quality Medical Publishing, 1997.

Berkow, R., ed. *The Merck Manual of Diagnosis and Therapy, 17th ed.* Merck & Co. Inc., 1999.

Bernard, Jan, and Miriam Schneider. *The True Work of Dying*. New York: Avon Books, 1996.

Brenner, David, and Eric Hall. *Making the Radiation Therapy Decision*. Los Angeles: Lowell House, 1997.

Brodin, Michael B. *The Encyclopedia of Medical Tests Pocket Books, 1997*. A 1982 book with the same title written by Pinckney and Pinckney should be passed over in favor of this newer book.

Callahan, Maggie, and Patricia Kelley. *Final Gifts: Understanding the Special Awareness, Needs and Communications of the Dying*. New York: Bantam Book, 1997.

Cancer Rates and Risks, 1996. The National Cancer Institute, (800) 4-CANCER.

Carlson, Richard. *Don't Sweat the Small Stuff...And It's All Small Stuff*. New York: Hyperion, 1997.

Cash, Connaght. *The Medicare Answer Book: What You and Your Family Need to Know Now!* Provincetown, Massachusetts: Race Point Press, 1997.

Cassell, Eric, MD. *The Healer's Art: A New Approach to the Doctor-Patient Relationship*. Philadelphia: J. B. Lippincott Co., 1979.

Clinical Pharmacology Online: *http://www.cponline.gsm.com/*.

Cohen, A., and S. Winawer, eds. *Cancer of the Colon, Rectum, and Anus.* New York: McGraw-Hill, Inc., 1995.

Cooper, Cary, and Maggie Watson. *Cancer and Stress: Psychological, Biological and Coping Studies.* New York: John Wiley & Sons, 1996.

Cousins, Norman. *Anatomy of an Illness as Perceived by the Patient.* New York: W. W. Norton, 1979.

Crane, Judy B. *How to Survive Your Hospital Stay.* Westlake Village, California: The Center Press, 1997.

Cukier, Daniel, and Virginia McCullough. *Coping with Radiation Therapy: A Ray of Hope.* Los Angeles: Lowell House, 1996.

Detlefs, Dale, Robert Myers, and J. R. Treanor. *1997 Mercer Guide to Social Security & Medicare.* William M. Mercer, Inc.

Dollinger, M., E. Rosenbaum, and G. Cable. *Everyone's Guide to Cancer Therapy.* Toronto, Ontario: Somerville House Books Ltd., 1991.

Drum, D. *Making the Chemotherapy Decision.* Los Angeles: Lowell House, 1997.

Dunn, Steve. "CancerGuide": *http://www.cancerguide.org.*

Enteen, Robert. *Health Insurance: How to Get it, Keep It, or Improve What You've Got.* New York: Paragon House, 1992.

The Family Internet web site: at: *http://familyinternet.com.*

Friedman, A., T. Klein, and H. Friedman. *Psychoneuroimmunology, Stress, and Infection.* New York: CRC Press, 1996.

Food and Drug Administration (FDA) web site: *http://www.fda.gov.*

Foster, George, and Barbara Anderson. *Medical Anthropology.* New York: John Wiley & Sons, 1978.

Furman, Joan, and David McNabb. *The Dying Time: Practical Wisdom for the Dying.* New York: Bell Tower, 1997.

Glaser, Ronald, and Janice Kiecolt-Glaser. *Handbook of Human Stress and Immunity.* New York: Academic Press, 1994.

Goleman, Daniel. *Emotional Intelligence.* New York: Bantam, 1995.

Gray, H. *Gray's Anatomy.* Philadelphia: Running Press, 1974.

Groopman, Jerome. *The Measure of Our Days.* New York: Viking (Penguin), 1997.

Hakin, Cliff. *When You Lose Your Job.* San Francisco: Berrett-Loehler Publishers, 1993.

Handler, Evan. *Time on Fire: My Comedy of Terrors.* New York: Little, Brown & Co., 1996.

Harpham, Wendy Schlessel. *After Cancer: A Guide to Your New Life.* New York: W. W. Norton, 1994.

Harpham, Wendy Schlessel. *Diagnosis: Cancer.* New York: W. W. Norton, 1998.

Harpham, Wendy Schlessel. *When a Parent Has Cancer: A Guide to Caring for Your Children.* HarperCollins, 1997.

HealthGate's "Be Well" web site: *http://www.healthgate.com/.*

Heymann, Jody, MD. *Equal Partners: A Physician's Call for a New Spirit of Medicine.* New York: Little, Brown & Co., 1995.

Hoffman, Barbara, ed. *A Cancer Survivor's Almanac.* The National Coalition for Cancer Survivorship. Minneapolis: Cronimed, 1996.

Humphry, Derek. *Final Exit: The Practicalities of Self-Deliverance and Assisted Suicide for the Dying.* The Hemlock Society, 1997.

Inlander, Charles B., ed. *People's Medical Society Health Desk Reference: Information Your Doctor Can't or Won't Tell You*. New York: Hyperion, 1996.

Inlander, Charles, and Michael Donio. *Medicare Made Easy*. Allentown, Pennsylvania: People's Medical Society, 1998.

Johnson, J., and L. Klein. *I Can Cope: Staying Healthy with Cancer*. Minneapolis: Chronimed, 1994.

Katz, Jay. *The Silent World of Doctor and Patient*. New York: The Free Press, 1984.

Keene, Nancy. *Childhood Leukemia*. Sebastopol, California: O'Reilly & Associates, 1997. Every medical and emotional topic of concern to parents of children undergoing treatment is discussed in this book.

Keene, Nancy. *Working with Your Doctor: Getting the Healthcare You Deserve*. Sebastopol, California: O'Reilly & Associates, 1997.

Keene, Nancy. *Your Child in the Hospital*. Sebastopol, California: O'Reilly & Associates, 1997. Covers all aspects of the child's experiences with hospitalization.

Kubler-Ross, Elisabeth. *Death: The Final Stage of Growth*. New York: Simon and Schuster, 1975.

Kubler-Ross, Elisabeth. *Living with Death and Dying*. New York: Touchstone (Simon and Schuster), 1981.

Kubler-Ross, Elisabeth. *On Death and Dying*. New York: Macmillan Publishing, 1969.

Kubler-Ross, Elisabeth. *To Live Until We Say Goodbye*. New York: Fireside (Simon and Schuster), 1978.

Kushner, Harold. *When Bad Things Happen to Good People*. G. K. Hall, 1982.

Lattanzi-Licht, Marcia, John Mahoney, and Galen Miller. *The Hospice Choice: In Pursuit of a Peaceful Death*. New York: Fireside (Simon and Schuster), 1998.

Lerner, Michael. *Choices in Healing: Integrating the Best of Conventional and Complimentary Approaches to Cancer*. Cambridge, Massachusetts: The MIT Press, 1996.

Levin, B. *Colorectal Cancer: A Thorough and Compassionate Resource for Patients and Their Families*. The American Cancer Society. New York: Random House, 1999.

Mayer, Musa. *Advanced Breast Cancer: A Guide to Living with Metastatic Disease*. Sebastopol, California: O'Reilly & Associates, 1998.

McAllister, Horowitz, and Gilden. *Cancer*. BasicBooks (HarperCollins), 1993.

McElroy, Susan. *Animals as Teachers and Healers*. New York: Ballantine, 1997.

McKay, J., N. Hirano, and M. Lampenfeld. *The Chemotherapy & Radiation Therapy Survival Guide*. New Harbinger Publications, 1998.

Mercy Medical Airlift: *http://www.mercymedical.org*.

Mid-South Imaging & Therapeutics: *http://www.msit.com*.

Miscovitz, P., and M. Betancourt. *What to Do If You Get Colon Cancer*. New York: John Wiley & Sons, 1997.

Morris, Desmond. *The Human Animal: A Personal View of the Human Species*. New York: Crown Publishers, 1994.

Motulsky, Harvey. *Intuitive Biostatistics*. New York: Oxford University Press, 1995.

Mullen, B., and K. McGinn. *The Ostomy Book*. Palo Alto, California: Bull Publishing, 1992.

Murphy, G., L. Morris, and D. Lange, eds. *Informed Decisions—The Complete Book of Cancer Diagnosis, Treatment, and Recovery*. The American Cancer Society. Viking, 1997.

The National Cancer Institute's *Physicians Data Query (PDQ) State-of-the-Art Treatment Statements for Physicians.* Many various cancer related topics.

The National Cancer Institute's web resources: *http://cancernet.nci.nih.gov.*

Nickel, Gudrun Maria, Esq. *Debtors' Rights.* Clearwater, Florida: Sphinx Publishing, 1998.

Nuland, Sherwin. *How We Die: Reflections on Life's Final Chapter.* New York: Alfred A. Knopf, 1993.

Oslon, Kaye, RN. *Surgery and Recovery: How to Reduce Anxiety and Promote Healthy Healing.* Traverse City, Michigan: Rhodes and Easton, 1998.

Pagana, Kathleen, and Timothy Pagana, eds. *Mosby's Diagnostic and Laboratory Test Reference,* 1992.

Pezim, M. *Colon & Rectal Cancer: All You Need to Know to Take an Active Part in Your Treatment.* Vancouver, British Columbia: Intelligent Patient Guide, 1992.

PharmInfoNet: *http://pharminfo.com.*

Phillips, Robert. *Coping with an Ostomy.* Wayne, New Jersey: Avery Publishing, 1986.

Phillips, Robin, ed. *Colorectal Surgery.* London: W. B. Saunders Co., 1998.

Porter, Steven L. *Save Your Home! How to Protect Your Home and Property from Foreclosure.* Colorado Springs: Java Publishing Co., 1990.

Radiation Therapy and You. The US National Cancer Institute, (800) 4-CANCER.

Ray, M. Catherine. *I'm With You Now: A Guide Through Incurable Illness for Patients, Families, and Friends.* New York: Bantam Books, 1997.

Rosenbaum, Edward, MD. *A Taste of My Own Medicine.* New York: Random House: 1988.

Rosenfeld, Isadore, MD. *Second Opinion: Your Medical Alternatives.* New York: Simon & Schuster, 1981.

RxMed: *http://www.rxmed.com.*

Schover, L. *Sexuality and Fertility After Cancer.* New York: John Wiley & Sons, 1997.

Schultz, Ellen E. "If You Use the Firm's Counselors, Remember Your Secrets Could Be Used Against You." *The Wall Street Journal,* May 26, 1994.

Shatsel, Philip. *Medical Tests and Diagnostic Procedures—A Patient's Guide to Just What the Doctor Ordered.* Harper and Row, 1990.

Shernoff, William M., Esq. *How to Make Insurance Companies Pay Your Claims and What to Do if They Don't.* Mamaroneck, New York: Hastings House, 1990.

Siebert, Al. *The Survivor Personality.* Portland, Oregon: Practical Psychology Press, 1994.

Social Security Handbook 1997, 13th ed., at: *http://www.ssa.gov/OP_Home/handbook/ssa-hbk.htm.*

Spiegel, David. *Living Beyond Limits.* New York: Fawcett Columbine, 1993.

Stauffer, Joseph, and Joseph C. Segen. *The Patient's Guide to Medical Tests: Everything You Need to Know About the Tests Your Doctor Prescribes, 4th ed.* Facts on File, 1997.

Stern, Ken. *Comprehensive Guide to Social Security and Medicare.* Hawthorne, New Jersey: The Career Press, 1995.

ThriveOnline: *http://www.thriveonline.com.*

University of Arizona's Biology Project: *http://www.biology.arizona.edu.*

University of California, Los Angeles, at: *http://anima.crump.ucla.edu.*

University of Washington, Seattle, Department of Pathology: *http://www.pathology. washington.edu.*

US News and World Report's annual "Best Hospitals" edition, 2400 N Street, NW, Washington, DC 20037-1196, (202) 955-2000.

Ventura, John. *Fresh Start! Surviving Money Troubles.* Dearborn Financial Publishing, Inc., 1992.

Wanebo, H., ed. *Surgery for Gastrointestinal Cancer: A Multidisciplinary Approach.* Philadelphia: Lippincott-Raven, 1997.

Weenolsen, Patricia. *The Art of Dying.* New York: St. Martin' s Press, 1996.

Westhem, Andrew, and Donald J. Korn. *Protecting What's Yours: How to Safeguard Your Assets and Maintain Your Personal Wealth.* New York: Carol Publishing Group, 1995.

Youngson, Robert, with the Diagram Group. *The Surgery Book.* New York: St. Martin's Press, 1993.

Zakarian, Beverly. *The Activist Cancer Patient.* New York: John Wiley & Sons, 1996.

Zukerman, Eugenia, and Julie Ingelfinger. *Coping with Prednisone—and Other Cortisone-Related Medicines.* New York: St. Martin's Press, 1997.

Index

B

bargaining, 68
barium enema (single- or double-contrast), 102–103
BAY 12-9566, 424
BCNU (carmustine), 424, 431
bilirubin, 79
biofeedback as stress reducer, 245
biological anticancer substances, 419–421
  cytokines, 119, 420–421, 428
  leukocyte therapy, 420, 432
  monoclonal antibodies, 119, 432, 433
  tumor vaccines, 120, 420, 435–436
biopsy samples, need for storage of, 136
blame at diagnosis, 20–21
blinded trial, 375
blood/blood product transfusions, 66–67, 77
blood test values, table of, 489–490
blood tests/counts, 78–81, 163, 489–490
body surface area, calculation of, table, 491–492
bolus infusion, 113
bone marrow ablation with stem cell support, 436
bone marrow aspiration/biopsy, 82–83
bone scan (scintigraphy), 83
bowel obstruction, 210–211, 332
bowel preparation before surgery, 140
brachytherapy, 117, 176, 183–184
breathing problems, 211
bronchoscopy, 91–92
bruising/bleeding, 211
Bryostatin 1, 429
Buspar (buspirone), 258

C

CA19-9, 79–80
Camptosar (irinotecan, CPT-11), 114, 205
  See also entries on specific side effects
cancer
  causes of, 40–41, 417
  prevention of, 422

resources, 467–478
  See also colorectal cancers
cancer personality, 241–242
Capecitabine (Xeloda), 114, 205
carboplatin, 424, 438
carcinoembryonic antigen (CEA), 6, 60–61, 79, 365–367, 434
Carcinoembryonic Antigen Peptide-1 (CAP), 436
caring for ostomies, 191–201
  appliances and supplies, 192–194
  attaching/reattaching the pouch, 197–198
  cleaning stoma and skin, 194–195
  discarding waste, 197
  emptying the pouch, 196
  enterostomal therapy (ET) nurse, role in, 191
  noises/gas, 199
  odor, 198–199
  resuming activities, 200–201
  skin barriers and seals, 195–196
  support groups helpful in, 201
  various sensations and observations possible, 199–200
carmustine (BCNU), 424, 431
case-control study, 376
cat scan (computed tomography/CT scan), 56, 89–91
catheters, 83–86, 318
causes of colorectal cancer, possible, 41–48, 417
CBC (complete blood count), 80, 163, 489–490
CEA (carcinoembryonic antigen), 6, 60–61, 79, 365, 434
cellular matrix exploitation, 441
central catheter/central line, 83–86, 318
chemoprotectants, 426
chemosensitization/potentiation, 427
  See also drug modulation; radiosensitization
chemotherapy
  drugs
    alkylating agents, 116, 424
    antimetabolites, 115–116, 426
    in breast milk, 359
    chemosensitization drugs, 116

depression/despair
    causes of, 68, 239
    at end of treatment, 324
    medications for, 258–259
    at recurrence, 370
    relationship to immune system
        function, 238
    symptoms of, 238–239
diagnosis of colorectal cancer
    emotional responses to, 16–21
    grading, 12, 15
    misdiagnosis/delayed diagnosis
        possible, 8–11
    second opinions in, 15, 24, 270
    staging, 12–15, 56–57, 494–495
    surgery in, 7–8
    symptoms, 1–4
    tests for, 5–11
        CEA blood testing, 6, 60–61,
            79, 365–366
        colonoscopy, 6–7, 86–89
    See also staging colorectal cancers;
        tests and procedures,
        specific
diarrhea, 213–214, 332–333
differentiation therapy, 429
difluorodeoxycytidine (Gemcitabine),
    426
disability income, 308, 310
    See also insurance
discarding waste, 197
dissociation, 18
dizziness, 216, 338
DNA. See genes and genetics
DNA adduct formation, 116, 429
doctors. See oncologists and surgeons
dolastatin 10, 435
dosages, calculation and verification of,
    172, 177, 180–181, 461–
    463, 491–492
double-blinded trial, 375–376
doxorubicin, 435
drug modulation, 429–430
    See also chemosensitization/
        potentiation
drugs
    anti-anxiety medications, 258
    antidepressant medications, 258–
        259

chemotherapy drugs, 205–206
    dosage, calculation and verification
        of, 172, 461–463, 492–
        493
    stress, medications for, 258–260
    See also chemotherapy; clinical trials
dry mouth, difficulty swallowing, 214–
    215
Dukes system (staging), 13, 56–57,
    494–495

E

Efudex, 114
electrolytes, 80
electromyelography (EMG), 76–77
embolization, 131, 437
EMLA (topical anesthetic), 72, 78–79
emotions
    end of treatment, responses to,
        318–327
    fear
        of abandonment at end of
            treatment, 320
        physical aspects of, 16–17
        possible usefulness of, 235
        at recurrence, 369
        of recurrence, 321
    during preparation for end of life,
        405–410
    prognoses, responses to, 67–69
    stress, responses to, 234–242
    from symptoms to diagnosis, 16–21
    workplace, reentering at end of
        treatment, responses to,
        326–327
employment issues, 311
    ADA (Americans with Disabilities
        Act), 311
    employee assistance programs
        (EAPs), 311
    FMLA (Family and Medical Leave
        Act), 311
    insurance, 307
    reentering workplace at end of
        treatment, 326–327
    resources, 483–484
    See also insurance
en bloc resection, 109

ileorectal (surgery), 110
ileostomy, 109, 187
  See also ostomies
imaging tools, 422
immune system
    complexity of response of, 52
    developing colorectal cancer, role
        in, 44
    impact of age on, 47
    stress and, 233–260
immunophenotype, 59–62
importation of foreign drugs, 392
impotence. *See* sexuality
incidence of colorectal cancer, 38
incontinence, 221, 336
indigestion, 222
infections, 153, 222, 337
infertility. *See* fertility
inherited forms of colorectal cancers,
        42–44
insomnia, 216–218
insurance
    COBRA, 305
    coverage for travel for care, 401
    ERISA, 305–306
    health and disability insurance,
        301–308
    HIPPA, 304–305
    HMO case managers,
        communication with, 267
    life insurance, 307
    limitations of on choice of
        oncologists and surgeons,
        25
    long-term care insurance, 307–308
    medical underwriting (coverage/
        benefits dependent on
        health), 302–303
    Medicare/Medicaid, 306
    payment for clinical trial or
        . investigational drug, 393–
        394
    resources, 483–485
    unemployment insurance, 307
    See also financial issues
interacting with medical personnel,
        261–273
    conflict resolution, 270–273
    by family and friends, 267–268

    issues in, 262–263
    suggestions for, 268–270
    when necessary, 263
    See also communication
interferons, 425, 428, 439
interleukins, 425, 428, 439
Internet
    Association of Cancer Online
        Resources, 293
    colorectal cancer support groups on
        the Web, 292–294
    oncologists, surgeons, treatment
        centers, use of in finding,
        26–28, 31–32
interstitial laser photocoagulation, 438
interstitial radiotherapy, 117, 176, 183
intestinal ganglioneuromatosis, 43
intra-operative electron beam irradiation
        (IOERT), 117
intra-operative radiotherapy, 175, 438
intraperitoneal chemotherapy, 169–170,
        439
intravenous chemotherapy, 168–169
intravenous pyelogram, 93
investigational new drugs (INDs), 392
    See also clinical trials
in vitro sensitivity-directed
        chemotherapy, 442
irinotecan (CPT-11, Camptosar), 114,
        205
    See also entries on specific side
        effects
ISIS 3521/5132, 426
isolated perfusion, 439

J

jaundice, 222–223
J-pouch, 110, 188
juvenile polyposis syndrome, 43

K

kidney damage, 222–223, 337
Kytril (granisetron), 224

raltitrexed (Tomudex, ICI D1694, ZD 1694), 206, 430, 435
randomized trial, 375
RASBI (radiation-associated small-bowel injury), 228
reading, as stress reducer, 254
recall sensitivities, 228, 340–341
recombinant viral vaccines, 434
record-keeping
    biopsy/tissue samples, storage of, 136, 312
    importance of, 312
    obtaining records for, 312–314
    organization of, 314
rectal cancer. *See* colorectal cancers
rectal pain, 223–224
rectal perforation, 228
rectum, 34
recurrence
    of aggressive/advanced tumors more likely, 364
    causes of, 363–364
    clinical, 362–363
    definition of, 15, 362
    detection of, 75–76, 362–363
    distinguished from aftereffects of treatment, 361
    emotional responses to, 369–372
    pathologic, 363
    sites of (local, regional, distant), 364–365
    time of occurrence, 367
    treatment options, 367–368
relapse. *See* recurrence
relaxation training, as stress reducer, 255
religion. *See* spirituality/faith/religious beliefs
rescue drugs, 117
research by patients/non-professionals
    chemotherapy dose, calculation of, 172, 461–463, 491–492
    clinical trials, finding, 386–388, 457–459
    drugs, information about, 461
    information needed to begin, 447
    Internet and web sites, 26–28, 31–32, 464–465
    medical libraries, 455–456

medical research papers, obtaining, 452–456
medical textbooks, obtaining, 456–457
Medline, 453–455
National Cancer Institute, obtaining information from, 451–452
not a substitute for care by professionals, x
perspectives and attitudes during, 448–450
reasons for doing, 446–447
resources, 467–488
search firm, hiring, 456
support groups, finding, 460
test results, interpretation of, 463, 481
tests and procedures, information about, 73–74, 463, 481
unproven remedies, assessment of, 464
ways of finding information, ix–x, 450–451
research by professionals
    current clinical trials, 374–396
    future trials, 441–445
    novel treatment techniques and devices, 436–440
    overview of trends in, 418–422
    prevention trials, 440–441
    progress of, 53–55
    See also clinical trials
resection, 107–112
    See also surgery
resuming activities after ostomy, 200–201
runny nose, 229

S

sadness at diagnosis, 20
scintigraphy (bone scan), 83
second and subsequent opinions, 15, 24, 270
second cancers, 341–342
self-help groups. *See* support and self-help groups
sessile polyps, 36

Colorectal Cancer Screening

For the general population

The American Cancer Society's recommendations for colorectal cancer screening among those over age 50 who have no family history of colorectal cancer or irritable bowel disease include:

- Annual fecal occult blood tests, combined with flexible sigmoidoscopy and digital rectal examination every 5 years, or

- Colonoscopy and digital rectal examination every 10 years, or

- Double contrast barium enema and digital rectal examination every 5 to 10 years.

Your doctor will advise you which combination of tests is most suitable for your circumstances.

For those with a family history of colorectal cancer

Anyone with a first-order relative (mother, father, sibling, child) having colon cancer should consider genetic testing to assess their risk, and should have screening tests earlier in life, and more often, than those in the general population.

For those with family cancer syndromes

Anyone with a known family colorectal cancer syndrome such as hereditary nonpolyposis colon cancer (HNPCC) or familial adenomatous polyps (FAP) should consult a physician regularly about screening. Depending on your family history, your doctor might recommend screening as early as age twenty.

For colorectal cancer survivors

All survivors of an episode of colorectal cancer should have remaining colonic and rectal tissue evaluated regularly on a schedule determined by an oncologist.

For those with irritable bowel disease

Anyone with a history of irritable bowel disease such as Crohn's disease or ulcerative colitis should be screened more often than the general population. Consult your doctor for the timing of screening tests that are appropriate for your circumstances.

About the Author

Lorraine Johnston first became involved with the cancer patient community while researching and advocating for family members. She is the wife of an eight-year lymphoma survivor and the daughter of a twenty-year lymphoma survivor. In the years since her husband's diagnosis, she has been involved in a number of support groups that offer emotional and practical support to cancer survivors.

In the course of her support group efforts, Lorraine has been interviewed by the *Philadelphia Inquirer* and by National Public Radio's *Marketplace* program regarding the best ways to find reliable medical information using a personal computer and various media such as the Internet. She attempts to dispel the myths that access to sound medical information is cloaked in secrecy and that medical literature is impossible to interpret. Using her lifelong love of biology and her degree in life sciences, she helps cancer survivors accurately evaluate the material they locate.

Lorraine's years of study have included many courses in psychology, but she found that nothing in her educational background prepared her adequately for facing the terror and heartbreak of cancer. One of her chief interests is helping the newly diagnosed as well as long-term survivors feel less lonely and less afraid as they confront their diagnoses and weigh their options.

Colon and Rectal Cancer: A Comprehensive Guide for Patients and Families is Lorraine's second book. Her first book was *Non-Hodgkin's Lymphomas: Making Sense of Diagnosis, Treatment, and Options*. She is currently working on her third book, *Lung Cancer*.

You can reach the author care of O'Reilly & Associates, Inc., by mail or email (*patientguides@oreilly.com*).

Colophon

Patient-Centered Guides are about the experience of illness. They contain personal stories as well as a mixture of practical and medical information. The faces on the covers of our Guides reflect the human side of the information we offer.

Edie Freedman designed the cover of *Colon and Rectal Cancer: A Comprehensive Guide for Patients and Families*, using Adobe Photoshop 5.0 and QuarkXPress 3.32 with Onyx BT and Berkeley fonts from Bitstream. The cover photo is from RubberBall and Photodisk stock photo archives and is used with their permission. Kathleen Wilson prepared the cover mechanical.

Alicia Cech designed the interior layout for the book, based on a series design by Edie Freedman and Nancy Priest. The interior fonts are Berkeley and Franklin Gothic.

Alicia Cech and Mike Sierra prepared the text, using QuarkXPress 3.32 and FrameMaker 5.5. Robert Romano and Rhon Porter created the illustrations that appear in the book, using Adobe Photoshop 5.0 and Macromedia FreeHand 8.0.

The text was copyedited by Lunaea Hougland and proofread by Abigail Myers. Nancy Wolfe Kotary, Claire Cloutier LeBlanc, and David Futato conducted quality assurance checks. Katherine J. Wilkinson wrote the index. Claire Cloutier LeBlanc and Judith Hoer were the interior compositors.

Patient-Centered Guides™

Questions Answered
Experiences Shared

We are committed to empowering individuals to evolve into informed consumers armed with the latest information and heartfelt support for their journey.

When your life is turned upside down, your need for information is great. You have to make critical medical decisions, often with what seems little to go on. Plus you have to break the news to family, quiet your own fears, cope with symptoms or treatment side effects, figure out how you're going to pay for things, and sometimes still get to work or get dinner on the table.

Patient-Centered Guides provide authoritative information for intelligent information seekers who want to become advocates of their own health. They cover the whole impact of illness on your life. In each book, there's a mix of:

- **Medical background for treatment decisions**
  We can give you information that can help you to intelligently work with your doctor to come to a decision. We start from the viewpoint that modern medicine has much to offer and also discuss complementary treatments. Where there are treatment controversies we present differing points of view.

- **Practical information**
  Once you've decided what to do about your illness, you still have to deal with treatments and changes to your life. We cover day-to-day practicalities, such as those you'd hear from a good nurse or a knowledgeable support group.

- **Emotional support**
  It's normal to have strong reactions to a condition that threatens your life or changes how you live. It's normal that the whole family is affected. We cover issues like the shock of diagnosis, living with uncertainty, and communicating with loved ones.

Each book also contains stories from both patients and doctors — medical "frequent flyers" who share, in their own words, the lessons and strategies they have learned when maneuvering through the often complicated maze of medical information that's available.

We provide information online, including updated listings of the resources that appear in this book. This is freely available for you to print out and copy to share with others, as long as you retain the copyright notice on the print-outs.

http://www.patientcenters.com

Other Books in the Series

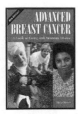

Advanced Breast Cancer
A Guide to Living with Metastatic Disease
By Musa Mayer
ISBN 1-56592-522-X, Paperback 6" x 9", 542 pages, $19.95

"An excellent book...if knowledge is power, this book will be good medicine."

—David Spiegel, MD, Stanford University,
Author, Living Beyond Limits

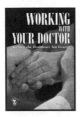

Working with Your Doctor
Getting the Healthcare You Deserve
By Nancy Keene
ISBN 1-56592-273-5, Paperback, 6" x 9", 382 pages, $15.95

"Working with Your Doctor fills a genuine need for patients and their family members caught up in this new and intimidating age of impersonal, economically-driven health care delivery."

—James Dougherty, MD, Emeritus Professor of Surgery,
Albany Medical College

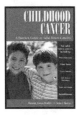

Childhood Cancer
A Parent's Guide to Solid Tumor Cancers
By Nancy Keene
ISBN 1-56592-531-9, Paperback, 6"x 9", 544 pages, $24.95

"I recommend [this book] most highly for those in need of high-level, helpful knowledge that will empower and help parents and caregivers to cope."

—Mark Greenberg, MD, Professor of Pediatrics,
University of Toronto

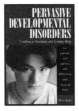

Pervasive Developmental Disorders
Finding a Diagnosis and Getting Help
By Mitzi Waltz
ISBN 1-56592-530-0, Paperback, 6" x 9", 592 pages, $24.95

"Mitzi Waltz's book provides clear, informative, and comprehensive information on every relevant aspect of PDD. Her in-depth discussion will help parents and professionals develop a clear understanding of the issues and, consequently, they will be able to make informed decisions about various interventions. A job well done!"

—Dr. Stephen M. Edelson, Director,
Center for the Study of Autism, Salem, Oregon

Patient-Centered Guides
Published by O'Reilly & Associates, Inc.
Our products are available at a bookstore near you.
For information: **800-998-9938 • 707-829-0515 • info@oreilly.com**
101 Morris Street • Sebastopol • CA • 95472-9902

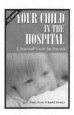

Your Child in the Hospital
A Practical Guide for Parents, Second Edition
By Nancy Keene and Rachel Prentice
ISBN 1-56592-573-4, Paperback, 5" x 8", 176 pages, $11.95

"When your child is ill or injured, the hospital setting can be over-whelming. Here is a terrific 'road map' to help keep families 'on track.'"

—James B. Fahner, MD, Division Chief,
Pediatric Hematology/Oncology, DeVos Children's Hospital,
Grand Rapids, Michigan

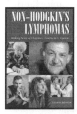

Choosing a Wheelchair
A Guide for Optimal Independence
By Gary Karp
ISBN 1-56592-411-8, Paperback, 5" x 8", 192 pages, $9.95

"I love the idea of putting knowledge often possessed only by profes-sionals into the hands of new consumers. Gary Karp has done it. This book will empower people with disabilities to make informed equip-ment choices."

—Barry Corbet, Editor, New Mobility Magazine

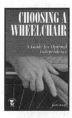

Non-Hodgkin's Lymphomas
Making Sense of Diagnosis, Treatment & Options
By Lorraine Johnston
ISBN 1-56592-444-4, Paperback, 6" x 9", 584 pages, $24.95

"When I gave this book to one of our patients, there was an instant, electric connection. A sense of enlightenment came over her while she absorbed the information. It was thrilling to see her so sparked with new energy and focus."

—Susan Weisberg, LCSW, Clinical Social Worker,
Stanford University Medical Center

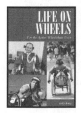

Life on Wheels
For the Active Wheelchair User
By Gary Karp
ISBN 1-56592-253-0, Paperback, 6" x 9", 576 pages, $24.95

"Gary Karp's Life On Wheels is a super book. If you use a wheelchair, you cannot do without it. It is THE wheelchair-user reference book."

—Hugh Gregory Gallagher, Author,
FDR's Splendid Deception

Patient-Centered Guides
Published by O'Reilly & Associates, Inc.
Our products are available at a bookstore near you.
For information: **800-998-9938 • 707-829-0515 • info@oreilly.com**
101 Morris Street • Sebastopol • CA • 95472-9902

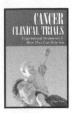

Cancer Clinical Trials
Experimental Treatments and How They Can Help You
By Robert Finn
ISBN 1-56592-566-1, Paperback, 5" x 8", 216 pages, $14.95

"I highly recommend this book as a first step in what will be for many a difficult, but crucially important, part of their struggle to beat their cancer."

—From the foreword by Robert Bazell, Chief Science
Correspondent for NBC News and Author,
Her-2: The Making of Herceptin, a Revolutionary
Treatment for Breast Cancer

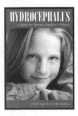

Hydrocephalus
A Guide for Patients, Families & Friends
By Chuck Toporek and Kellie Robinson
ISBN 1-56592-410-X, Paperback, 6" x 9", 384 pages, $19.95

"Toporek, a medical editor, and wife Robinson, a writer and hydrocephalus patient, fill a void of information on hydrocephalus (water on the brain) for the lay reader. Highly recommended for public and academic libraries."

—Library Journal

"In this book, the authors have provided a wonderful entry into the world of hydrocephalus to begin to remedy the neglect of this important condition. We are immensely grateful to them for their groundbreaking effort."

—Peter M. Black, MD, PhD, Franc D. Ingraham Professor of
Neurosurgery, Harvard Medical School,
Neurosurgeon-in-Chief, Brigham and Women's Hospital,
Children's Hospital, Boston, Massachusetts

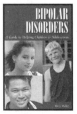

Bipolar Disorders
A Guide to Helping Children & Adolescents
By Mitzi Waltz
ISBN 1-56592-656-0, Paperback, 6 x 9, 450 pages, $24.95

"As bipolar disorders are becoming more commonly diagnosed in children and adolescents, a readable, informative guide for these youths and their families is certainly needed. This book certainly fits the bill. It covers all of the major topics that are of greatest importance to guide parents and families on the topic of pediatric bipolarity ..."

—Robert L. Findling, MD, Director, Division of Child and
Adolescent Psychiatry, Co-director, Stanley Clinical Research
Center, Case Western Reserve University/ University
Hospitals of Cleveland

Patient-Centered Guides
Published by O'Reilly & Associates, Inc.
Our products are available at a bookstore near you.
For information: **800-998-9938** • **707-829-0515** • **info@oreilly.com**
101 Morris Street • Sebastopol • CA • 95472-9902